# Hepatocellular Carcinoma in Adults and Children

*Editor*

ADRIAN REUBEN

# CLINICS IN
# LIVER DISEASE

www.liver.theclinics.com

*Consulting Editor*
NORMAN GITLIN

May 2015 • Volume 19 • Number 2

**ELSEVIER**

1600 John F. Kennedy Boulevard • Suite 1800 • Philadelphia, Pennsylvania, 19103-2899

http://www.theclinics.com

**CLINICS IN LIVER DISEASE Volume 19, Number 2**
**May 2015 ISSN 1089-3261, ISBN-13: 978-0-323-39340-9**

Editor: Kerry Holland
Developmental Editor: Meredith Clinton

*Clinics in Liver Disease* (ISSN 1089-3261) is published quarterly by Elsevier Inc., 360 Park Avenue South, New York, NY 10010-1710. Months of issue are February, May, August, and November. Business and Editorial Offices: 1600 John F. Kennedy Blvd., Ste. 1800, Philadelphia, PA 19103-2899. Customer Service Office: 3251 Riverport Lane, Maryland Heights, MO 63043. Periodicals postage paid at New York, NY and additional mailing offices. Subscription prices are $295.00 per year (U.S. individuals), $145.00 per year (U.S. student/resident), $401.00 per year (U.S. institutions), $395.00 per year (international individuals), $200.00 per year (international student/resident), $498.00 per year (international instituitions), $340.00 per year (Canadian individuals), $200.00 per year (Canadian student/resident), and $498.00 per year (Canadian institutions). Foreign air speed delivery is included in all *Clinics* subscription prices. All prices are subject to change without notice. **POSTMASTER:** Send address changes to *Clinics in Liver Disease*, Elsevier Health Sciences Division, Subscription Customer Service, 3251 Riverport Lane, Maryland Heights, MO 63043. **Customer Service: Telephone: 1-800-654-2452 (U.S. and Canada); 314-447-8871 (outside U.S. and Canada). Fax: 314-447-8029. E-mail: journalscustomer service-usa@elsevier.com (for print support); journalsonlinesupport-usa@elsevier.com (for online support).**

*Reprints.* For copies of 100 or more of articles in this publication, please contact the Commercial Reprints Department, Elsevier Inc., 360 Park Avenue South, New York, NY 10010-1710. Tel.: 212-633-3874; Fax: 212-633-3820; E-mail: reprints@elsevier.com.

*Clinics in Liver Disease* is covered in *MEDLINE/PubMed (Index Medicus)*, Science Citation Index Expanded, Journal Citation Reports/Science Edition, and Current Contents/Clinical Medicine.

# Contributors

## CONSULTING EDITOR

**NORMAN GITLIN, MD, FRCP (LONDON), FRCPE (EDINBURGH), FACG, FACP**
Formerly, Professor of Medicine, Chief of Hepatology, Emory University; Currently, Consultant, Atlanta Gastroenterology Associates, Atlanta, Georgia

## EDITOR

**ADRIAN REUBEN, BSc, MBBS, FRCP, FACG, FAASLD**
Professor Emeritus, Division of Gastroenterology and Hepatology, Department of Medicine, Medical University of South Carolina, Charleston, South Carolina

## AUTHORS

**BENYAM D. ADDISSIE, MD**
Instructor, Division of Gastroenterology and Hepatology, Mayo Clinic College of Medicine, Rochester, Minnesota

**AIJAZ AHMED, MD**
Division of Gastroenterology and Hepatology, Stanford University School of Medicine; Associate Professor of Medicine, Medical Director, Liver Transplant Program, Palo Alto, California

**MOHAMED E. AKOAD, MD**
Department of Transplantation and Hepatobiliary Diseases, Lahey Hospital and Medical Center, Burlington, Massachusetts

**MUNAZZA ANIS, MD**
Attending Physician, Department of Radiology, Hunter Holmes McGuire VAMC, Richmond, Virginia

**ZIV BEN ARI, MD**
Liver Disease Center; Liver Research Laboratory, Sheba Medical Center, Ramat Gan, Israel; Sackler School of Medicine, Tel Aviv University, Tel Aviv, Israel

**RACHEL M. BROWN, MBChB, FRCPath**
Consultant Pathologist, Department of Cellular Pathology, Queen Elizabeth Hospital Birmingham, University Hospitals Birmingham NHS Foundation Trust, Birmingham, United Kingdom

**ELIZABETH M. BRUNT, MD**
Professor, Department of Pathology and Immunology, Washington University School of Medicine, St Louis, Missouri

**KUSH DESAI, MD**
Section of Interventional Radiology, Division of Interventional Oncology, Department of Radiology, Northwestern University, Chicago, Illinois

**ROBERT G. GISH, MD**
Liver Transplant Program, Palo Alto, California; Medical Director, Hepatitis B Foundation, Doylestown, Pennsylvania

**OLIVIER GOVAERE, MSc, PhD**
Translational Cell and Tissue Research, Department of Imaging and Pathology, KULeuven and University Hospitals Leuven, Leuven, Belgium

**ALI HABIB, BA**
Section of Interventional Radiology, Division of Interventional Oncology, Department of Radiology, Northwestern University, Chicago, Illinois

**RYAN HICKEY, MD**
Section of Interventional Radiology, Division of Interventional Oncology, Department of Radiology, Northwestern University, Chicago, Illinois

**APARNA KALYAN, MD**
Instructor, Northwestern Medicine Developmental Therapeutics Institute (NMDTI); Division of Hematology and Oncology, Robert H. Lurie Medical Research Center, Northwestern University, Chicago, Illinois

**DEIRDRE KELLY, FRCPCH, FRCP, FRCPI, MD**
Professor of Paediatric Hepatology, The Liver Unit, Birmingham Children's Hospital, Birmingham, United Kingdom

**LAURA KULIK, MD**
Associate Professor, Division of Hematology and Oncology, Robert H. Lurie Medical Research Center; Division of Hepatology and Gastroenterology, Northwestern University, Chicago, Illinois

**ROBERT LEWANDOWSKI, MD**
Section of Interventional Radiology, Division of Interventional Oncology, Department of Radiology, Northwestern University, Chicago, Illinois

**W. THOMAS LONDON, MD**
Fox Chase Cancer Center, Philadelphia, Pennsylvania

**KATHERINE A. McGLYNN, PhD, MPH**
Division of Cancer Epidemiology and Genetics, National Cancer Institute, Bethesda, Maryland

**BRENDAN M. McGUIRE, MD**
Medical Director of Liver Transplant and Professor of Medicine, The University of Alabama School of Medicine, Birmingham, Alabama

**BRUCE MORLAND, MBChB, MRCP, DM, FRCPCH**
Consultant Paediatric Oncologist, Oncology Department, Birmingham Children's Hospital, Birmingham, United Kingdom

**HALLA NIMEIRI, MD**
Assistant Professor, Northwestern Medicine Developmental Therapeutics Institute (NMDTI); Division of Hematology and Oncology, Robert H. Lurie Medical Research Center, Northwestern University, Chicago, Illinois

**MAZEN NOUREDDIN, MD**
Assistant Professor of Clinical Medicine, Division of Gastrointestinal and Liver Diseases, USC Keck School of Medicine, Los Angeles, California

**JESSICA L. PETRICK, PhD, MPH**
Division of Cancer Epidemiology and Genetics, National Cancer Institute, Bethesda, Maryland

**MEREDITH E. PITTMAN, MD**
Fellow, Department of Pathology, Johns Hopkins Medical Institutions, Baltimore, Maryland

**ELIZABETH A. POMFRET, MD, PhD**
Chair, Department of Transplantation and Hepatobiliary Diseases, Lahey Hospital and Medical Center, Burlington, Massachusetts

**MARY E. RINELLA, MD**
Associate Professor of Medicine, Division of Gastroenterology and Hepatology, Northwestern University Feinberg School of Medicine, Chicago, Illinois

**LEWIS R. ROBERTS, MB ChB, PhD, FACP**
Professor, Division of Gastroenterology and Hepatology, Mayo Clinic College of Medicine, Rochester, Minnesota

**TANIA ROSKAMS, MD, PhD**
Translational Cell and Tissue Research, Department of Imaging and Pathology, KULeuven and University Hospitals Leuven, Leuven, Belgium

**MICHAL SAFRAN, PhD**
Liver Disease Center; Liver Research Laboratory, Sheba Medical Center, Ramat Gan, Israel

**RIAD SALEM, MD, MBA**
Chief, Vascular and Interventional Radiology; Vice-Chair, Image-Guided Therapy, Section of Interventional Radiology; Director, Division of Interventional Oncology, Department of Radiology, Northwestern University, Chicago, Illinois

**KHALID SHARIF, FRCS Paed, FCPS Paed Surg (Pak)**
Hepatobiliary and Transplant Surgeon, The Liver Unit, Birmingham Children's Hospital, Birmingham, United Kingdom

**HEATHER N. SIMPSON, MD**
Assistant Professor of Medicine, The University of Alabama School of Medicine, Birmingham, Alabama

**BARTLEY THORNBURG, MD**
Section of Interventional Radiology, Division of Interventional Oncology, Department of Radiology, Northwestern University, Chicago, Illinois

**ELLA WEITZMAN, MD**
Liver Disease Center, Sheba Medical Center, Ramat Gan, Israel; Sackler School of Medicine, Tel Aviv University, Tel Aviv, Israel

**ROBERT J. WONG, MD, MS**
Assistant Clinical Professor of Medicine, Division of Gastroenterology and Hepatology, Alameda Health System-Highland Hospital, Oakland, California

# Contents

> Liver cancer is the second leading cause of global cancer mortality. The major risk factors for hepatocellular carcinoma (HCC) are being addressed with success by prevention efforts. Vaccination against hepatitis B virus has reduced incidence of HCC in Taiwan and is partly responsible for lower rates in China. New infections with hepatitis C virus are low in developed countries because of prevention of posttransfusion infections and reduced exposure to HCV by drug users. Aflatoxin exposure has been reduced by better grain storage and dietary changes. Obesity, metabolic syndrome, and diabetes are increasing in developed and developing countries and will lead to more cases of HCC.

> Hepatocellular carcinoma can be diagnosed on a needle biopsy of the liver; however, uncertainty may arise because of the inherent complexity of liver histology. This article aims to provide practicing pathologists with tools for the approach to mass-directed liver biopsies clinically concerning for hepatocellular carcinoma. The examination of routine hematoxylin-eosin stains and the use of ancillary histochemical and immunohistochemical stains are discussed. Sections reviewing liver carcinoma with biphenotypic differentiation and the challenge of dysplastic nodules are included.

> Different approaches predict the outcome for patients with hepatocellular carcinoma (HCC). The expression of biliary-hepatic progenitor cell markers generally correlates with poor prognosis. This article focuses on the pathogenesis of HCC, how differentiation or dedifferentiation leads to a phenotype switch, and heterogeneity in the same tumor. A tumor cell decides its fate based on a complex interplay of signaling pathways. Interaction with the microenvironment decides whether it will invade, proliferate, or enter survival mode. Several signaling pathways contribute to stemness features, reflecting a small chemoresistant subpopulation of the tumor that expresses biliary-hepatic progenitor cell markers.

additional data discussed in the context of transplantation. As rapid innovation occurs in the realm of oncology, interventional oncology represents a safe, effective alternative that continues to generate impressive data that could potentially change treatment paradigms.

Treatment of advanced hepatocellular carcinoma (HCC) remains challenging, particularly with the limited systemic therapy options. Sorafenib remains the only approved, targeted molecule for the treatment of advanced HCC. Although a survival benefit was demonstrated with sorafenib, it remains only true in the population of patients with Child-Turcotte-Pugh class A disease. Sorafenib also has distinct side effects that require close monitoring. Newer tyrosine kinase inhibitors and angiogenic inhibitors have been evaluated with disappointing results, particularly in phase III trials. Herein we review the pertinent trials for targeted therapy in HCC to date.

Liver tumors are relatively rare in childhood, but may be associated with a range of diagnostic, genetic, therapeutic, and surgical challenges sufficient to tax even the most experienced clinician. This article outlines the epidemiology, etiology, pathologic condition, initial workup, and management of hepatocellular carcinoma in children and adolescents.

# CLINICS IN LIVER DISEASE

**NOW AVAILABLE FOR YOUR iPhone and iPad**

# Preface

# Hepatocellular Carcinoma in Adults and Children

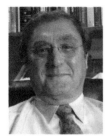

Adrian Reuben, BSc, MBBS, FRCP, FACG, FAASLD
*Editor*

Hepatocellular carcinoma (HCC) was once thought to be singularly uncommon, thanks to persuasion by the renowned nineteenth-century German pathologist, Rudolph Virchow (1821-1902) that "Primary cancer is rare in organs prone to metastases."[1] His equally renowned contemporary, the Canadian clinician, William Osler, whose influence extended well into the twentieth century, attested to the scarcity of HCC, since barely a handful of cases was seen among several thousand admissions at Johns Hopkins Hospital,[2] of which he was a founding professor. This was the same William Osler, who subscribed for a while to Guido Banti's notion that splenomegaly is the cause of portal hypertension and not its consequence.[3,4]

Even after the first description of HCC by Gaspard-Laurent Bayle in the eighteenth century, as reported by Frerichs,[5] and the collection of 1616 verified cases by Rosenberg and Ochsner in 1948,[6] HCC was considered to be essentially a disease of Africans and Asians, which indeed it is, rather than a Western phenomenon. The incidence of HCC may well be increasing in the West, but 75% of cases worldwide still occur in Asia, of which two-thirds are in China. In 2012, a daunting 782,000 cases were diagnosed globally, with a fearsome case-fatality rate of 95% (ie, 746,000 deaths).[7] HCC is now one of the commonest malignancies on the planet (fifth in men and ninth in women) and the second most frequent cause of cancer mortality. In the United States, the 2014 preliminary estimates are of 33,190 cases of liver and intrahepatic bile duct cancer, leading to 23,000 (69%) fatalities.[8]

In their opening article on the Global Epidemiology of Liver Cancer, Katherine McGlynn, Jessica Petrick, and Thomas London set the scene for the rest of the current issue of *Clinics in Liver Disease*. Although this and each succeeding article are self-contained, readers might want to refer to the earlier *Clinics in Liver Disease* issue on HCC [2011;15(2)] for details that are still relevant but not found in this update. The editorial tenet underlying the current volume was to provide the clinician with guidance and explanations that are useful in everyday practice, based on contemporary

Clin Liver Dis 19 (2015) xiii–xvi
http://dx.doi.org/10.1016/j.cld.2015.02.001
1089-3261/15/$ – see front matter © 2015 Published by Elsevier Inc.

scientific research, published evidence, and, where germane, the credible experience of seasoned experts. It seems serendipitous that almost half of the contributors to this volume are women and many are minorities but, in fact, it is a welcome reflection of modern academia.

Disturbing as the global statistics are, all is not doom and gloom. HCC incidences are falling in some parts of the world in response to preventative measures to combat Hepatitis B virus (HBV) infection, the introduction of conditions to reduce aflatoxin B1 generation (**Fig. 1**), and, in Japan, the waning of the Hepatitis C virus (HCV) epidemic there.

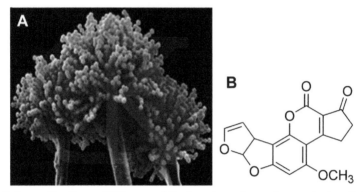

Fig. 1. (*A*) *Aspergillus flavus*. (*B*) Source of the hepatocarcinogenic mycotoxin, aflatoxin B1.

Although mortality has not yet fallen in the United States, incidence rates may actually have stabilized recently. As a reliable cure of HCV becomes feasible for those who have access to the new direct-acting antiviral medications, it is now conceivable that the peak incidence of HCV-associated HCC predicted for the United States in 2019-2020 may turn out to be an overestimate. A striking feature of the global epidemiology of HCC is its diversity with respect to geographic distribution, gender-association, and risk factors that must be accounted for in surveillance programs and staging systems, as described succinctly in lucid detail by Heather Simpson and Brendan McGuire, and in a creative classification by Benyam Addisie and Lewis Roberts, respectively. Munazza Anis updates us ably on the improved diagnostic imaging criteria for HCC and the newly proposed structured approach to reporting, so-called LI-RADS (Liver Imaging-Reporting and Data System), that should be applicable wherever dynamic contrast computer-assisted or MRI is performed, notably in transplant centers. In this context, the discussion by Robert Wong, Aijaz Ahmed, and Robert Gish of the vagaries of serum α-fetoprotein (AFP) is most pertinent, as the applicability of this time-honored diagnostic test and other serologic biomarkers remains controversial; this article provides a useful exhaustive background with which to understand the arguments in favor of and against the use of AFP for screening and diagnosis.

The heterogeneity of HCC impacts therapy, be it potentially curative, as described by Mohamed Akoad and Elizabeth Pomfret in their review of surgical resection and liver transplantation, or palliative and/or adjunctive, as given by locoregional intervention, which is described in encyclopedic detail by Ali Habib, Kush Desai, Ryan Hickey, Bartely Thomburg, Robert Lewandowski, and Riad Salem. Although treatment with sorafenib is well-tolerated and has some efficacy in advanced disease, and it established the proof of principle for oral systemic therapy, this form of care has yet to reach its potential, as updated realistically by Aparna Kalyan, Halla Nimeiri, and Laura Kulik, including descriptions of promising single and combination manipulations in the future.

The description by Olivier Govaere and Tania Roskams of HCC pathogenesis at the molecular and cellular levels is remarkable for its scientific elegance, but most notable is its emphasis on the molecular profiles, namely, the expression of biliary and progenitor cell markers, that can be linked to prognosis. The complementary article by Meredith Pittman and Elizabeth Brunt shows that classic hepatopathology is still a living and evolving discipline. Clinicians would do well to share the microscope with their *Pathology Partners* to understand better the heterogeneity of HCC and how this can be relevant to prognosis and the utilization and outcomes of different therapies. The causes and pathogenesis of HCC are further explored in great detail by the focused treatises on the oncogenic viruses, HBV and HCV, by Ziv Ben-Ari, Ella Weitzman, and Michal Safran, and on the interrelationships and common pathways shared with obesity, diabetes, and nonalcoholic fatty liver disease, penned by Mazen Noureddin and Mary Rinella. That cirrhosis due to oncogenic viruses and steatohepatitis, respectively, can lead to HCC is no surprise; neither is its development in noncirrhotic HBV infection. What is disturbing, however, is that HCC appears to occur sometimes in noncirrhotic HCV infection or fatty liver disease, which has important implications for understanding pathogenesis, as reviewed in the two aforementioned articles, and because it may challenge our surveillance practice.

At this juncture, it is worth noting that up to 20% of HCC worldwide occurs in the absence of cirrhosis, which is of especial relevance to the last article, concerning HCC in children by Deidre Kelly, Khalid Sharif, Rachel Brown, and Bruce Morland. In contrast with the causes in adults, only one-third of HCCs in children are associated with cirrhosis, in whom an additional set of risk factors, hereditary and genetic, therefore come into play, particularly $\alpha$-1-antitrypsin deficiency, glycogen storage disease III, tyrosinemia, and progressive familial intrahepatic cholestasis type 2 that results from a mutation of the *ABCB11* gene, resulting in deficiency of the hepatocyte canalicular membrane bile acid transporter (ie, the Bile Salt Export Pump). The rare fibrolamellar type of HCC that is seen in older children and young adults generally occurs in the absence of cirrhosis and, rather than being associated with elevated AFP, vitamin $B_{12}$ binding proteins (especially transcobalamin I) are useful disease biomarkers. These pediatric predispositions to HCC may extend into adult life, and this serves to remind practitioners to be watchful that HCC may complicate other common metabolic disorders, such as hereditary hemochromatosis, and rare defects like many of the porphyrias.

It has been an honor to have been invited to edit this issue of *Clinics in Liver Disease* and a privilege to have worked with such reasonable, talented, and knowledgeable authors; the education has been incomparable.

Given the pace at which the field of HCC studies is advancing scientifically and clinically, I predict that another *Clinics in Liver Disease* update will be needed every 3 years in perpetuity.

Adrian Reuben, BSc, MBBS, FRCP, FACG, FAASLD
Division of Gastroenterology and Hepatology
Department of Medicine
Medical University of South Carolina
Suite 249 MSC 702, 114 Doughty Street
Charleston, SC 29425, USA

E-mail address:
reubena@musc.edu

## REFERENCES

1. Virchow R. Die Krankhaften Geschwülste: Dreissig Vorlesungen, Gehalten Während des Wintersemesters 1862-1863, an der Universitat zu Berlin, vol. 1. Berlin: Augustus Hirschwald; 1863. p. 1.
2. Osler W. New growths in the liver. Chapter 6. In: The principles and practice of medicine. Section III: Diseases of the digestive system. VIII. Diseases of the liver. New York: D. Appleton and Company; 1892. p. 451.
3. Osler W. On splenic anemia. Am J Med Sci 1900;119:54–73, 1902;124:751–800.
4. Osler WM, T. 3rd edition. Modern medicine: its theory and practice, vols. 1–2. Philadelphia: Lea and Febiger; 1925.
5. Frerichs FT. 1. Historical account. In: Murchison C, editor. A clinical treatise of diseases of the liver, vol. III. New York: W.Wood and Co; 1879. p. 41–3.
6. Rosenberg DML, Ochsner A. Primary carcinoma of the liver; an analysis of 55 autopsied cases, the record of a case with resection, and a review of the recent literature. Surgery 1948;24:1036–68.
7. International Agency for Research on Cancer. GLOBOCAN 2012: Estimated cancer incidence, mortality and prevalence worldwide in 2012. Available at: http://www.globocan.iarc.fr. Accessed January 15, 2015.
8. American Cancer Society: Facts and figures 2014. Atlanta, GA. Available at: http://www.cancer.gov. Accessed January 15, 2015.

# Global Epidemiology of Hepatocellular Carcinoma

## An Emphasis on Demographic and Regional Variability

Katherine A. McGlynn, PhD, MPH[a],*, Jessica L. Petrick, PhD, MPH[a],
W. Thomas London, MD[b]

## KEYWORDS

- Incidence • Hepatitis B virus • Hepatitis C virus • Aflatoxin • Diabetes • Alcohol
- Chemoprevention • Coffee

## KEY POINTS

- HCC incidence has decreased in Japan and China; it has plateaued in the United States; incidence has increased in many other countries.
- Neonatal and early childhood vaccination against HBV has reduced chronic HBV infection rates in Asian countries to very low levels; in people younger than age 30 in Taiwan, HCC rates have fallen 80%.
- The identification of the HBV cell receptor and new approaches to degrading cccDNA will result in curative therapies for HBV infection.
- The discovery of sofosbuvir and similar curative drugs for HCV infection coupled with currently effective methods of preventing new infections will greatly reduce the risk of HCC.

## INTRODUCTION

Primary liver cancer is the sixth most commonly occurring cancer in the world and the second largest contributor to cancer mortality.[1] Globally, the most common histology (approximately 80%) is hepatocellular carcinoma (HCC), a tumor of the parenchymal cells of the liver. The second most common histology (approximately 15%) is intrahepatic cholangiocarcinoma, which arises in the cholangiocytes of the intrahepatic bile ducts. Large geographic disparities in incidence and mortality of all types of liver cancer exist.

This work was supported by funding of the National Institutes of Health Intramural Research Program.

The authors have no conflicts to disclose.

[a] Division of Cancer Epidemiology and Genetics, National Cancer Institute, 9609 Medical Center Drive, Bethesda, MD 20892, USA; [b] Fox Chase Cancer Center, Philadelphia, PA 19111, USA

* Corresponding author.

E-mail address: mcglynnk@mail.nih.gov

## INCIDENCE AND MORTALITY

The highest incidence rates of liver cancer in the world are in Asia and Africa (**Fig. 1**).[1] Approximately 75% of liver cancer occurs in Asia, with China accounting for more than 50% of the world's burden. The country with the single highest incidence rate, however, is Mongolia, with an age-standardized rate per 100,000 persons of 78.1.[2] In contrast, the lowest incidence rates in the world occur in countries of Northern Europe, the Middle East, Oceania, and North and South America, whereas countries in Central Europe have intermediate rates. Even within specific geographic regions, however, there is great variability. For example, in Asian countries with cancer registries, the age-standardized rates of males range from 2.0 in Bhopal and Dindigul, India, to 77.5 in Qidong City, China.[1]

In the interval between 1983 to 1987 and 2003 to 2007, liver cancer incidence increased in many areas of the world, notably in India, Oceania, and North and South America, as well as in most European countries (**Figs. 2** and **3**). Recently, however, incidence in the United States has stabilized with little annual change in rate between 2009 and 2011 (**Fig. 4**).[3] In contrast, incidence rates have declined in some Asian countries, Spain, and Italy. The decreasing incidence rates seen in China are likely caused by programs to reduce aflatoxin $B_1$ ($AFB_1$) exposure and hepatitis B virus (HBV) transmission and other public health efforts.[4] In Japan, the decreasing incidence of HCC is related to declining rates of hepatitis C virus (HCV) infection in the population.[5]

In the United States, the 5-year relative survival for liver cancer is only 14%.[6] Prognosis is even poorer in less developed regions, thus incidence and mortality rates are roughly equivalent in all countries. In the United States, mortality, unlike incidence, has not yet begun to stabilize; the annual percentage increase in rates was approximately 2.2 between 2000 and 2011.[3] In some countries, mortality can seem to be even higher than incidence because the liver is a common site for metastases and secondary liver cancer can be mistakenly counted as primary liver cancer.

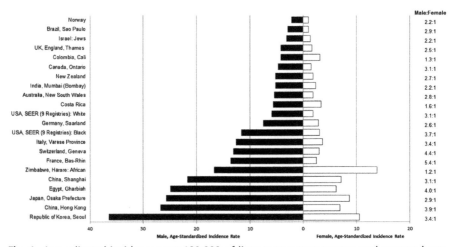

**Fig. 1.** Age-adjusted incidences per 100,000 of liver cancer among men and women by region, 2003 to 2007. Age-adjusted to world standard. SEER, Surveillance, Epidemiology, and End Results. (*Data from* Ferlay J, Parkin DM, Curado MP, et al. Cancer incidence in five continents, volumes I to X: IARC CANCERBase No. 10 [Internet]. Available at: http://ci5.iarc.fr. Accessed November 12, 2014.)

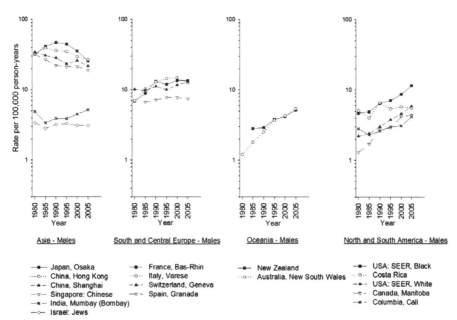

**Fig. 2.** Age-adjusted trends in liver cancer incidence among men by region, 1978-1982, to 2003-2007. Age-adjusted to the world standard. (*Data from* Ferlay J, Parkin DM, Curado MP, et al. Cancer incidence in five continents, volumes I to X: IARC CANCERBase No. 10 [Internet]. Available at: http://ci5.iarc.fr. Accessed November 12, 2014.)

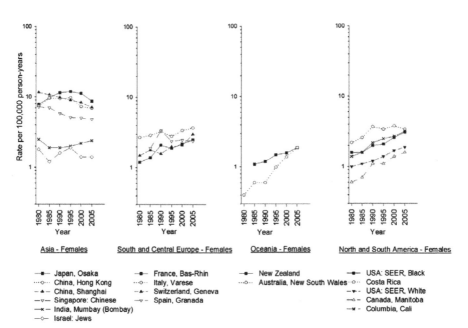

**Fig. 3.** Age-adjusted trends in liver cancer incidence among women by region, 1978-1982, to 2003-2007. Age-adjusted to the world standard. (*Data from* Ferlay J, Parkin DM, Curado MP, et al. Cancer incidence in five continents, volumes I to X: IARC CANCERBase No. 10 [Internet]. Available at: http://ci5.iarc.fr. Accessed November 12, 2014.)

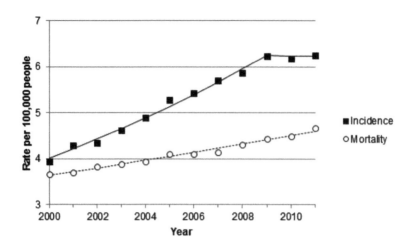

| Incidence/Mortality | Trend 1 | 95% CI | Trend 2 | 95% CI | Joinpoint[a] |
|---|---|---|---|---|---|
| Incidence | 5.0[a] | (4.5, 5.6) | -0.2 | (-4.7, 4.6) | 2009 |
| Mortality | 2.2[a] | (2.0, 2.4) | | | |

**Fig. 4.** Age-adjusted Surveillance, Epidemiology and End Results liver cancer incidence and US liver cancer mortality rates by year, 2000-2011. Age-adjusted to the US standard. CI, confidence interval. Trend indicates annual percent change. Joinpoint regression defines when a trend changes. [a]Slope of trend differs from zero (P<.05).

### Gender and Racial/Ethnic Differences in Rates

Gender disparity in incidence is notable in almost all countries, with rates among males being two- to three-fold higher than rates among females (see **Fig. 1**). High-rate areas do not, however, have greater gender disparity than other areas. In fact, the greatest disparity in incidence occurs in Central European countries where some registries have rates among males four- to five-fold higher than rates among females. The gender disparity in rates is not well understood, although most liver cancer risk factors are more prevalent in men than women. It has also been hypothesized that differences in sex steroid hormones, immune responses, and epigenetics could be related to the higher rates among men.

In addition to gender differences, racial/ethnic disparity within multiethnic populations is also notable. In the United States between 2006 and 2010, Asians/Pacific Islanders had the highest incidence rate per 100,000 (11.7), followed by Hispanics (9.5), blacks (7.5), and whites (4.2).[7] Rates of liver cancer among persons of the same ethnicity also vary by geographic location. For example, liver cancer rates among Chinese populations outside China are lower than the rates reported by Chinese registries. As with gender differences, racial/ethnic differences are likely caused by variability in the prevalence of risk factors between racial/ethnic groups and between geographic locations.

## HEPATOCELLULAR CARCINOMA RISK FACTORS AND PREVENTION

The dominant risk factors for HCC vary in high- and low-rate regions. In most high-rate countries of Asia and Africa, chronic HBV infection and $AFB_1$ exposure are the major risk factors. In contrast, HCV infection, excessive alcohol consumption, and diabetes/obesity/metabolic syndrome play more important roles in low-rate areas. Exceptions to these patterns are seen in Japan and Egypt, where the dominant risk factor is HCV infection. Of the two HCC-related viruses, HBV is responsible for 75% to 80% of virus-associated HCC, whereas HCV is responsible for 10% to 20%.[8] In addition to the major risk factors, certain inherited metabolic disorders, such as hemochromatosis, $\alpha_1$-antitrypsin deficiency, tyrosinemia, and several porphyrias also increase risk. The rarity of these disorders, however, results in them contributing little to risk at the population level.

The global pattern of HCC incidence is related to the history of the major HCC risk factors and the length of time the factors have been present in human populations. Evidence suggests that HBV entered human populations about 33,600 years ago,[9] whereas HCV dates back less than 1000 years and only became globally widely dispersed during the twentieth century.[10] Alcohol consumption has been a common exposure among humans during all recorded history, whereas high rates of obesity, diabetes, and metabolic syndrome are phenomena of the late twentieth century.

### Hepatitis B Virus

In 1994, the International Agency for Research on Cancer (IARC) classified HBV as carcinogenic to humans.[11] Currently, about 5% of the world's population (240–350 million people) are chronically infected.[12] The evidence supporting the causal association of HBV with HCC is substantive. Countries with a chronic HBV infection prevalence of greater than 2% have increased incidence and mortality rates of HCC.[13] Case-control studies in all regions of the world have shown that chronic HBV infection is significantly more common among HCC cases than controls with odds ratios ranging between 5:1 and 65:1.[11] Similarly, prospective studies of HBV carriers have consistently demonstrated high relative risks for HCC, ranging from 5 to 103.[11] In high-rate HCC areas where HBV infection is common, approximately 70% of HBV infections are acquired in the perinatal period or in early childhood.[13,14] HBV DNA is integrated into the genome of liver tissues in almost all HCC cases who are HBV carriers. Investigators have also detected HBV DNA sequences in 10% to 20% of HCC tumors from patients who were seronegative for hepatitis B surface antigen.[15]

Among chronic carriers of HBV, risks of HCC vary by several factors, the major one being serum HBV DNA levels (viral load).[16,17] Although there is no discrete cut-off level, having greater than $10^5$/mL viral copies confers a 2.5- to three-fold greater risk over an 8- to 10-year follow-up period, than does having a lower viral load. Eight major HBV genotypes (A to H) and several subgenotypes have been reported.[18] In multiple population-based studies, genotype C has been associated with a higher risk of HCC than genotypes A2, Ba, Bj, and D.[19] In studies that controlled for genotype, double mutations in the basal core promoter of the HBV genome were independent predictors of increased risk. Mutations in the precore region of the viral genome have also been associated with risk, although less consistently so.[20] The lifetime risk of HCC among HBV carriers is estimated to be 10% to 25%. Estimates suggest that annually, 780,000 chronically infected people die from HCC and chronic liver disease and, eventually, 35 to 87 million of the 240 to 350 million current HBV carriers will die of HCC.[21]

Prevention of chronic HBV infection via vaccination drastically reduces the risk of HCC,[22] although the vaccine is ineffective in 5% of individuals because of a variety of conditions related to vaccine (eg, site of administration and storage conditions) and host (eg, obesity, age, pre-exisiting comorbidities).[23,24] On the population level, it is anticipated that the widespread neonatal vaccination that started in the mid-1980s in most east Asian countries will result in a 70% to 85% decrease in the incidence of HBV-related HCC.[22] In Taiwan, 30 years after the initiation of universal newborn vaccination, HBV carrier rates in persons younger than age 30 have fallen from 10-17% to 0.7-1.7%[25] and rates of HCC have fallen 80%.[26] Similar low rates of hepatitis B surface antigen prevalence are being achieved in China[27] and Singapore,[25,28] thus declines in HCC incidence similar to Taiwan's can be expected. Currently, all countries in Asia and Eastern Europe have integrated newborn HBV vaccination into their routine vaccination programs and are delivering three immunization doses. Perinatal transmission of HBV in Africa is rare[14] and vaccination, without a birth dose, is now routine in greater than 50% of sub-Saharan African countries. To eradicate HBV, new therapies for chronic infections need to be devised. With the identification of the cell receptor for HBV[29] and new approaches to targeting cccDNA, the minichromosome of HBV,[30] such drugs will soon become a reality.

### Hepatitis C Virus

HCV was identified in 1989.[31] Reliable serologic tests for antibody to HCV (anti-HCV) became available in 1990, and in 1994 IARC classified HCV as carcinogenic to humans.[11] Phylogenetic analysis of HCV has identified at least six major genotypes (1–6) and numerous subtypes (denoted by lowercase letters).[32,33] Evidence indicates that HCV existed as a long-term, low-level, endemic virus before the twentieth century, but spread worldwide by several transmission routes starting around 1900.[34] How HCV was maintained as an endemic infection before the twentieth century is uncertain.[35] The highest rates of chronic HCV infection in the world occur in northern Africa, particularly Egypt, where the rate is estimated at 18%.[36] In Asia, the HCV infection rate is highest in Mongolia (10%),[36] whereas rates in Europe (0.5%–2.5%) are similar to the United States (1.8%), but higher than Canada (0.1%–0.8%), which has one of the world's lowest rates.

The population dispersal times of HCV in Japan are consistent with the introduction of antischistosomal therapy using intravenous antimony sodium tartrate beginning in the 1920s.[37,38] Molecular clock studies of HCV in Egypt have also suggested spread via intravenous antischistosomal therapy.[39] Antischistosomal campaigns likely also spread HBV but the risk of an adult becoming a chronic HBV carrier after infection is low (approximately 10%), whereas the risk of an adult developing a chronic HCV infection after exposure is high (approximately 80%).

Molecular analysis of HCV genotype 1a in the United States suggests that the virus first entered the population around 1910 and became more widely disseminated in the 1960s.[37] The reason for spread of HCV in the 1960s is less clear, but the timing of the dissemination is consistent with the estimates derived from mathematical modeling.[40,41] Although several models infer that HCC incidence could hit the very high levels seen earlier in Japan, other studies suggest that the long-term risk of HCC among HCV-infected Americans will be lower.[42] Because HCV circulated in the US blood supply for fewer years than it did in Japan, and newer, more effective antiviral agents are being used to treat HCV infection, the long-term effect of HCV on HCC rates is likely to be less dramatic in the United States than in Japan. In 2010, it was estimated that the peak of the HCV-related HCC epidemic in the United States would occur in 2019 with 14,000 cases per year.[43] However, recent dramatic developments in treatment of HCV may affect this estimate. Until 2014, HCV infection was difficult to eradicate. With the discovery of sofosbuvir[44] and other antiviral drugs, almost all HCV infection could be cured.[45] These medications are currently very expensive, but their price will decrease as more drugs come on the market and with widespread use, the incidence of HCV-related HCC should rapidly decline.

## Aflatoxin

Aflatoxin, a mycotoxin produced by molds of the *Aspergillus* species (*Aspergillus flavus* and *Aspergillus parasiticus*), contaminates maize, groundnuts, and tree nuts in warm, humid environments and is a known hepatic carcinogen. $AFB_1$, the most potent aflatoxin, has been classified by IARC as a group 1 human carcinogen.[46] The regions of the world with the highest levels of $AFB_1$ exposure are sub-Saharan Africa, Southeast Asia, and China. Within these areas, higher levels are found among rural than urban populations,[47] among males than females,[48,49] and among persons chronically infected with HBV.[49] Exposure to $AFB_1$ is associated with a signature DNA mutation in the p53 cancer suppressor gene at the third base of codon 249 (p53 249ser mutation).

There is a synergistic association between $AFB_1$ and HBV in increasing risk of HCC. Compared with persons with neither risk factor, the risk of HCC is reported to be four-fold greater among persons with elevated levels of $AFB_1$, seven-fold greater among chronic HBV carriers, and 60-fold greater among persons with both factors.[50,51] Evidence suggests that there is also a synergistic effect between $AFB_1$ and HCV infection.[52] $AFB_1$ exposure, however, is more common in areas where HBV is the dominant virus. A recent examination of the population attributable risk of $AFB_1$ in high rate areas reported that between 8.8% and 21% of liver cancer could be attributed to $AFB_1$.[53]

In general, in areas of the world where $AFB_1$ exposure is high, chronic HBV infection is highly prevalent. Because little can be done to alter the HBV chronic infection state, eradicating $AFB_1$ from the food supply is an important strategy to reduce HCC incidence.[54] In areas of the world where $AFB_1$ eradication programs have been implemented, such as China, notable reductions in HCC rates have been documented.[55]

## Alcohol Consumption

Although the relationship of alcohol consumption to HCC has been widely studied, deciphering the association has been challenging because heavy consumption frequently leads to chronic liver disease, which results in a cessation of consumption before the development of cancer. In general, however, past studies in low-rate populations have found alcohol to increase risk of HCC, whereas studies from high-rate areas have been less consistent.[56] The disparity between low- and high-rate regions may have been caused by lower mean alcohol consumption in high-rate populations and/or differences in the interaction between alcohol with other risk factors. Evidence suggests that HBV and HCV, in conjunction with alcohol, have synergistic effects on HCC risk.[57–59] Based on the accumulated evidence, IARC concluded in 1988 that alcohol consumption was causally related to liver cancer,[60] whereas a 2007 World Cancer Research Fund/American Institute for Cancer Research report concluded that alcohol consumption was a probable cause of liver cancer.[61] A recent meta-analysis of 19 prospective studies estimated a 16% increased risk of liver cancer among consumers of three or more drinks per day and a 22% increased risk among consumers of six or more drinks per day.[62]

Between 1960 and 2000, per capita consumption declined in European, North American, and African countries. During the same interval, consumption levels increased in Southeast Asia and Western Pacific countries. Because excessive alcohol consumption has historically been a more important HCC risk factor in low-rate HCC areas, declines in consumption suggest a favorable effect on HCC rates in those areas. However, increasing consumption in Southeast Asia and the Western Pacific countries is a concern. For example, high alcohol consumption among men in Mongolia is thought to be contributing to that country's very high HCC rate.[63]

### Obesity, Diabetes Mellitus, and Metabolic Syndrome

The related metabolic disorders of obesity, type II diabetes, and metabolic syndrome, with its hepatic manifestation of nonalcoholic fatty liver disease, have been increasing in frequency in many countries. Studies of each of the conditions have indicated that they are significantly related to the development of HCC. Meta-analyses of diabetes and HCC have consistently estimated relative risks of 2.0 to 2.5 and have found the relationship is consistent across various populations and is independent of other risk factors.[64–67] Several studies, as summarized in recent reviews, have reported that obesity is also related to liver cancer.[68] In comparing normal weight persons with overweight and obese persons, a meta-analysis of 11 cohort studies found significant liver cancer risks among overweight (odds ratio = 1.17) and obese (odds ratio = 1.87) persons.[69] Similarly, a meta-analysis of four studies of metabolic syndrome and HCC estimated a significant relative risk of 1.81.[70]

Although the relative risks of diabetes, obesity, and metabolic syndrome do not approach those of HCV or HBV, they are far more prevalent conditions than HCV and HBV in developed countries. In developing countries, the prevalence of diabetes is growing much faster than it is in developed countries.[71] It has been estimated that there are currently 285 million persons in the world, or 6.4% of the global population, with diabetes.[71] Furthermore, the prevalence is projected to increase by 69% in developing countries, and 20% in developed countries, by the year 2030. Similarly, increases in body mass index have been documented in many countries since 1980.[72] Given the increasing prevalence of these conditions, the proportion of HCC related to obesity, diabetes, and metabolic syndrome will likely grow in the future.

### Tobacco

The effect of cigarette smoking on risk of HCC has been widely examined in studies from high- and low-rate countries.[56] Inconsistent findings in studies of the same populations, and the correlation of smoking with other risk factors, such as alcohol, have made the relationship between tobacco and HCC difficult to define. In 2004, however, IARC concluded that there was sufficient evidence that tobacco smoking caused liver cancer.[73] This same position was adopted by the 2014 US Surgeon General's report.[74] A recent meta-analysis estimated that there was a 1.5-fold increased risk of HCC among current smokers, a risk similar to that imposed by obesity.[75]

### Coffee and Tea

Recent meta-analyses have examined the association between coffee[76] and tea[77] and risk of HCC. Based on 16 studies, the coffee meta-analysis found a significant 40% reduced risk of HCC among consumers.[76] Based on 12 studies, tea was associated with a nonsignificant 23% reduced risk.[77] Since the publication of these results, an additional study from Europe reported 72% and 59% significantly reduced risks associated with coffee and tea, respectively.[78] The sole study of coffee from the United States, thus far, reported a significant 41% decreased risk of HCC.[79]

Compounds in coffee that potentially have chemopreventive effects include diterpenes (ie, cafestol and kahweol), chlorogenic acid, and caffeine.[80] Diterpenes are lipids that inhibit enzyme expression and enzymatic activity, induce detoxifying enzymes, and regulate signaling pathways.[81] Chlorogenic acid is a polyphenol that increases activity of detoxifying enzymes.[82] Caffeine has antioxidant properties and increases metabolic rate and energy expenditure, which could potentially regulate weight and reduce the risk of developing metabolic syndrome.[83] Similarly, tea contains bioactive compounds, including caffeine and polyphenolic compounds. One specific polyphenol, (–)-epigallocatechin-3-gallate, has shown promise as a chemopreventive by inhibiting enzymatic activities, cell invasion, angiogenesis, and metastasis.[84]

## CHEMOPREVENTION
### Statins

Statins (3-hydroxy-3-methylglutaryl coenzyme A reductase inhibitors) are commonly prescribed cholesterol-lowering medications used for the prevention of cardiovascular disease.[85] Statins may also have anticarcinogenic effects[86] related to inhibited angiogenesis, enhanced apoptosis, and metastasis inhibition.[87] Promising evidence that statins may decrease risk of HCC has been reported in observational studies in Taiwan.[88–92] Two general population studies reported significant inverse associations between statins and HCC with odds ratios of 0.53[88] and 0.44.[90] In addition, significant inverse associations were reported in studies of HBV-positive persons[92] and HCV-positive persons[91] and in association with individual statins.[89] In contrast, early results from low-rate HCC areas reported null associations.[93,94] Subsequent studies from these areas, however, have provided support for an inverse association. Studies from the US Veterans Affairs' population have found inverse associations among men with diabetes[95] and HCV infection,[96] whereas studies conducted among members of US health maintenance organizations[97,98] and a large Swedish record-linkage study also reported significant inverse associations.[99] Meta-analyses of these results concluded that an inverse relationship exists.[100,101] Collectively, the evidence suggests that statin use could contribute to a decline in HCC incidence.

### Antidiabetic Medications

The relationship between diabetes and HCC has suggested that antidiabetic medication use could modify HCC risk. Metformin, a widely prescribed antidiabetic drug that reduces levels of circulating glucose and insulin, is frequently prescribed as a first-line treatment. As diabetes progresses, individuals often transition to use of other oral hypoglycemic drugs and ultimately to insulin.

Three recent meta-analyses of metformin and HCC have evaluated the results of published studies and have reported significantly decreased risks with odds ratios between 0.24 and 0.50.[102–104] All studies included in the meta-analyses, however, compared use of metformin with the use of other antidiabetic drugs. The close correlation of the drugs with duration and severity of disease, however, has made the interpretation of these results unclear. Such comparisons are likely to overestimate the protective effect of metformin, an early disease treatment, and overestimate the risk imposed by insulin, a treatment of last resort. In a study published after the meta-analyses were conducted, data from the United Kingdom were used to compare metformin use with use of no medication and the results found no association between metformin and risk of HCC.[105] Similarly, there was no increased risk with use of insulin. These results suggest that metformin may not be a good candidate for chemoprevention of HCC.

### Aspirin

Nonsteroidal anti-inflammatory drugs (NSAIDs), including aspirin and nonaspirin NSAIDs, are widely used as analgesic drugs, and low-dose aspirin is commonly used in the chemoprevention of cardiovascular and cerebrovascular disease.[106] In vitro studies and animal experiments suggest that NSAIDs also have chemopreventive and therapeutic benefit for HCC.[107–109] However, results of early human studies of

NSAID use and HCC[110,111] were inconsistent. More recently, a US cohort study reported a 37% reduced risk of HCC in association with NSAID use.[112] Aspirin-only users had a 49% reduced risk of HCC, whereas there was no effect of nonaspirin NSAIDs. The protective effect of aspirin was consistent across frequency (daily, monthly, and weekly) of use. Because daily aspirin use was likely to involve a low-dose formulation for cardiovascular chemoprotection, these data suggest that the same low-dose may be associated with a lower risk of HCC. Experimental and in vivo evidence for a protective effect of NSAIDs against liver cancer offer biologic plausibility for this association. NSAIDs modulate the risk of inflammation by inhibiting the cyclooxygenase enzymatic pathways necessary for synthesis of prostaglandins.[113] This inhibition, and decreases in epithelial proliferation and angiogenesis, coupled with increased apoptosis, results in the reduction of the inflammatory response, which has implications for prevention.[114] It has also been suggested that aspirin and NSAIDs in general might play a protective role in hepatic carcinogenesis through other noncyclooxygenase inhibitory pathways[109,115] and down regulation of proinflammatory cytokines.[116]

## SUMMARY

As the second greatest cause of cancer mortality in the world, liver cancer is a huge contributor to the world's cancer burden, but it is a preventable disease. Vaccination against HBV will have a dramatic effect on HCC incidence in coming generations. New infections with HCV have declined in most countries since the early 1990s and new curative treatments for HCV infection should have a major impact when their use becomes more widespread. Aflatoxin eradication programs and decreasing levels of alcohol consumption in some populations may also have favorable effects on HCC rates. The epidemic of obesity, diabetes, and metabolic syndrome in many areas, however, may prevent very steep declines in HCC rates that would otherwise be possible.

## REFERENCES

1. Ferlay J, Parkin DM, Curado MP, et al. Cancer incidence in five continents, volumes I to X: IARC CANCERBase No. 10 [Internet]. 2014. Available at: http://ci5.iarc.fr. Accessed November 25, 2014.
2. Ferlay J, Soerjomataram I, Ervik M, et al. GLOBOCAN 2012 v1.0, Cancer Incidence and Mortality Worldwide: IARC CancerBase No. 11 [Internet]. Lyon (France): International Agency for Research on Cancer. 2013. Available at: http://globocan.iarc.fr. Accessed November 12, 2014.
3. Altekruse SF, Henley SJ, Cucinelli JE, et al. Changing hepatocellular carcinoma incidence and liver cancer mortality rates in the United States. Am J Gastroenterol 2014;109(4):542–53.
4. Gao S, Yang WS, Bray F, et al. Declining rates of hepatocellular carcinoma in urban Shanghai: incidence trends in 1976-2005. Eur J Epidemiol 2012;27(1):39–46.
5. Tanaka H, Imai Y, Hiramatsu N, et al. Declining incidence of hepatocellular carcinoma in Osaka, Japan, from 1990 to 2003. Ann Intern Med 2008;148(11):820–6.
6. Surveillance, Epidemiology, and End Results (SEER) Program (www.seer.cancer.gov) SEER*Stat Database: Incidence - SEER 18 Regs Research Data + Hurricane Katrina Impacted Louisiana Cases, Nov 2013 Sub (1973–2011) Total U.S., National Cancer Institute, DCCPS, Surveillance Research

Program, Surveillance Systems Branch, based on the November 2013 submission. 2014.

7. Surveillance, Epidemiology and End Results (SEER) Program. SEER*Stat Database: North American Association of Central Cancer Registries (NAACCR) Incidence-CiNA Analytic File, 1995–2009. Bethesda, MD: National Cancer Institute, Division of Cancer Control and Population Sciences, Surveillance Research Program, Surveillance Systems Branch. 2012.

8. Perz JF, Armstrong GL, Farrington LA, et al. The contributions of hepatitis B virus and hepatitis C virus infections to cirrhosis and primary liver cancer worldwide. J Hepatol 2006;45(4):529–38.

9. Paraskevis D, Magiorkinis G, Magiorkinis E, et al. Dating the origin and dispersal of hepatitis B virus infection in humans and primates. Hepatology 2013;57(3):908–16.

10. Simmonds P. Reconstructing the origins of human hepatitis viruses. Philos Trans R Soc Lond B Biol Sci 2001;356(1411):1013–26.

11. International Agency for Research on Cancer. Hepatitis viruses. Lyon (France): International Agency for Research on Cancer; 1994.

12. Ott JJ, Stevens GA, Groeger J, et al. Global epidemiology of hepatitis B virus infection: new estimates of age-specific HBsAg seroprevalence and endemicity. Vaccine 2012;30(12):2212–9.

13. Centers for Disease Control and Prevention. Hepatitis B. 2010. Available at: http://wwwnc.cdc.gov/travel/yellowbook/2010/chapter-2/hepatitis-b.aspx. Accessed November 5, 2014.

14. Marinier E, Barrois V, Larouze B, et al. Lack of perinatal transmission of hepatitis B virus infection in Senegal, West Africa. J Pediatr 1985;106(5):843–9.

15. Ming L, Thorgeirsson SS, Gail MH, et al. Dominant role of hepatitis B virus and cofactor role of aflatoxin in hepatocarcinogenesis in Qidong, China. Hepatology 2002;36(5):1214–20.

16. Chen G, Lin W, Shen F, et al. Past HBV viral load as predictor of mortality and morbidity from HCC and chronic liver disease in a prospective study. Am J Gastroenterol 2006;101(8):1797–803.

17. Chen CJ, Yang HI, Iloeje UH. Hepatitis B virus DNA levels and outcomes in chronic hepatitis B. Hepatology 2009;49(Suppl 5):S72–84.

18. McMahon BJ. The natural history of chronic hepatitis B virus infection. Hepatology 2009;49(Suppl 5):S45–55.

19. McMahon BJ. Natural history of chronic hepatitis B. Clin Liver Dis 2010;14(3): 381–96.

20. Sumi H, Yokosuka O, Seki N, et al. Influence of hepatitis B virus genotypes on the progression of chronic type B liver disease. Hepatology 2003;37(1):19–26.

21. World Health Organization. Hepatitis B. 2010. Available at: http://www.who.int/immunization/topics/hepatits_b/en/index.html. Accessed November 3, 2014.

22. Goldstein ST, Zhou F, Hadler SC, et al. A mathematical model to estimate global hepatitis B disease burden and vaccination impact. Int J Epidemiol 2005;34(6): 1329–39.

23. World Health Organization. Fact sheet no. 204, Hepatitis B. World Health Organization; 2014. Available at: http://www.who.int/mediacentre/factsheets/fs204/en/. Accessed December 3, 2014.

24. Filippelli M, Lionetti E, Gennaro A, et al. Hepatitis B vaccine by intradermal route in non responder patients: an update. World J Gastroenterol 2014;20(30):10383–94.

25. Chang MH, You SL, Chen CJ, et al. Decreased incidence of hepatocellular carcinoma in hepatitis B vaccinees: a 20-year follow-up study. J Natl Cancer Inst 2009;101(19):1348–55.

26. Chiang CJ, Yang YW, You SL, et al. Thirty-year outcomes of the national hepatitis B immunization program in Taiwan. JAMA 2013;310(9):974–6.
27. Liang X, Bi S, Yang W, et al. Evaluation of the impact of hepatitis B vaccination among children born during 1992-2005 in China. J Infect Dis 2009;200(1):39–47.
28. Ang LW, Cutter J, James L, et al. Seroepidemiology of hepatitis B virus infection among adults in Singapore: a 12-year review. Vaccine 2013;32(1):103–10.
29. Yan H, Peng B, Liu Y, et al. Viral entry of hepatitis B and D viruses and bile salts transportation share common molecular determinants on sodium taurocholate cotransporting polypeptide. J Virol 2014;88(6):3273–84.
30. Ding S, Robek MD. Cytidine deamination and cccDNA degradation: a new approach for curing HBV? Hepatology 2014;60(6):2118–21.
31. Choo QL, Kuo G, Weiner AJ, et al. Isolation of a cDNA clone derived from a blood-borne non-A, non-B viral hepatitis genome. Science 1989;244(4902):359–62.
32. Simmonds P. Genetic diversity and evolution of hepatitis C virus: 15 years on. J Gen Virol 2004;85(Pt 11):3173–88.
33. Simmonds P, Holmes EC, Cha TA, et al. Classification of hepatitis C virus into six major genotypes and a series of subtypes by phylogenetic analysis of the NS-5 region. J Gen Virol 1993;74(Pt 11):2391–9.
34. Pybus OG, Barnes E, Taggart R, et al. Genetic history of hepatitis C virus in East Asia. J Virol 2009;83(2):1071–82.
35. Pybus OG, Markov PV, Wu A, et al. Investigating the endemic transmission of the hepatitis C virus. Int J Parasitol 2007;37(8–9):839–49.
36. Bostan N, Mahmood T. An overview about hepatitis C: a devastating virus. Crit Rev Microbiol 2010;36(2):91–133.
37. Tanaka Y, Hanada K, Mizokami M, et al. Inaugural Article: a comparison of the molecular clock of hepatitis C virus in the United States and Japan predicts that hepatocellular carcinoma incidence in the United States will increase over the next two decades. Proc Natl Acad Sci U S A 2002;99(24):15584–9.
38. Iida F, Iida R, Kamijo H, et al. Chronic Japanese schistosomiasis and hepatocellular carcinoma: ten years of follow-up in Yamanashi Prefecture, Japan. Bull World Health Organ 1999;77(7):573–81.
39. Frank C, Mohamed MK, Strickland GT, et al. The role of parenteral antischistosomal therapy in the spread of hepatitis C virus in Egypt. Lancet 2000;355(9207):887–91.
40. Armstrong GL, Alter MJ, McQuillan GM, et al. The past incidence of hepatitis C virus infection: implications for the future burden of chronic liver disease in the United States. Hepatology 2000;31(3):777–82.
41. Salomon JA, Weinstein MC, Hammitt JK, et al. Empirically calibrated model of hepatitis C virus infection in the United States. Am J Epidemiol 2002;156(8):761–73.
42. Seeff LB, Miller RN, Rabkin CS, et al. 45-year follow-up of hepatitis C virus infection in healthy young adults. Ann Intern Med 2000;132(2):105–11.
43. Davis GL, Alter MJ, El-Serag H, et al. Aging of hepatitis C virus (HCV)-infected persons in the United States: a multiple cohort model of HCV prevalence and disease progression. Gastroenterology 2010;138(2):513–21, 521.e1–6.
44. Sofia MJ, Bao D, Chang W, et al. Discovery of a beta-d-2'-deoxy-2'-alpha-fluoro-2'-beta-C-methyluridine nucleotide prodrug (PSI-7977) for the treatment of hepatitis C virus. J Med Chem 2010;53(19):7202–18.

45. Sulkowski MS, Gardiner DF, Rodriguez-Torres M, et al. Daclatasvir plus sofosbuvir for previously treated or untreated chronic HCV infection. N Engl J Med 2014; 370(3):211–21.
46. IARC. Overall evaluations of carcinogenicity: an updating of IARC monographs volumes 1 to 42. Supplement 7. Lyon (France): International Agency for Research on Cancer; 1987.
47. Wild CP, Hall AJ. Primary prevention of hepatocellular carcinoma in developing countries. Mutat Res 2000;462(2–3):381–93.
48. Plymoth A, Viviani S, Hainaut P. Control of hepatocellular carcinoma through hepatitis B vaccination in areas of high endemicity: perspectives for global liver cancer prevention. Cancer Lett 2009;286(1):15–21.
49. Sun CA, Wu DM, Wang LY, et al. Determinants of formation of aflatoxin-albumin adducts: a seven-township study in Taiwan. Br J Cancer 2002;87(9):966–70.
50. Qian GS, Ross RK, Yu MC, et al. A follow-up study of urinary markers of aflatoxin exposure and liver cancer risk in Shanghai, People's Republic of China. Cancer Epidemiol Biomarkers Prev 1994;3(1):3–10.
51. Ross RK, Yuan JM, Yu MC, et al. Urinary aflatoxin biomarkers and risk of hepatocellular carcinoma. Lancet 1992;339(8799):943–6.
52. Kuang SY, Lekawanvijit S, Maneekarn N, et al. Hepatitis B 1762T/1764A mutations, hepatitis C infection, and codon 249 p53 mutations in hepatocellular carcinomas from Thailand. Cancer Epidemiol Biomarkers Prev 2005;14(2):380–4.
53. Liu Y, Wu F. Global burden of aflatoxin-induced hepatocellular carcinoma: a risk assessment. Environ Health Perspect 2010;118(6):818–24.
54. Wild CP, Gong YY. Mycotoxins and human disease: a largely ignored global health issue. Carcinogenesis 2010;31(1):71–82.
55. Chen JG, Egner PA, Ng D, et al. Reduced aflatoxin exposure presages decline in liver cancer mortality in an endemic region of China. Cancer Prev Res (Phila) 2013;6(10):1038–45.
56. London WT, McGlynn KA. Liver Cancer. In: Schottenfeld D, Fraumeni JF, editors. Cancer epidemiology and prevention. New York: Oxford University Press; 2006. p. 763–86.
57. Donato F, Tagger A, Gelatti U, et al. Alcohol and hepatocellular carcinoma: the effect of lifetime intake and hepatitis virus infections in men and women. Am J Epidemiol 2002;155(4):323–31.
58. Kuper H, Tzonou A, Kaklamani E, et al. Tobacco smoking, alcohol consumption and their interaction in the causation of hepatocellular carcinoma. Int J Cancer 2000;85(4):498–502.
59. Yuan JM, Govindarajan S, Arakawa K, et al. Synergism of alcohol, diabetes, and viral hepatitis on the risk of hepatocellular carcinoma in blacks and whites in the U.S. Cancer 2004;101(5):1009–17.
60. International Agency for Research on Cancer. Alcohol drinking. Lyon (France): International Agency for Research on Cancer; 1988.
61. World Cancer Research Fund/American Institute for Cancer Research. Food, nutrition, physical activity, and the prevention of cancer: a global perspective. Washington, DC: American Institute for Cancer Research; 2007.
62. Turati F, Galeone C, Rota M, et al. Alcohol and liver cancer: a systematic review and meta-analysis of prospective studies. Ann Oncol 2014;25(8):1526–35.
63. Alcorn T. Mongolia's struggle with liver cancer. Lancet 2011;377(9772):1139–40.
64. Chen J, Han Y, Xu C, et al. Effect of type 2 diabetes mellitus on the risk for hepatocellular carcinoma in chronic liver diseases: a meta-analysis of cohort studies. Eur J Cancer Prev 2015;24:89–99.

65. El-Serag HB, Richardson PA, Everhart JE. The role of diabetes in hepatocellular carcinoma: a case-control study among United States veterans. Am J Gastroenterol 2001;96(8):2462–7.
66. Wang C, Wang X, Gong G, et al. Increased risk of hepatocellular carcinoma in patients with diabetes mellitus: a systematic review and meta-analysis of cohort studies. Int J Cancer 2012;130(7):1639–48.
67. Wang P, Kang D, Cao W, et al. Diabetes mellitus and risk of hepatocellular carcinoma: a systematic review and meta-analysis. Diabetes Metab Res Rev 2012; 28(2):109–22.
68. Saunders D, Seidel D, Allison M, et al. Systematic review: the association between obesity and hepatocellular carcinoma: epidemiological evidence. Aliment Pharmacol Ther 2010;31(10):1051–63.
69. Larsson SC, Wolk A. Overweight, obesity and risk of liver cancer: a meta-analysis of cohort studies. Br J Cancer 2007;97(7):1005–8.
70. Jinjuvadia R, Patel S, Liangpunsakul S. The association between metabolic syndrome and hepatocellular carcinoma: systemic review and meta-analysis. J Clin Gastroenterol 2014;48(2):172–7.
71. Shaw JE, Sicree RA, Zimmet PZ. Global estimates of the prevalence of diabetes for 2010 and 2030. Diabetes Res Clin Pract 2010;87(1):4–14.
72. James WP. The epidemiology of obesity: the size of the problem. J Intern Med 2008;263(4):336–52.
73. IARC. Tobacco smoke and involuntary smoking. IARC Monogr Eval Carcinog Risks Hum 2004;83:1–1438.
74. The health consequences of smoking: 50 years of progress. A report of the Surgeon General. Available at: http://www.surgeongeneral.gov/library/reports/ 50-years-of-progress/. Accessed December 10, 2014.
75. Lee YC, Cohet C, Yang YC, et al. Meta-analysis of epidemiologic studies on cigarette smoking and liver cancer. Int J Epidemiol 2009;38(6):1497–511.
76. Bravi F, Bosetti C, Tavani A, et al. Coffee reduces risk for hepatocellular carcinoma: an updated meta-analysis. Clin Gastroenterol Hepatol 2013;11(11): 1413–21.e1.
77. Fon Sing M, Yang WS, Gao S, et al. Epidemiological studies of the association between tea drinking and primary liver cancer: a meta-analysis. Eur J Cancer Prev 2011;20(3):157–65.
78. Bamia C, Lagiou P, Jenab M, et al. Coffee, tea and decaffeinated coffee in relation to hepatocellular carcinoma in a European population: multicentre, prospective cohort study. Int J Cancer 2014. http://dx.doi.org/10.1002/ijc.29214.
79. Setiawan VW, Wilkens LR, Lu SC, et al. Association of coffee intake with reduced incidence of liver cancer and death from chronic liver disease in the US multiethnic cohort. Gastroenterology 2014;148(1):118–25.
80. Cavin C, Holzhaeuser D, Scharf G, et al. Cafestol and kahweol, two coffee specific diterpenes with anticarcinogenic activity. Food Chem Toxicol 2002;40(8): 1155–63.
81. Muriel P, Arauz J. Coffee and liver diseases. Fitoterapia 2010;81(5):297–305.
82. Boettler U, Sommerfeld K, Volz N, et al. Coffee constituents as modulators of Nrf2 nuclear translocation and ARE (EpRE)-dependent gene expression. J Nutr Biochem 2011;22(5):426–40.
83. Ludwig IA, Clifford MN, Lean ME, et al. Coffee: biochemistry and potential impact on health. Food Funct 2014;5(8):1695–717.
84. Yang CS, Wang X, Lu G, et al. Cancer prevention by tea: animal studies, molecular mechanisms and human relevance. Nat Rev Cancer 2009;9(6):429–39.

85. Baigent C, Blackwell L, Emberson J, et al. Efficacy and safety of more intensive lowering of LDL cholesterol: a meta-analysis of data from 170,000 participants in 26 randomised trials. Lancet 2010;376(9753):1670–81.
86. Chan KK, Oza AM, Siu LL. The statins as anticancer agents. Clin Cancer Res 2003;9(1):10–9.
87. Gazzerro P, Proto MC, Gangemi G, et al. Pharmacological actions of statins: a critical appraisal in the management of cancer. Pharmacol Rev 2012;64(1):102–46.
88. Chiu HF, Ho SC, Chen CC, et al. Statin use and the risk of liver cancer: a population-based case-control study. Am J Gastroenterol 2011;106(5):894–8.
89. Lai SW, Liao KF, Lai HC, et al. Statin use and risk of hepatocellular carcinoma. Eur J Epidemiol 2013;28(6):485–92.
90. Leung HW, Chan AL, Lo D, et al. Common cancer risk and statins: a population-based case-control study in a Chinese population. Expert Opin Drug Saf 2013; 12(1):19–27.
91. Tsan YT, Lee CH, Ho WC, et al. Statins and the risk of hepatocellular carcinoma in patients with hepatitis C virus infection. J Clin Oncol 2013;31(12):1514–21.
92. Tsan YT, Lee CH, Wang JD, et al. Statins and the risk of hepatocellular carcinoma in patients with hepatitis B virus infection. J Clin Oncol 2012;30(6):623–30.
93. Friis S, Poulsen AH, Johnsen SP, et al. Cancer risk among statin users: a population-based cohort study. Int J Cancer 2005;114(4):643–7.
94. Marelli C, Gunnarsson C, Ross S, et al. Statins and risk of cancer: a retrospective cohort analysis of 45,857 matched pairs from an electronic medical records database of 11 million adult Americans. J Am Coll Cardiol 2011;58(5):530–7.
95. El-Serag HB, Johnson ML, Hachem C, et al. Statins are associated with a reduced risk of hepatocellular carcinoma in a large cohort of patients with diabetes. Gastroenterology 2009;136(5):1601–8.
96. Khurana V, Saluja A, Caldito G, et al. Statins are protective against hepatocellular cancer in patients with hepatitis C virus infection: half a million U.S. veterans' study. Gastroenterology 2005;128:A714.
97. Friedman GD, Flick ED, Udaltsova N, et al. Screening statins for possible carcinogenic risk: up to 9 years of follow-up of 361,859 recipients. Pharmacoepidemiol Drug Saf 2008;17(1):27–36.
98. McGlynn KA, Divine GW, Sahasrabuddhe VV, et al. Statin use and risk of hepatocellular carcinoma in a U.S. population. Cancer Epidemiol 2014;38(5):523–7.
99. Bjorkhem-Bergman L, Backheden M, Soderberg Lofdal K. Statin treatment reduces the risk of hepatocellular carcinoma but not colon cancer-results from a nationwide case-control study in Sweden. Pharmacoepidemiol Drug Saf 2014; 23(10):1101–6.
100. Pradelli D, Soranna D, Scotti L, et al. Statins and primary liver cancer: a meta-analysis of observational studies. Eur J Cancer Prev 2012;22(3):229–34.
101. Singh S, Singh PP, Singh AG, et al. Statins are associated with a reduced risk of hepatocellular cancer: a systematic review and meta-analysis. Gastroenterology 2013;144(2):323–32.
102. Franciosi M, Lucisano G, Lapice E, et al. Metformin therapy and risk of cancer in patients with type 2 diabetes: systematic review. PLoS one 2013;8(8):e71583.
103. Singh S, Singh PP, Singh AG, et al. Anti-diabetic medications and risk of pancreatic cancer in patients with diabetes mellitus: a systematic review and meta-analysis. Am J Gastroenterol 2013;108(4):510–9 [quiz: 520].
104. Zhang H, Gao C, Fang L, et al. Metformin and reduced risk of hepatocellular carcinoma in diabetic patients: a meta-analysis. Scand J Gastroenterol 2013; 48(1):78–87.

105. Hagberg KW, McGlynn KA, Sahasrabuddhe VV, et al. Anti-diabetic medications and risk of primary liver cancer in persons with type II diabetes. Br J Cancer 2014;111(9):1710–7.

106. Conaghan PG. A turbulent decade for NSAIDs: update on current concepts of classification, epidemiology, comparative efficacy, and toxicity. Rheumatol Int 2012;32(6):1491–502.

107. Cervello M, Foderaa D, Florena AM, et al. Correlation between expression of cyclooxygenase-2 and the presence of inflammatory cells in human primary hepatocellular carcinoma: possible role in tumor promotion and angiogenesis. World J Gastroenterol 2005;11(30):4638–43.

108. Fodera D, D'Alessandro N, Cusimano A, et al. Induction of apoptosis and inhibition of cell growth in human hepatocellular carcinoma cells by COX-2 inhibitors. Ann N Y Acad Sci 2004;1028:440–9.

109. Leng J, Han C, Demetris AJ, et al. Cyclooxygenase-2 promotes hepatocellular carcinoma cell growth through Akt activation: evidence for Akt inhibition in celecoxib-induced apoptosis. Hepatology 2003;38(3):756–68.

110. Cibere J, Sibley J, Haga M. Rheumatoid arthritis and the risk of malignancy. Arthritis Rheum 1997;40(9):1580–6.

111. Coogan PF, Rosenberg L, Palmer JR, et al. Nonsteroidal anti-inflammatory drugs and risk of digestive cancers at sites other than the large bowel. Cancer Epidemiol Biomarkers Prev 2000;9(1):119–23.

112. Sahasrabuddhe VV, Gunja MZ, Graubard BI, et al. Nonsteroidal anti-inflammatory drug use, chronic liver disease, and hepatocellular carcinoma. J Natl Cancer Inst 2012;104(23):1808–14.

113. Knights KM, Mangoni AA, Miners JO. Defining the COX inhibitor selectivity of NSAIDs: implications for understanding toxicity. Expert Rev Clin Pharmacol 2010;3(6):769–76.

114. Jankowska H, Hooper P, Jankowski JA. Aspirin chemoprevention of gastrointestinal cancer in the next decade. a review of the evidence. Pol Arch Med Wewn 2010;120(10):407–12.

115. Kern MA, Schubert D, Sahi D, et al. Proapoptotic and antiproliferative potential of selective cyclooxygenase-2 inhibitors in human liver tumor cells. Hepatology 2002;36(4 Pt 1):885–94.

116. Imaeda AB, Watanabe A, Sohail MA, et al. Acetaminophen-induced hepatotoxicity in mice is dependent on Tlr9 and the Nalp3 inflammasome. J Clin Invest 2009;119(2):305–14.

# Anatomic Pathology of Hepatocellular Carcinoma

## Histopathology Using Classic and New Diagnostic Tools

Meredith E. Pittman, MD[a], Elizabeth M. Brunt, MD[b],*

### KEYWORDS

- Hepatocellular carcinoma • Liver biopsy • Dysplastic nodule
- Immunohistochemistry • Glypican-3 • Glutamine synthetase • Arginase-1
- Biphenotypic

### KEY POINTS

- The diagnosis of hepatocellular carcinoma requires careful evaluation of architecture and cytology on the H&E stained slide.
- Ancillary stains are helpful when applied in a systematic manner.
- High-grade dysplastic nodules are precursors to hepatocellular carcinoma, but a definitive diagnosis may not be possible by needle biopsy alone.

## INTRODUCTION

The liver biopsy for a clinical concern of hepatocellular carcinoma (HCC) can be very straightforward for the pathologist or can present one of the more challenging specimens in surgical pathology, even for specialists. Despite ever-improving imaging techniques, such studies cannot always address the origin or the malignant potential of a hepatic lesion and thus a biopsy is performed. A concurrent biopsy of nonlesional liver for comparison is helpful when provided. This article is a guide through liver biopsy evaluation from the perspective of pathologists using routine stains available in most laboratories. The understanding is that such a biopsy is only carried out under highly specialized circumstances.[1]

## CLINICAL DATA

Patient demographics and clinical history are important when reviewing a mass-directed biopsy. Specifically, patient gender and age provide the first breakpoints in

[a] Department of Pathology, Johns Hopkins Medical Institutions, 401 North Broadway, Baltimore, MD 21231, USA; [b] Department of Pathology and Immunology, Washington University School of Medicine, 660 South Euclid Avenue, St Louis, MO 63110, USA
* Corresponding author.
*E-mail address:* EBrunt@path.wustl.edu

Clin Liver Dis 19 (2015) 239–259
http://dx.doi.org/10.1016/j.cld.2015.01.003
1089-3261/15/$ – see front matter © 2015 Elsevier Inc. All rights reserved.

the diagnostic algorithm for a differential diagnosis.[2] Men are at 3-fold risk for developing HCC in the United States, and risk for most adult liver carcinomas increases with age. Pediatric liver malignancies are separate considerations, not further discussed in this article. Knowledge of possible underlying chronic liver disease (CLD) is the next step in the decision tree. In a patient with known CLD or cirrhosis, the working diagnosis of a new nodule favors primary liver carcinoma over either metastatic liver disease or benign tumor of the liver because up to 90% of HCC cases occur in patients with underlying CLD[3] and benign liver tumors are very unusual in cirrhosis.

It is important for the pathologist to correlate histologic features with imaging studies (see elsewhere in this issue by Anis for further discussion). The most useful tool for a pathologist remains the routine hematoxylin-eosin (H&E) stain and, in most cases, it is the careful study of the H&E that will lead to the diagnosis or guide additional work-up.

## HEMATOXYLIN-EOSIN STAIN EVALUATION OF THE DIRECTED BIOPSY FOR HEPATOCELLULAR CARCINOMA
### Liver Biopsy in Hepatocellular Carcinoma: Yes or No?

Unlike other solid organs, consideration of biopsy for malignancy in the cirrhotic liver continues to be controversial. The most recent iteration of the controversy[4] highlights the use of the newer targeted molecular therapies in many other organs, which require tumor tissue analysis but do not exist for HCC. Pathologists have responded to these arguments in the past and will continue because several important considerations in the discussion remain.[5]

For cirrhotic patients, current practice guidelines[1] dictate that when imaging findings of a 1 to 2 cm lesion are atypical, the lesion should be biopsied (see later discussion).

### Architecture

The initial assessment determines the presence of the lesion in the biopsy tissue, which begins with overall evaluation of parenchymal architecture. Unaccompanied arteries and lack of complete portal tracts indicate that lesional tissue is present (**Fig. 1**). The hepatocyte and cord growth patterns also highlight the lesion. Some HCCs have sheet-like compact growth, others have a pseudoglandular pattern with a dilated canaliculus in the center (**Fig. 2**), and others recapitulate the trabecular formations of hepatic cords or plates.

A well-differentiated HCC may initially appear, on low-power microscopy, to be normal hepatic parenchyma and, in this case, loss of the normal liver cell plates from 1 to 2 cell nuclei across (normal) to 3 or more nuclei in a single cord (neoplastic) is a feature of malignancy. Whereas normal liver should have narrow cords of hepatocytes running in parallel, even well-differentiated HCC tissue has a somewhat disorganized pattern secondary to the increased thickness of the hepatocyte cords (**Fig. 3**). These altered patterns of growth are an indication of lesional tissue. A reticulin stain may be an additional aid in these types of cases.

### Cytology

Although architecture is often the most helpful tool in recognizing the presence of an HCC, cytologic clues are present in HCC as well. One may appreciate 2 different populations of cells, and the neoplastic population may take various appearances. Up to one-third of HCCs are steatotic and the presence of a fatty nodule in a background of nonfatty liver is suggestive of a lesion. In fact, HCC may show any cytologic or nuclear features of its benign counterparts, including steatosis, steatohepatitis, Mallory-Denk bodies, hyaline globules, and intranuclear inclusions.

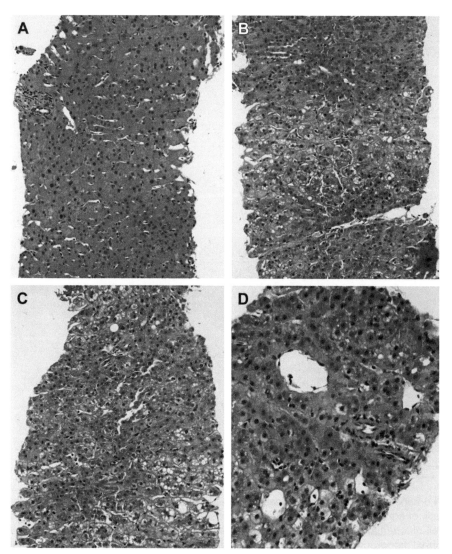

**Fig. 1.** Architectural changes in neoplastic liver. (*A*) Nonneoplastic liver core with portal tract and unremarkable hepatocytes (H&E stain, ×10). (*B–D*) Well-differentiated HCC with no visible portal tracts, variation in hepatocytes, and unpaired arteries (B, C, H&E stain, ×10; D, H&E stain, ×20).

Steatohepatitic-HCC is reportedly more common in livers with background findings of steatohepatitis from metabolic syndrome or alcoholic liver disease.[6] Clear cell change is not an uncommon feature of HCC and, rarely, even giant cells may be present; however, iron accumulation is notably not seen in HCC, even in livers with hereditary hemochromatosis (**Figs. 4** and **5**). Nuclear alterations of malignancy may also occur. Nuclear pleomorphism can occur as a feature of regeneration in the liver; therefore, hepatopathologists rely on mitoses and specifically abnormal mitoses as features of some HCCs. Abnormal mitotic figures are neither common nor necessary in small and well-differentiated HCC.

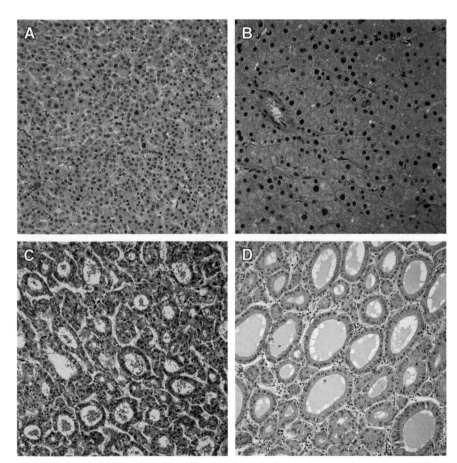

**Fig. 2.** HCC growth: (*A* and *B*) sheet-like and (*C* and *D*) pseudoacinar (H&E stain, ×10).

Edmondson and Steiner's[7] classification of HCC, published in 1954, remains the basis of current classifications of well-, moderately- and poorly differentiated HCCs. Well-differentiated HCC, grade I, is characterized by tumor cells that closely resemble normal hepatocytes with relatively abundant eosinophilic cytoplasm but slightly enlarged nuclei in a thin trabecular pattern. Moderately differentiated HCC, grade II, has an increased nuclear-to-cytoplasmic ratio and often increasing nuclear hyperchromasia. Pseudoglandular structures are frequent. Poorly differentiated HCC, grade III, has larger and more hyperchromatic nuclei. This grade may have giant cells. Grade IV, also known as poorly differentiated, has a very high nuclear-to-cytoplasmic ratio (**Fig. 6**). It is important to realize that HCC may have several different architectural and cytologic features and forms of differentiation within any given lesion.

### Stroma

HCC is most commonly a stroma-poor malignancy. The normal liver does not have a true basement membrane to be invaded, nor does HCC produce a desmoplastic response as many other invasive carcinomas do. The description and proof of stromal alteration and invasion came through the careful observations of our Japanese colleagues.[8] Loss of the keratin (K) 7 (also known as cytokeratin [CK] 7)–positive or

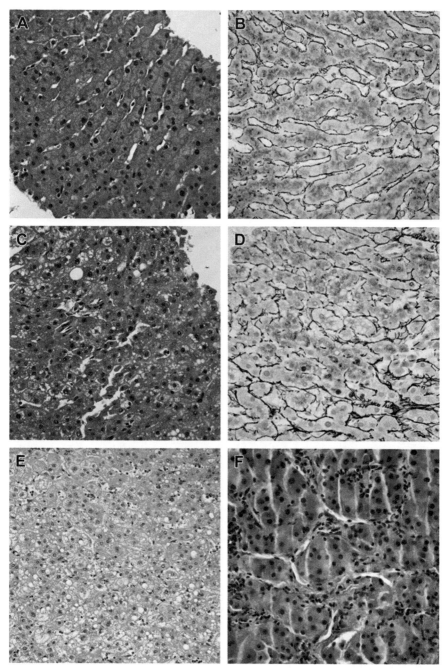

**Fig. 3.** Organization of the hepatic cords in HCC. (*A*) Nonneoplastic liver with normal liver plates (1–2 nuclei thick) parallel to each other; sinusoids are easily visible (H&E stain, ×20). (*B*) The reticulin lines the cords in nonneoplastic liver (Sweet's reticulin, ×20). (*C*) Well-differentiated HCC without clearly identifiable cords or sinusoids (H&E stain, ×20). (*D*) Loss of reticulin in HCC. Some cords are wide with 3 to 4 nuclei in a cord (Sweet's reticulin, ×20). (*E* and *F*) HCC with broad trabeculae, disorganized hepatic cords (H&E stain, ×20).

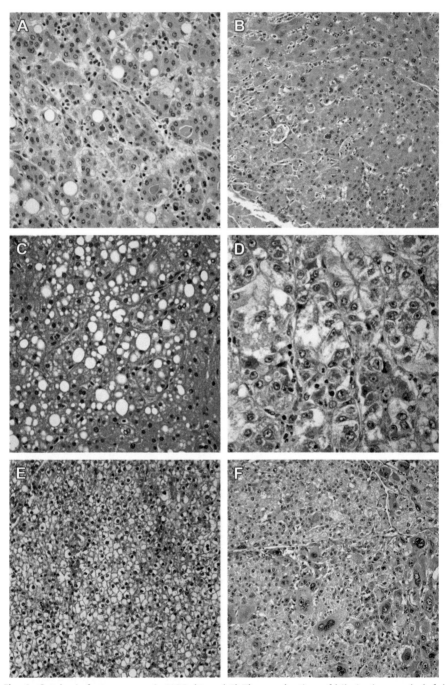

**Fig. 4.** Cytologic features seen in HCC. (*A* and *B*) The production of bile is always a helpful clue that the lesion is of hepatocellular origin (H&E stain, ×10). (*C*) Steatosis (H&E stain, ×10), (*D*) Mallory-Denk bodies (H&E stain, ×20), (*E*) clear cell change (H&E stain, ×4), and (*F*) giant cells in HCC (H&E stain, ×4).

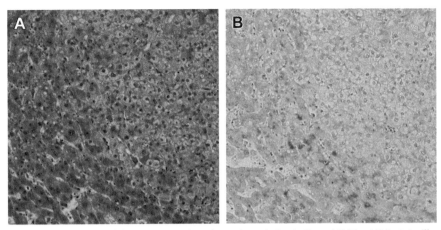

**Fig. 5.** A dysplastic nodule as an iron-free focus in a cirrhotic liver. (*A*) The H&E stain illustrates a nodule-in-nodule with pushing margins (H&E stain, ×10); (*B*) this same nodule does not retain iron, as seen on a Prussian blue stain (Modified Perls', ×10).

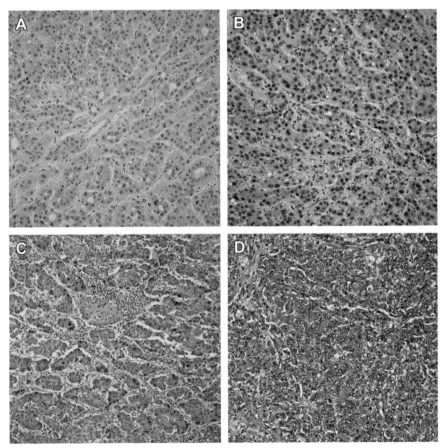

**Fig. 6.** Cytologic differentiation of HCC. (*A* and *B*) Moderately differentiated HCC. (*C* and *D*) Poorly differentiated HCC (H&E stain, ×10).

K19 (CK19)–positive ductular reaction around cirrhotic nodules during the process of intranodular hepatocarcinogenesis is a step in this process of stromal invasion.[9,10] Two distinct variants of HCC do have abundant stroma and these variants can be recognized on needle biopsy.

The first variant, scirrhous HCC, is rare. These tumors are firm and have abundant eosinophilic stroma that dissects through the neoplastic hepatocytes in large bands. Because of the dense fibrosis and altered morphology of the tumor cells, which form clusters, strands, and tubules, the differential diagnosis includes intrahepatic cholangiocarcinoma and primary liver carcinoma with biphenotypic differentiation. In fact, if appropriate immunohistochemistry (IHC) stains are not done, the latter diagnosis may be missed. At least focally, the cellular regions of scirrhous HCC should have hepatocellular features and look similar to nonscirrhous HCC.[11] This tumor has also been reported to be associated with hypercalcemia clinically (**Fig. 7**).[12]

The second stromal-rich HCC variant is fibrolamellar HCC (FLC). This tumor has distinct gross and microscopic appearances. Grossly, these may resemble focal nodular hyperplasia with a central scar. Microscopically, they are characterized by fibrotic bands of eosinophilic, lamellated collagen of varying size that are apparent at low-power dissecting through groups of large neoplastic hepatocytes with deeply eosinophilic, granular cytoplasm. The cells have open nuclei with vesicular chromatin and a single, large, eosinophilic, and hyperchromatic nucleolus (**Fig. 8**). The diagnosis of FLC rests more on the hepatocytic cells than the stroma. FLC typically occurs as a single tumor in noncirrhotic livers in younger individuals[13] but has been reported as a component of mixed FLC-HCC, a tumor with features of FLC and conventional HCC in cirrhosis in older individuals.[14]

## FURTHER WORK-UP OF SUSPECTED HEPATOCELLULAR CARCINOMA

Although careful evaluation of the H&E stained slide is the best initial tool when evaluating a hepatic biopsy, confirmation of the diagnosis by ancillary special and IHC stains is frequently necessary. The optimum panel of stains varies depending on the tissue present and the clinical situation.

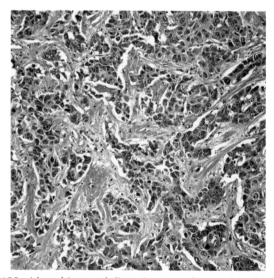

**Fig. 7.** Scirrhous HCC with architectural distortion secondary to the sclerotic stroma. Biphenotypic primary liver carcinoma is in the differential diagnosis (H&E stain, ×10).

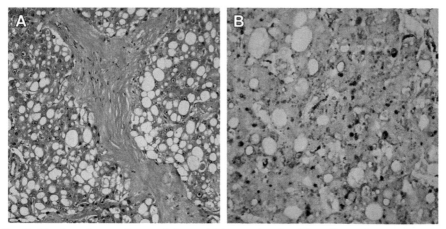

**Fig. 8.** Fibrolamellar carcinoma. (*A*) In addition to bands of lamellar collagen, the large neoplastic eosinophilic cells have prominent vesicular nuclei and nucleoli; intracytoplasmic eosinophilic inclusions are also present. The amount of steatosis is unusual (H&E stain, ×10). (*B*) CD68 immunostain has a granular pattern within the neoplastic cells (Anti-CD 68 immunohistochemistry, ×10).

### Scenario 1: Metastasis Versus Primary Liver Carcinoma

Metastatic disease is far more common than primary liver carcinoma in the noncirrhotic liver. This section is not meant as a complete review of the metastases common to the liver.[15] Instead, it highlights stains that are useful in confirming hepatocellular or primary liver carcinoma with hepatobiliary-biphenotypic differentiation. The initial staining panel includes markers of hepatocellular differentiation, followed by markers of biliary and progenitor-stem cell differentiation. The former include the canalicular markers, polyclonal carcinoembryonic antigen (pCEA), and/or canalicular immunostaining of neprilysin (CD10). In addition, cytoplasmic glypican-3 (GPC-3), arginase (Arg), and hepatocyte paraffin 1 (Hep Par 1) can be helpful (**Fig. 9**).

pCEA is a glycoprotein found in fetal and adult epithelial cells and cytoplasmic staining is present in a variety of adenocarcinomas,[15] including cholangiocarcinoma. In HCC, however, pCEA has a very distinctive canalicular pattern of immunoreactivity with a sensitivity approaching 100%.[16,17] The less differentiated the HCC, however, the more membranous the staining pattern becomes. CD10 is also reactive to hepatocyte canaliculi and may be as sensitive as pCEA.[18] It is often worthwhile doing both CD10 and pCEA because vagaries of fixation may result in one reacting better than the other in any given HCC. CD10 also has the benefit of differentiating clear cell HCC from clear cell renal cell carcinoma.

GPC-3, an oncofetal protein and member of the glycosyl-phosphatidylinositol–anchored cell-surface heparan sulfate proteoglycans, is overexpressed in HCC, as well as germ cell tumors and malignant melanoma.[19] Glypican-3 staining in HCC has been reported with a sensitivity around 80% in most studies and it is likely to be reactive in both a poorly differentiated HCC and well-differentiated HCC.[15,20–23] Because reactivity is not homogeneous throughout the tumor, a negative result should not exclude HCC. The staining pattern may be granular or dot-like cytoplasmic or diffuse cytoplasmic with or without membranous enhancement.[21,23,24]

Arg-1 is a urea cycle enzyme with expression in nonneoplastic human liver and the antibody to Arg-1 shows immunolabeling of normal hepatocytes throughout the lobule.[25] Like glypican-3, Arg-1 has also been reported as a sensitive marker for

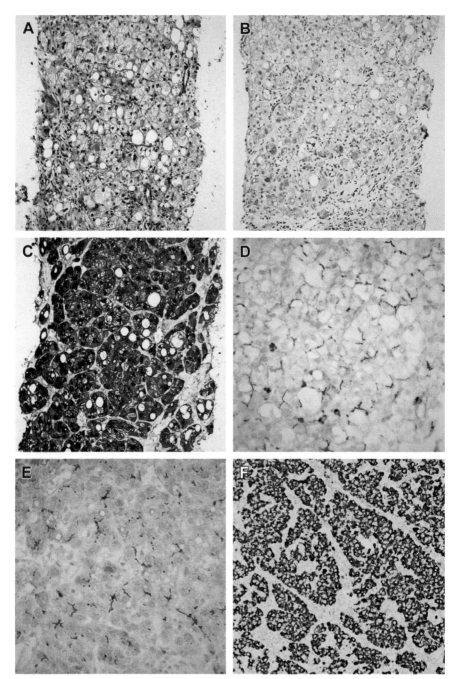

**Fig. 9.** Photomicrographs (*A–D*) are taken from one HCC. (*A*) Extensive clear cell change as well as steatosis (H&E stain, ×10), (*B*) weak but positive GPC-3 (anti-GPC-3 immunohistochemistry, ×10), (*C*) strong Arg-1 (anti-Arg-1 immunohistochemistry, ×10), and (*D*) canalicular pCEA immunostain all confirm hepatocellular differentiation (anti-pCEA immunohistochemistry, ×10). Other helpful confirmatory stains are (*E*) canalicular CD10 (anti-CD10 immunohistochemistry, ×10) and (*F*) cytoplasmic Hepatocyte Paraffin 1 (anti-hepatocyte (Hep-par 1), ×10).

hepatocellular differentiation in carcinoma (~90%) and reactivity may be seen even in poorly differentiated HCC. The staining of Arg-1 may be patchy within the tumor and the pattern is reported as cytoplasmic with or without nuclear reactivity.[26]

### Scenario 2: Hepatocellular Carcinoma Versus Other Hepatocellular Lesion

If the sampled mass appears hepatocellular by H&E and/or some of the markers previously discussed, a different set of stains may be helpful in determining the malignant potential of the lesion. Two of the most useful ancillary stains for this scenario are the reticulin histochemical stain and CD34 immunohistochemical stain. As previously discussed, the proliferation of neoplastic cells in HCC disrupts the liver plate architecture and, therefore, contributes to disruption (loss) of the normal reticulin network that outlines the liver cell plates. The reticulin pattern in HCC is both decreased (but not entirely lost) and disorganized (**Fig. 10**). Caution must be taken not to overinterpret reticulin disruption in the setting of steatosis as a sign of neoplasia.[27]

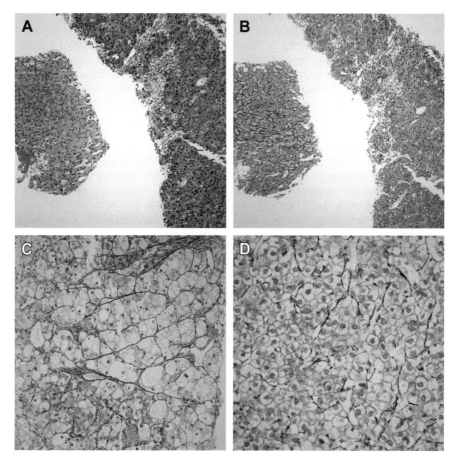

**Fig. 10.** Reticulin loss in HCC. (*A* and *B*) H&E and reticulin stained slides showing nonneoplastic liver on the left with HCC on the right. Note the loss of reticulin and the disorganized growth of the neoplasm (A, H&E stain, ×10; B, Sweet's reticulin, ×10). (*C*) A reticulin stain from the HCC (also shown in **Fig. 9**); note the widened hepatocellular plates (Sweet's reticulin, ×20). (*D*) A reticulin stain from the clear cell HCC (also shown in **Fig. 4**) illustrates dramatic loss of reticulin (Sweet's reticulin, ×20).

As reticulin is lost in HCC, CD34 sinusoidal expression is increased. Normally, the sinusoidal endothelial cells label with CD34, in the cells adjacent to the portal tracts or emanating from cirrhotic septa. Capillarization of endothelium occurs in HCC because these cells are exposed to higher oxygen tension, after which complete sinusoidal reactivity is observed. Of note, incomplete CD34 reactivity in a core needle biopsy is not necessarily evidence against HCC; however, complete CD34 reactivity is strong evidence for an HCC.[17] Two caveats regarding CD34 are that hepatocellular adenomas may show areas of complete sinusoidal reactivity, as may the surfaces of cirrhotic nodules. For these reasons, although the sinusoidal CD34 reactivity of HCC is characteristic, CD34 cannot be used as a stand-alone stain for HCC. This differential diagnosis remains challenging and clinical correlation is required (**Fig. 11**).

The findings from H&E, reticulin, and CD34 have been incorporated into a helpful classification tool by Quaglia, and colleagues.[28] The presence of necrosis, cellular atypia, trabeculae more than 4 cells thick (by H&E or reticulin), mitotic figures, or diffuse capillarization of the sinusoids by CD34, are all helpful features of HCC. When at least 3 of these features are present, the nodule is very likely to be HCC.[28]

As previously discussed, glypican-3 is a marker of hepatocellular differentiation but this antibody can also be useful in determining the malignant potential of a lesion. Glypican-3 was originally developed to distinguish hepatocellular adenoma from HCC.[19,29] Strong GPC-3 staining can be seen HCC but should not occur in adenoma. This antibody is not a perfect tool, however, and patchy reactivity may also occur in nonneoplastic liver. Staining has been shown in up to 80% of nonneoplastic liver with very active hepatitis C, as well as in approximately 50% of high-grade dysplastic nodules (HGDNs).[30] Nevertheless, the combination of strong GPC-3 along with typical CD34 sinusoidal reactivity is typical of an HCC (**Fig. 12**).[20]

Another IHC stain that is useful in differentiating hepatocellular lesions is glutamine synthetase (GS), a target of β-catenin signaling.[31] In normal liver, GS labels a thin rim of zone 3 hepatocytes next to the terminal hepatic venule. Instead, up to 70% of HCCs show diffuse and cytoplasmic GS cellular labeling (**Fig. 13**).[32]

FLC, as previously discussed, is a distinct neoplasm with respect to conventional HCC, and has a unique immunohistochemical staining profile. The IHC markers

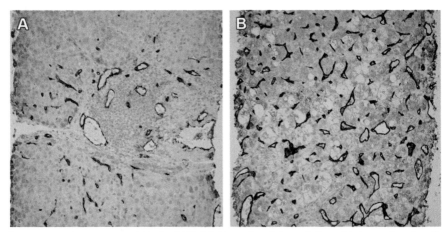

**Fig. 11.** CD34 immunoreactivity in HCC. (*A*) Normal staining of sinusoids immediately adjacent to a portal tract. (*B*) Diffuse capillarization of the sinusoids with CD34 reactivity to endothelium throughout the sinusoids (Anti-CD 34 Immunohistochemistry, ×10).

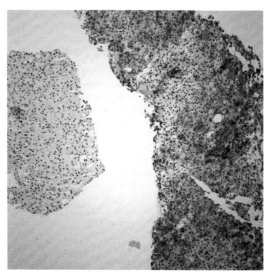

**Fig. 12.** GPC-3 in HCC (*right*); negative in nonneoplastic liver (*left*) (also shown in **Fig. 9**). GPC-3 can have various and inhomogeneous reactivity (Anti-GPC-3 immunohistochemistry, ×10).

include hepatocellular (Hep Par-1, pCEA, glypican-3), biliary (K7, epithelial membrane antigen), progenitor cell (K19, epithelial cell adhesion molecule [EpCAM]), stem cell (CD133, CD44), and macrophage (CD68) markers. The presence of CD68-positive granular or dot-like pattern in a diffuse manner can be useful in the diagnosis of FLC (see **Fig. 8**).[33]

### Scenario 3: Primary Liver Carcinoma Versus Mixed Hepatobiliary-Biphenotypic Carcinoma

The presence of greater than 5% of K19 positivity in tumor cells in otherwise standard HCC is recognized as a poor prognostic marker. Possible reasons for this have been explored in a recent study.[34] These tumors, however, differ from another form of primary liver carcinoma (see later discussion).

Liver pathologists in large centers around the world are encountering tumors of mixed hepatobiliary phenotype with greater frequency. These are no longer the oddity they once were thought to be, yet their exact derivation is still poorly understood: be it from a common stem cell or from dedifferentiation of a malignant hepatocellular tumor.[35] Regardless, these tumors are increasingly encountered because they are atypical on imaging in both cirrhotic and noncirrhotic livers.[36] The terminology for these tumors remains under discussion among international working parties[37] but the current terminology is that of the 2010 World Health Organization (WHO) (**Box 1**).[38]

These tumors can be recognized, in the simplest terms, by demonstration of both hepatocellular and biliary phenotypes. This dual phenotype may be expressed in separate parts of the same tumor or it may be present in an intermingling of cell types, or by dual phenotypic expression of one cell type. This duality may be demonstrated with any of the markers noted previously for hepatocellular differentiation and with markers for K7 and K19 for biliary differentiation and progenitor-stem cell differentiation. Although some biphenotypic tumors declare themselves with poorly formed glands within a dense stromal component, others do not have the helpful stroma, Some simply appear as a ductular reaction and are associated with HCC elsewhere.

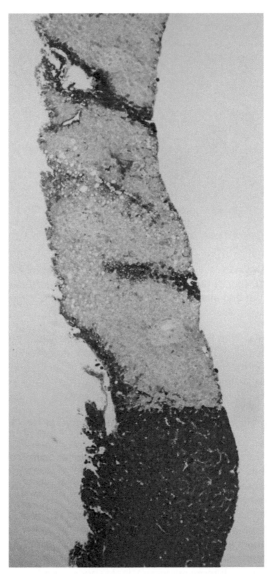

**Fig. 13.** GS immunoreactivity in HCC. The nonneoplastic hepatocytes label with GS around the terminal hepatic venule in zone 3. The bottom portion of the core biopsy is HCC, which has a diffuse pattern of immunoreactivity. Diffuse GS immunoreactivity can also be noted in β-catenin activated adenomas, thus, clinical context, including gender and knowledge of background liver disease, is important. In focal nodular hyperplasia, GS immunoreactivity is along vascular septa and results in a geographic map-like pattern that is easily recognized in a whole section but can be more difficult to appreciate on biopsy (Anti-glutamine synthetase immunohistochemistry, ×10).

These latter tumors, referred to as cholangiolocellular carcinoma, may recapitulate a ductal plate. Sheets of otherwise routine HCC or cholangiocarcinoma may show hints of biphenotypic differentiation with appropriate immunohistochemical staining (**Fig. 14**).

---

**Box 1**
**WHO Classification of combined hepatocellular-cholangiocarcinoma**

*Combined hepatocellular-cholangiocarcinoma, classic type*

- Contains typical HCC and typical cholangiocarcinoma
- pCEA and CD10 can confirm hepatocellular differentiation
- Mucin, K7, and K19 can highlight the adenocarcinoma component
- No stem-progenitor cells should be seen

*Combined hepatocellular-cholangiocellular carcinoma with stem-cell features, typical subtype*

- Mature appearing hepatocytes with peripheral clusters of hyperchromatic cells
- Peripheral cells react with K7, K19, NCAM, KIT, and/or EpCAM, the profile of stem-progenitor cells

*Combined hepatocellular-cholangiocarcinoma with stem-cell features, intermediate-cell subtype*

- Tumor cells have features of both hepatocytes and cholangiocytes on H&E
- Trabeculae, nests, or strands are formed; no well-formed glands are seen
- Cells are reactive for both hepatocyte and biliary markers

*Combined hepatocellular-cholangiocarcinoma with stem-cell features, cholangiolocellular type*

- Small cells grow in tubular, cord-like, anastomosing antler pattern, a recapitulation of the canals of Hering
- Cells are reactive for K19, KIT, NCAM (neural cell adhesion molecule), and EpCAM (stem-progenitor phenotype)
- Formerly categorized as a subtype of cholangiocarcinoma

*Adapted from* Theise ND, Nakashima O, Park YN, et al. Combined hepatocellular-cholangiocarcinoma. In: Bosman FT, Carneiro F, Hruban RH, et al, editors. WHO Classification of Tumors of the Digestive System. 4th edition. Lyon (France): IARC; 2010. p. 225–7; with permission.

---

## PRECURSOR LESIONS AND EARLY HEPATOCELLULAR CARCINOMA IN CIRRHOSIS

HCC arises from a multistep progression of genetic and epigenetic alterations. These alterations are currently undergoing rigorous investigation. Correlations with histologic findings have validated the earliest molecular findings of dysplastic nodules (DNs) and early HCC (eHCC).[39,40]

### Dysplastic Foci and Nodules

Dysplastic foci and DNs, first defined by an international working party nearly 2 decades ago[41] and updated 14 years later,[42] are premalignant lesions. The nodules are well-defined and circumscribed, whereas foci are less well defined. These lesions arise in the setting of CLD, most often in cirrhosis. They can be identified on gross examination of the liver as distinct from other cirrhotic nodules because of color or bulging. Histologically they are graded as either low or high. These lesions are generally small (<1 cm) but can become quite large. The smaller lesions may be difficult to detect by imaging and accurate characterization using current imaging modalities is challenging. As these lesions transition to complete malignancy, they may or may not have the vascular characteristics and capsular formation of HCC.

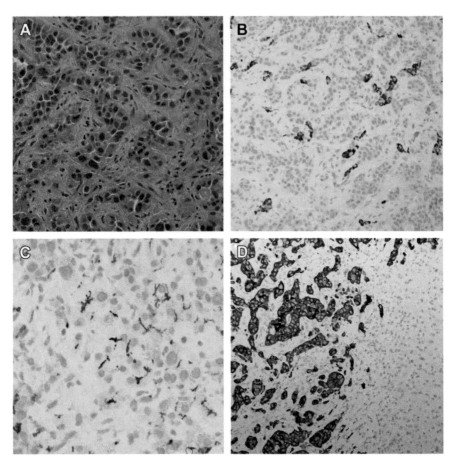

**Fig. 14.** A biphenotypic primary liver carcinoma. (A) H&E shows a tumor made up of pleomorphic cells growing in tubules (H&E stain, ×10). The malignant cells show a dual phenotype with expression of (B) Hep Par 1 (Anti-hepatocyte (Hep-par 1), immunohistochemistry, ×10), (C) CD10 (Anti-CD 10 immunohistochemistry, ×20), and (D) K19 (or CK19) (Anti-K19 immunohistochemistry, ×10).

Many lines of evidence point to DNs being true precursors to HCC. First, there is the morphologic evidence. Pathologists have noted that in a nodular liver there can exist a distinct HGDN that then has an HCC growing within, the so-called nodule-in-nodule formation (**Fig. 15**). The presence of overtly malignant foci in a background of cirrhosis or dysplasia is visual confirmation.[43] Additional morphologic evidence comes from the perinodular stroma, in which gradual loss of K19-positive ductular reaction parallels the progression from cirrhotic nodule to DN to HCC.[10] Second, there is epidemiologic evidence that cirrhotic patients with HGDNs are 4 times as likely to develop HCC as cirrhotic patients without DN.[44] Finally, molecular studies have shown that DN and HCC share genetic alterations, although DN has fewer mutations than HCC.[39,45]

Interobserver agreement for the diagnosis of a low-grade DN (LGDN) is quite low.[42] In general, a LGDN can be recognized by its monotonous cell population when compared with the surrounding cirrhotic liver. Although a LGDN has mildly increased cell density, the cells are not obviously small. Architectural and cytologic atypia are minimal, and pseudoglandular architecture is uncommon. Portal tracts are commonly

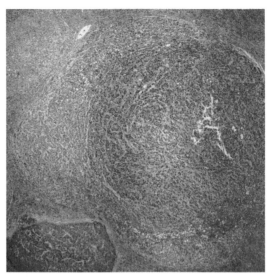

**Fig. 15.** A nodule of HCC arising within a dysplastic nodule, the so-called nodule-in-nodule pattern. The right center shows a clonal nodule growing within and distinct from the background nodule surrounding it (H&E stain, ×4).

present within LGDN, particularly the large, so-called macroregenerative, nodules. LGDNs carry a low risk of transformation to HCC.

In contrast, HGDNs have many but not all features of HCC. They stand out from surrounding cirrhotic nodules because of architectural or cytologic features; therefore, although they may be less monotonous than LGDN, they are clearly clonal. Small cell change may be prominent but other alterations not present in surrounding cirrhotic nodules may occur as well, including steatosis, deep eosinophilia, and steatohepatitis. Iron loss in otherwise iron-rich cirrhosis is a strong feature of HGDN (see **Fig. 5**). Occasional unpaired arteries may occur, but diffuse CD34 positivity would place the diagnosis of HGDN in doubt and raise a concern of HCC. Portal tracts are uncommon but no invasion of the surrounding portal tracts is seen. HGDN is a frequent differential diagnosis in a needle biopsy for the nodule with atypical features by imaging. Small cell change, in which the hepatocyte nuclei align themselves along the sinusoids and the cells appear crowded due to an increasing nuclear-to-cytoplasmic ratio, is a sign of dysplasia in hepatocellular lesions. Some investigators have proposed terms such as small cell dysplasia[46] or increased nuclear density[47] to describe the features.

### Small Hepatocellular Carcinoma

According to the International Consensus Group for Hepatocellular Neoplasia (ICGHN) in 2009, small HCC are those less than 2 cm, the size less than which radiologists may have difficulty classifying a lesion as definitive HCC.[42,48] Two types of small HCC defined by the ICGHN are eHCC and progressed HCC.

eHCC, referred to by some investigators as small well-differentiated HCC of the vaguely nodular type,[8,44] has increased cell density, irregular hepatic plates, decreased numbers (or loss of) portal tracts, unpaired arteries, and (occasionally) diffuse fatty change (noted in up to 50% of eHCC). eHCC is not well-circumscribed or encapsulated but is somewhat nodular by imaging and gross evaluation. By histopathologic evaluation, neoplastic hepatocytes tend to grow in an infiltrative pattern along the existing hepatocyte cords.[44] The definitive diagnosis can be made with

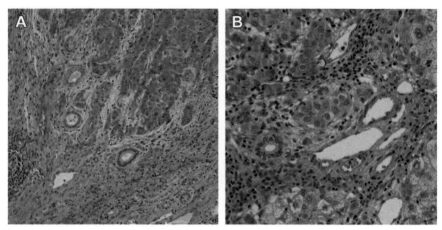

**Fig. 16.** Stromal invasion by HCC. No ductular reaction is present. (*A*) Overtly malignant hepatocytes making bile (H&E stain, ×10) (*B*) invading into a large portal tract (H&E stain, ×20).

identification of stromal invasion of a portal tract or septum (**Fig. 16**). Useful adjuncts for diagnosing stromal invasion are either the loss of K7 or K19 ductular cells, or the presence of GS-positive tumor cells.[10,44]

A panel of immunostains has been proposed and shown to help differentiate DN from eHCC and includes glypican-3, GS, and heat shock protein 70 (HSP70). HSP70 is an antiapoptotic protein that is overexpressed in HCC (**Fig. 17**). LGDNs and regenerative nodules should always be negative for the panel of GPC-3, GS, and HSP70. If 2 of these 3 stains are positive, in any combination, the sensitivity and specificity for the detection of eHCC are approximately 60% and 100%, respectively.[31,32] Two positive stains, therefore, support the diagnosis of HCC but negative results do not unequivocally rule it out. Diffusely positive CD34 is a useful adjunct in this situation.

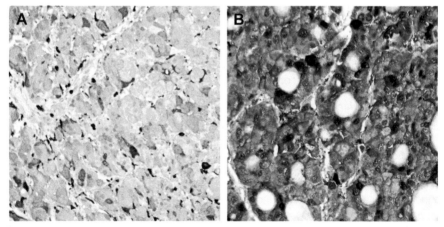

**Fig. 17.** HSP70 in HCC. (*A*) The staining may be patchy, as in this metastatic HCC to the lung, (*B*) or very strong and diffuse. When positive in conjunction with GS or GPC-3, this stain is evidence of malignancy (anti-HSP70 immunohistochemistry, ×10). (*Courtesy of* Dr Dora Lam-Himlin, Mayo Clinic, AZ, USA.)

In contrast to eHCC, progressed HCC is a smaller than 2 cm nodule that is obvious on the gross examination and clearly neoplastic by histologic evaluation. These HCCs, although small, are nodular, typically encapsulated, well-demarcated from the surrounding parenchyma, and usually moderately differentiated. Progressed HCC may already show microvascular invasion.[42]

## SUMMARY

As the incidence of HCC continues to increase, especially with the epidemic of liver disease related to obesity and the metabolic syndrome, and as imaging techniques become more sophisticated, the number of detectable hepatocellular lesions that require biopsy may also increase. The interpretation of mass-directed needle biopsies will remain a challenge as samples become smaller and pathologists are asked to do more with less tissue. As shown in this article, many of the most important histologic findings will likely be on the routine H&E stained slide. Only after careful evaluation of this tissue should further immunohistochemical work-up or molecular testing be performed. Pathologists who correlate clinical history, imaging findings, and a good core needle biopsy will usually have the ability to confidently and correctly diagnose a malignant hepatocellular neoplasm.

## REFERENCES

1. Bruix J, Sherman M. American Association for the Study of Liver Diseases. Management of hepatocellular carcinoma: an update. Hepatology 2011;53: 1020–2.
2. Brunt EM. Histopathologic features of hepatocellular carcinoma. Clin Liver Dis 2012;1:194–9.
3. Forner A, Llovet JM, Bruix J. Hepatocellular carcinoma. Lancet 2012;379: 1245–55.
4. Sherman M, Bruix J. Biopsy for liver cancer: how to balance research needs with evidence based clinical practice. Hepatology 2014;61(2):433–7.
5. Schirmacher P, Bedossa P, Roskams T, et al. Fighting the bushfire in HCC trials. J Hepatol 2011;55:276–7.
6. Salomao M, Remotti H, Vaughan R, et al. The steatohepatitic variant of hepatocellular carcinoma and its association with underlying steatohepatitis. Hum Pathol 2012;43:737–46.
7. Edmondson HA, Steiner PE. Primary carcinoma of the liver. A study of 100 cases among 48,900 necropsies. Cancer 1954;7:462–503.
8. Kojiro M, Roskams T. Early hepatocellular carcinoma and dysplastic nodules. Semin Liver Dis 2005;25:133–42.
9. Park YN, Kojiro M, Di Tommaso L, et al. Ductular reaction is helpful in defining early stromal invasion, small hepatocellular carcinomas, and dysplastic nodules. Cancer 2007;109:915–23.
10. Lennerz JK, Chapman WC, Brunt EM. Keratin 19 epithelial patterns in cirrhotic stroma parallel hepatocarcinogenesis. Am J Pathol 2011;179:1015–29.
11. Krings G, Ramachandran R, Jain D, et al. Immunohistochemical pitfalls and the importance of glypican 3 and arginase in the diagnosis of scirrhous hepatocellular carcinoma. Mod Pathol 2013;26:782–91.
12. Albar JP, De Miguel F, Esbrit P, et al. Immunohistochemical detection of parathyroid hormone-related protein in a rare variant of hepatic neoplasm (sclerosing hepatic carcinoma). Hum Pathol 1996;27:728–31.

13. Ang CS, Kelley RL, Choti MA, et al. Clinicopathologic characteristics and survival outcomes of patients with fibrolamellar carcinoma: data from the fibrolamellar carcinoma consortium. Gastrointest Cancer Res 2013;6:3–9.

14. Malouf GG, Brugieres L, Le Deley MC, et al. Pure and mixed fibrolamellar hepatocellular carcinomas differ in natural history and prognosis after complete surgical resection. Cancer 2012;118:4981–90.

15. Kakar S, Gown AM, Goodman ZD, et al. Best practices in diagnostic immunohistochemistry: hepatocellular carcinoma versus metastatic neoplasms. Arch Pathol Lab Med 2007;131:1648–54.

16. Morrison C, Marsh W, Frankel WL. A comparison of CD10 to pCEA, MOC-31, and hepatocyte for the distinction of malignant tumors in the liver. Mod Pathol 2002; 15(12):1279–87.

17. Goodman ZD. Neoplasms of the liver. Mod Pathol 2007;20(Suppl 1):S49–60.

18. Borscheri N, Roessner A, Rocken C. Canalicular immunostaining of neprilysin (CD10) as a diagnostic marker for hepatocellular carcinomas. Am J Surg Pathol 2001;25:1297–303.

19. Capurro M, Wanless IR, Sherman M, et al. Glypican-3: a novel serum and histochemical marker for hepatocellular carcinoma. Gastroenterology 2003;125:89–97.

20. Libbrecht L, Severi T, Cassiman D, et al. Glypican-3 expression distinguishes small hepatocellular carcinomas from cirrhosis, dysplastic nodules, and focal nodular hyperplasia-like nodules. Am J Surg Pathol 2006;30:1405–11.

21. Coston WM, Loera S, Lau SK, et al. Distinction of hepatocellular carcinoma from benign hepatic mimickers using Glypican-3 and CD34 immunohistochemistry. Am J Surg Pathol 2008;32:433–44.

22. Ligato S, Mandich D, Cartun RW. Utility of Glypican-3 in differentiating hepatocellular carcinoma from other primary and metastatic lesions in FNA of the liver: an immunocytochemical study. Mod Pathol 2008;21:626–31.

23. Shafizadeh N, Ferrell LD, Kakar S. Utility and limitations of glypican-3 expression for the diagnosis of hepatocellular carcinoma at both ends of the differentiation spectrum. Mod Pathol 2008;21:1011–8.

24. Wang XY, Degos F, Dubois S, et al. Glypican-3 expression in hepatocellular tumors: diagnostic value for preneoplastic lesions and hepatocellular carcinomas. Hum Pathol 2006;37:1435–41.

25. Multhaupt H, Fritz P, Schumacher K. Immunohistochemical localization of arginase in human liver using monoclonal antibodies against human liver arginase. Histochemistry 1987;87:465–70.

26. Yan BC, Gong C, Song J, et al. Arginase-1: a new immunohistochemical marker of hepatocytes and hepatocellular neoplasms. Am J Surg Pathol 2010;34: 1147–54.

27. Singhi AD, Jain D, Kakar S, et al. Reticulin loss in benign fatty liver: an important diagnostic pitfall when considering a diagnosis of hepatocellular carcinoma. Am J Surg Pathol 2012;36:710–5.

28. Quaglia A, Jutand MA, Dhillon A, et al. Classification tool for the systematic histological assessment of hepatocellular carcinoma, macroregenerative nodules, and dysplastic nodules in cirrhotic liver. World J Gastroenterol 2005;11: 6262–8.

29. Wanless IR. Liver biopsy in the diagnosis of hepatocellular carcinoma. Clin Liver Dis 2005;9(2):281–5.

30. Abdul-Al HM, Makhlouf HR, Wang G, et al. Glypican-3 expression in benign liver tissue with active hepatitis C: implications for the diagnosis of hepatocellular carcinoma. Hum Pathol 2008;39:209–12.

31. Tremosini S, Forner A, Boix L, et al. Prospective validation of an immunohisto-chemical panel (glypican 3, heat shock protein 70 and glutamine synthetase) in liver biopsies for diagnosis of very early hepatocellular carcinoma. Gut 2012; 61:1481–7.

32. Di Tommaso L, Franchi G, Park YN, et al. Diagnostic value of HSP70, glypican 3, and glutamine synthetase in hepatocellular nodules in cirrhosis. Hepatology 2007;45:725–34.

33. Ross HM, Daniel HD, Vivekanandan P, et al. Fibrolamellar carcinomas are positive for CD68. Mod Pathol 2011;24:390–5.

34. Govaere O, Komuta M, Berkers J, et al. Keratin 19: a key role player in the invasion of human hepatocellular carcinomas. Gut 2014;63:674–85.

35. Dubois-Pot-Schneider H, Fekir K, Coulouarn C, et al. Inflammatory cytokines promote the retrodifferentiation of the tumor-derived hepatocyte-like cells to progenitor cells. Hepatology 2014;60:2077–90.

36. Fowler KJ, Sheybani A, Paker RA 3rd, et al. Combined hepatocellular and cholangiocarcinoma (biphenotypic) tumors: imaging features and diagnostic accuracy of contrast-enhanced CT and MRI. Am J Roentgenol 2013;201:332–9.

37. Brunt EM, Paradis V, Sempoux C, et al. Biphenotypic (hepatobiliary) primary liver carcinomas: the work in progress. Future Medicine Review, in press.

38. Theise ND, Nakashima O, Park YN, et al. Combined hepatocellular-cholangiocarcinoma. In: Bosman FT, Carneiro F, Hruban RH, et al, editors. WHO classification of tumours of the digestive system. 4th edition. Lyon (France): IARC; 2010. p. 225–7.

39. Nault JC, Calderaro J, Di Tommaso L, et al. Telomerase reverse transcriptase promoter mutation is an early somatic genetic alteration in the transformation of premalignant nodules in hepatocellular carcinoma on cirrhosis. Hepatology 2014;60: 1983–92.

40. Roskams T, Kojiro M. Pathology of early hepatocellular carcinoma: conventional and molecular diagnosis. Semin Liver Dis 2010;30(1):17–25.

41. International Working Party. Terminology of nodular hepatocellular lesions. Hepatology 1995;22:983–93.

42. International Consensus Group for Hepatocellular Neoplasia. Pathologic diagnosis of early hepatocellular carcinoma: a report of the international consensus group for hepatocellular neoplasia. Hepatology 2009;49:658–64.

43. Libbrecht L, Desmet V, Roskams T. Preneoplastic lesions in human hepatocarcinogenesis. Liver Int 2005;25:16–27.

44. Park YN. Update on precursor and early lesions of hepatocellular carcinomas. Arch Pathol Lab Med 2011;135(6):704–15.

45. Maggioni M, Coggi G, Cassani B, et al. Molecular changes in hepatocellular dysplastic nodules on microdissected liver biopsies. Hepatology 2000;32:942–6.

46. Watanabe S, Okita K, Harada T, et al. Morphologic studies of the liver cell dysplasia. Cancer 1983;51(12):2197–205.

47. Ferrell L. Liver pathology: cirrhosis, hepatitis, and primary liver tumors. Update and diagnostic problems. Mod Pathol 2000;13(6):679–704.

48. Mitchell DG, Bruix J, Sherman M, et al. LI-RADS (Liver Imaging Reporting and Data System): summary, discussion, consensus of the LI-RADS management working group and future directions. Hepatology 2014. http://dx.doi.org/10. 1002/hep.27304.

# Pathogenesis and Prognosis of Hepatocellular Carcinoma at the Cellular and Molecular Levels

 CrossMark

Olivier Govaere, MSc, PhD*, Tania Roskams, MD, PhD*

## KEYWORDS

- Hepatic progenitor cell features • Cell of origin • Phenotype switching
- Tumor behavior • Chemoresistant cancer stem cells • Prognosis
- Microenvironment

## KEY POINTS

- Survival gene signature data sets that classify human hepatocellular carcinomas (HCCs) based on worse prognosis show a high expression of biliary-hepatic progenitor cell markers.
- Mechanisms of differentiation and/or dedifferentiation give rise to heterogeneity in human HCCs, reflecting the cell of origin.
- The plasticity of HCCs strongly depends on the interaction with the microenvironment.
- The expression of biliary-hepatic progenitor cell markers in HCCs linked with stemness features is a way to survive in a hostile environment.

## INTRODUCTION

Liver cancer is the fifth most diagnosed cancer worldwide with an increasing incidence each year, making it the second leading cause of cancer-related death globally.[1] Hepatocellular carcinoma (HCC) represents the major histologic type of primary liver cancer, accounting for 70% to 85% of the total liver cancer burden worldwide, and has a phenotype resembling hepatocytes histologically, when examined microscopically on hematoxylin-eosin stain (H&E) specimens.[2,3] Although advances in imaging and surgery have improved the prognosis of HCC patients, HCC remains an ominous tumor because of high rates of metastases and recurrence.[4,5] About 80% of HCCs arise in a background of long-lasting chronic liver disease. To understand the pathogenesis of

This research was supported by a grant from the Belgian Federal Science Policy Office (Interuniversity Attraction Poles program, P7/47-HEPRO). The authors have no conflict of interest to report.

Translational Cell and Tissue Research, Department of Imaging and Pathology, KULeuven and University Hospitals Leuven, Minderbroedersstraat 12, Leuven B3000, Belgium

* Corresponding authors.

E-mail addresses: olivier.govaere@med.kuleuven.be; tania.roskams@med.kuleuven.be

HCC, therefore, it is important to know what is happening in the chronically diseased liver. In normal, healthy circumstances the hepatocytes have a low turnover rate and a life expectancy of more than a year.[6] In response to parenchymal cell loss due to injuries such as partial hepatectomy or toxic injury, the liver can regenerate by proliferation of the main epithelial cell compartments (hepatocytes and cholangiocytes), followed by the proliferation of mesenchymal cell types (hepatic stellate cells) and endothelial cells. When the injury is too severe or when the hepatocytes become senescent (in part the result of ongoing proliferation during 20 to 30 years of chronic disease), activation and proliferation of a reserve compartment, the hepatic progenitor cells (HPCs), is observed.[7,8] This activation of HPCs is seen as a ductular reaction, which comprises an expansion of a transit amplifying cell compartment of small biliary cells located in the Hering canal, consisting of stem cell progeny that are destined to undergo terminal differentiation.[9,10] These small biliary cells can differentiate into biliary epithelial cells (cholangiocytes) or hepatocytes, depending on the underlying liver disease cause and which cell type is damaged the most. With differentiation toward hepatocytes, the HPCs gradually lose their biliary features. Keratin (K) 19, sex determining region Y-box 9 (SOX9), and tumor-associated calcium signal transducer 2 (TACSTD2 or TROP2) are some of the first markers they lose, followed by K7 and epithelial cell adhesion molecule (EPCAM), and an up-regulation of the HIPPO pathway and NUMB, an inhibitor of the Notch pathway (**Fig. 1**).[11–15] The regenerating liver is an ambient setting full of inflammation, stress, and signal-cell interactions pushing the HPCs toward a certain cell fate but also regulating apoptosis or senescence of the hepatocytes and forming scar tissue.[16] This background is a vivid and complex substrate in which HCCs arise. This article focuses on the pathogenesis of HCC at the cellular and molecular levels and, more specifically, on the mechanisms of differentiation and dedifferentiation in relation to their possible cells of origin and how the microenvironment plays an important role in tumor behavior and tumor heterogeneity.

## PREDICTING TUMOR BEHAVIOR: A HIGH-THROUGHPUT APPROACH

In recent years, many research groups have linked molecular profiles with the prognosis of patients diagnosed with HCC. Although the molecular classification of HCCs is described in more detail in other publication, the authors would like to pause and highlight a few publications that are key to the understanding of human HCC behavior.[17–19] In 2004, Thorgeirsson and colleagues,[20] in collaboration with the authors' group, identified 2 different gene expression patterns, based on microarray analysis, in a set of 92 human HCC samples. The subclass, linked with a lower overall survival, showed a strong correlation with several survival genes involving hypoxia inducible factor 1a.[20] In extension of this research and using a larger data set of 139 HCC samples, models for predicting the risk of recurrence and the prognosis were constructed by integrating gene expression data from rat fetal hepatoblasts and from rat hepatocytes with human HCC profiles.[21] Patients whose tumors shared a similar gene expression pattern to that of fetal hepatoblasts and showed a higher expression for biliary-HPC markers (eg, *KRT19*, *KRT7*) had a poor overall outcome. During the succeeding years, many publications described the potential clinical use of gene signatures as prognostic markers for patients diagnosed with or treated for an HCC (**Table 1**).[22–28] Recently, a molecular scoring system based on the expression of only 5 genes (*HN1*, *RAN*, *RAMP3*, *KRT19*, and *TAF9*) was shown to predict the outcome of patients after resection of HCC.[29]

Stratifying human HCCs based on specific biliary-HPC markers and generating gene expression profiles of these subclasses, has been another approach to

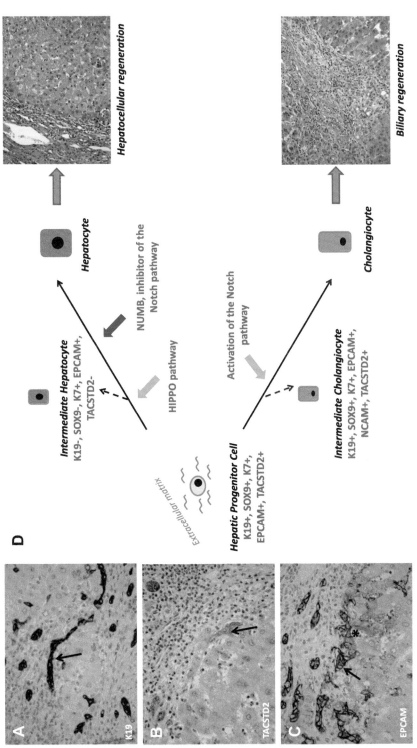

**Fig. 1.** Differentiation of HPCs toward hepatocytes or cholangiocytes. (*A–C*) Activation of human HPCs is seen as ductular reaction (*arrow*). On differentiation toward hepatocytes, the HPCs gradually lose their biliary markers. K19 and TACSTD2/TROP2 are some of the markers they lose first (*A, B*), whereas EPCAM can still be found in intermediate hepatocytes (*C, asterisk*). Magnification 400×. (*D*) Schematic overview of markers and pathways involved in the differentiation of HPCs to mediate hepatocellular or cholangiocellular regeneration, depending on the underlying cause (H&E magnification 200×).

**Table 1**
Selection of hepatocellular carcinoma gene signatures predicting worse prognosis

| Gene Signature | Description | Selection of Up-Regulated Biliary-HPC Genes | Author/Year |
|---|---|---|---|
| LIVER_CANCER_SURVIVAL_DN[a] | Genes highly expressed in human HCC with poor survival | KRT19, LAMB1, ANXA3, S100A6 | Lee et al,[20] 2004 |
| LIVER_CANCER_HEPATOBLAST[a] | Genes overexpressed in human HCC with hepatoblast property | KRT19, KRT7 | Lee et al,[21] 2006 |
| LIVER_CANCER_SUBCLASS_G1_UP[a] | Up-regulated genes in human HCC subclass G1, defined by unsupervised clustering | SOX9, S100A14 | Boyault et al,[22] 2007 |
| LIVER_CANCER_RECURRENCE_UP[a] | Genes positively correlated with recurrence in patients with hepatitis B–related HCCs | TACSTD2, NOTCH2, JAG1, S100A6, SOX9 | Woo et al,[23] 2008 |
| LIVER_CANCER_SUBCLASS_PROLIFERATION_UP[a] | Genes up-regulated in the proliferation subclass of HCCs; characterized by increased proliferation, high levels of serum AFP and chromosomal instability | S100P, LAMB1 | Chiang et al,[24] 2008 |
| LIVER_CANCER_SUBCLASS_S1[a] | Genes from subtype S1 signature of HCCs: aberrant activation of the WNT signaling pathway | LAMB1 | Hoshida et al,[25] 2009 |
| KRT19 rat signature | Genes up-regulated in K19 positive rat HCCs | Epcam | Andersen et al,[43] 2010 |
| Notch mouse signature | Genes highly expressed in liver tumors obtained from mice overexpressing the Notch intracellular domain | Sox9, Hnf1b, Hes1, Epcam | Villanueva et al,[31] 2012 |
| KRT19 human signature | Genes associated with high KRT19 expression in human HCCs | KRT19, KRT7, TACSTD2, JAG1, LAMB1, LAMC2 | Govaere et al,[44] 2014 |

[a] As found on http://www.broadinstitute.org/gsea/msigdb.
*Data from* Refs.[20–25,31,43,44]

understand tumor behavior. Yamashita and colleagues[30] classified human HCCs into 4 subtypes based on the HPC marker EPCAM and the patients' α-fetoprotein serum level, which could be linked with prognosis and unique molecular features. Villanueva and colleagues[31] generated the Notch signature, which proved to be strongly correlated with previously reported signatures that predict a clinically aggressive behavior and showed a role for the Notch pathway in HCC tumor initiation. The protein expression of biliary-HPC markers K19 and K7 in human HCCs was already described back in 1988, using an immunohistochemical approach.[32] Many publications that followed reported the clinicopathological relevance of K19 expression as a prognostic marker for patients diagnosed with an HCC.[33–42] Andersen and colleagues[43] used the gene signature from rat K19-positive HCCs as a predictive model for poor prognosis in patients diagnosed with an HCC. Recently, Govaere and colleagues[44] unraveled the underlying molecular phenotype of the K19-positive HCCs in human by using microarrays and microRNA profiling. Gene set enrichment analysis showed that genes positively correlated with keratin (KRT)19 gene expression linked with several other poor prognostic cancer-related data sets, including poor survival HCC subtype, proliferation HCC subtype, and subtype S1 signature with aberrant Wnt activation.[20,24,25] Overall, survival gene signature data sets that classify human HCCs based on worse prognosis show a high expression of biliary-HPC markers.

## CELL OF ORIGIN AND THE DIVERSITY IN HEPATOCELLULAR CARCINOMAS

How do HCCs acquire biliary-HPC features? Two hypotheses give possible explanations for this phenomenon: the processes of differentiation or dedifferentiation. Either HCCs arise from hepatocytes and the biliary-HPC features occur due to dedifferentiation mechanisms during cancer progression, or HCCs express biliary-HPC features as a reflection of their cell of origin (arising from an HPC or the progeny of an HPC). Hepatocytes display enormous plasticity. In chronic biliary diseases (eg, primary biliary cirrhosis and primary sclerosing cholangitis), the small bile ducts are inflamed and are slowly being destroyed, leading to the so-called vanishing bile duct syndrome. In these diseases, bile flow is hampered (ie, there is cholestasis) and there is intracellular accumulation of bile salts in the hepatocytes.[45] The periportal hepatocytes are the first cells that feel the toxic influence of the bile and in defense they dedifferentiate, becoming cholestatic hepatocytes, and express biliary-HPC markers such as K7 or JAG1 (a ligand of the Notch pathway) (**Fig. 2**). Also, in chronic hepatic venous congestion when there is parenchymal hypoxia, hepatocytes can express K7 and even K19.[46–49] Chen and colleagues[50] provided in vitro support for the concept of dedifferentiation by showing that healthy isolated rat hepatocytes can dedifferentiate into HPCs. Using an N-diethylnitrosamine–induced HCC mouse model, Santos and colleagues[51] showed that the expression of K7 or K19 occurred in end-stage HCC lesions rather than in early lesions, suggesting that dedifferentiation is a time-dependent process in HCC carcinogenesis. In daily clinical practice, the dedifferentiation process can be seen in late-stage human HCCs, which display a high degree of nuclear pleomorphism and anaplasia (personal observations, see **Fig. 2**).

On the other hand, HPCs could also be responsible for the heterogeneity found in HCCs. They have an enormous capacity to survive in an environment with reactive oxygen species, growth factors, and chronic inflammation, and thus are a potential target for carcinogenesis as well. The description of specific subsets of primary liver carcinomas with stemness features (characteristics typical for stem cells) and/or HPC features (eg, cholangiocellular carcinoma), with mixed HCC-cholangiocellular carcinoma features, supports the hypothesis of HPCs being the cell of origin for at

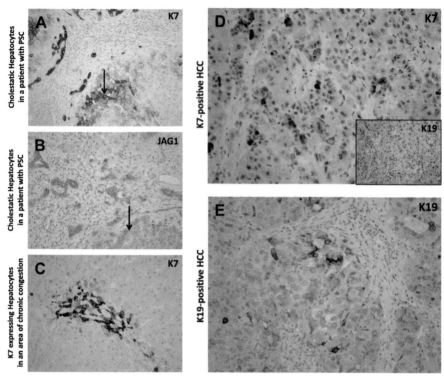

**Fig. 2.** Dedifferentiation during human chronic liver disease and HCC. (*A, B*) In human chronic biliary diseases (eg, primary sclerosing cholangitis [PSC]) hepatocytes can express biliary markers as a defense mechanism in response to the hampered bile flow. Arrow indicates cholestatic hepatocytes expressing K7 (*A*) or JAG1 (*B*). (*C*) Also in chronic congestion with parenchymal hypoxia, hepatocytes can express K7. (*D*) Late-stage human HCC, displaying a high degree of nuclear pleomorphism and anaplasia, which is positive for K7 though negative for K19 (*inset*), suggesting a process of dedifferentiation. (*E*) An example of a K19-positive HCC with less nuclear pleomorphism and anaplasia. The range of cell phenotypes found in the HCC resembles the differentiation of HPCs toward hepatocytes, suggestive that this tumor finds its origin in an HPC.

least a part of the hepatic carcinomas.[52,53] As mentioned previously, on differentiation toward hepatocytes, HPCs gradually lose their biliary markers and start to express typical hepatocyte markers and inhibitors of pathways necessary for biliary differentiation (eg, NUMB, inhibitor of the Notch pathway).[13,54,55] Thus, HPCs gives rise to a progeny of intermediate and mature hepatocytes to sustain parenchymal cell loss. This concept is sometimes referred to as the streaming liver because it is thought that the offspring of the HPCs have to migrate toward the damaged area, generating a continuous flow of cells.[56,57] The diversity of cell phenotypes (arising either via differentiation or dedifferentiation) that is seen in chronic liver disease could explain the heterogeneity found in human HCCs (**Fig. 3**).

## PLASTICITY OF HEPATOCELLULAR CARCINOMA DEPENDS ON THE MICROENVIRONMENT

Differentiation or dedifferentiation of a hepatic cell strongly depends on the interactions with its microenvironment and the range of signals the cell receives. This is also the case

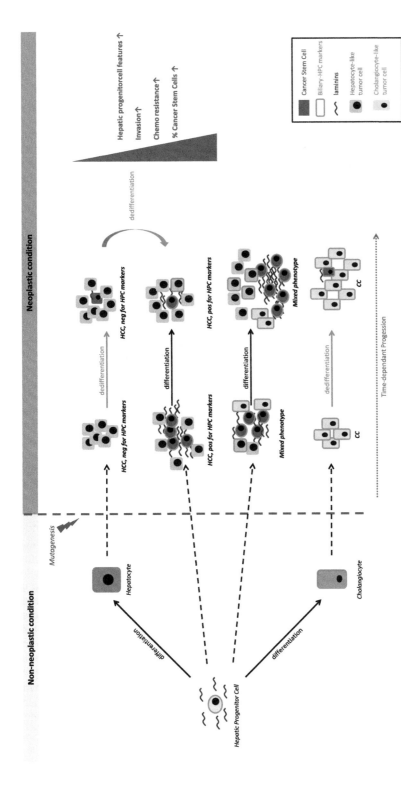

**Fig. 3.** Overview of how cell of origin and time-dependent dedifferentiation can contribute to different phenotypes found in hepatic cancer.

in human HCCs. HCC behavior is not that straightforward: the phenotype of a tumor cell cannot by itself completely explain how a tumor might react. The cross-talk between tumor cells and their microenvironment is crucial in determining the actions of those cells, even through interactions with the nonneoplastic surrounding liver tissue.[58] Using formalin-fixed paraffin-embedded tissue samples from patients diagnosed with HCC, Hoshida and colleagues[59] showed that the gene signature from the tissue adjacent to the tumor correlated with survival, rather than the gene signature from the HCCs themselves. Next, the authors will highlight some signaling pathways and mechanisms that relate to cell–microenvironment interactions and explain how these pathways help determine cell behavior in both HCC and in the regenerating liver. Laminins are constructed of 3 nonidentical peptide chains ($\alpha$, $\beta$, and $\gamma$) and are involved in many physiologic processes by interacting with integrin receptors.[60] In human liver disease, laminins have been reported to be part of the basement membrane surrounding the HPCs to help them remain in an undifferentiated state, sustaining the biliary-HPC features.[61] Using lineage tracing mouse models, Español-Suñer and colleagues[62] showed that HPC-mediated hepatocyte regeneration improved on reduction of laminin deposition. In a rat model of hepatocellular regeneration, the expression of the laminin gene subtypes $\beta 1$ and $\beta 2$ strongly correlated with *Krt19* expression.[63] In human HCCs, the laminin $\beta 1$ chain and the $\gamma 2$ chain have been linked with the *KRT19* signature, which could imply that laminin expression is important in sustaining the biliary-HPC features (as seen in the surrounding liver tissue) (see **Fig. 3**).[44] Laminin $\beta 1$ (*LAMB1*) expression was also noted in a few other gene signatures of poor prognosis (see **Table 1**). Using HCC cell lines in vitro, laminin $\beta 1$ expression was shown to be increased during epithelial to mesenchymal transition (EMT), a process in which tumor cells acquire a more invasive phenotype and lose some of their epithelial traits.[64,65] In a small set of hepatitis C virus–associated HCCs, an increase in DNA copy numbers for laminin $\gamma 2$ has been reported, implicating an association with HCC development.[66] Laminin $\gamma 2$ expression has also been linked with occurrence of metastases and a worse prognosis in patients diagnosed with HCC. In vitro coating experiments elucidated a role for laminin 332 (the protein that consists of the $\alpha 3$, the $\beta 3$, and the $\gamma 2$ chains) in the migration, proliferation, and resistance to targeted therapy for HCC cells.[67–70] The downstream pathway that is activated depends, not only on the laminin subtype but also to which integrin receptor and coreceptor the laminin binds. By binding to the alpha3 integrin receptor subunit, laminin 332 can induce proliferation through phosphorylation of the ERK1/2 pathway, whereas HCC cells that display a high expression of alpha6 integrin and CD151 undergo EMT in response to laminin 332, through hyperactivation of phosphatidylinositol-3-kinase.[69,71] Transforming growth factor (TGF)-$\beta 1$, a profibrotic cytokine that promotes the transition of hepatic stellate cells to myofibroblasts, has been reported to activate the beta1 integrin receptor subunit, causing noninvasive HCC cells to behave invasively.[72] Different sources for TGF-$\beta 1$ production have been suggested. Activated hepatic stellate cells or myofibroblasts have been shown to attenuate autocrine secretion of TGF-$\beta 1$, indicating the importance of tumor-stroma interaction, whereas tumor-associated macrophages have been reported as another source for TGF-$\beta 1$, promoting EMT and stemness features in HCC cells.[73–77] Whereas the TGF-$\beta$ cascade has an important role in inducing an invasive phenotype in HCCs, platelet-derived growth factor (PDGF) has been shown to be an important player in maintaining the invasive phenotype of HCCs at the tumor border.[78] PDGF treatment of immortalized mouse hepatocytes stimulated laminin $\beta 1$ expression, thereby underlining the crosstalk between the TGF-$\beta$–PDGF and the laminin pathway.[79] Govaere and colleagues[44] reported that PDGF receptor alpha is elevated in K19-positive HCCs and HPCs (which are surrounded by laminins) (**Fig. 4**). The PDGF receptor has been implicated as a potential

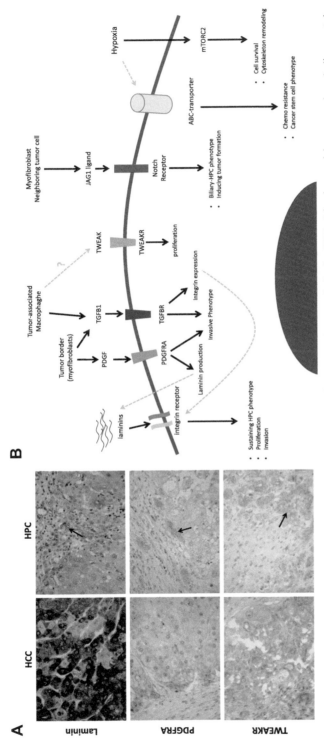

**Fig. 4.** Human HCCs mimic HPC behavior. Panel A shows how certain human HCCs can mimic the HPC niche (*arrows*) by expressing similar proteins: laminins, PDGFRA or TWEAKR. Magnification 400×. Panel B displays a schematic overview of the effect some pathways can have. Dotted green arrows indicate possible interactions between pathways.

target in the treatment of human HCCs because its inhibition could suppress the invasive phenotype (see **Fig. 4**).[80,81] Besides laminins and the PDGF receptor, there are other similarities between HPCs and HCCs. TWEAK is a member of the tumor necrosis factor family and has been reported to have a mitogenic effect on the progenitor cell compartment in mice.[82,83] Using engraftment mouse models, Bird and colleagues[84] showed that bone marrow-derived macrophages are responsible for TWEAK production and that they can induce progenitor cell activation, even in healthy livers. Activation of the TWEAK receptor, also known as Fn14, in HCC cell lines in vitro had a mild effect on their proliferation.[85] **Fig. 4** shows an example of the TWEAK receptor expressed in human HCC and HPCs. Whether tumor-associated macrophages are responsible for TWEAK production in human HCCs still remains unclear. However, in a phase I trial in a subject with melanoma there seemed to be a strong link because inhibition of TWEAK signaling caused tumor regression together with a strong decrease of the tumor macrophage content.[86]

## STEMNESS, A WAY TO SURVIVE IN A HOSTILE ENVIRONMENT

Besides self-renewal, differentiation, and tumor-initiation capacity, chemoresistance is one of the traits that defines stemness in cancer.[87,88] Tumor cells that show an increase in stemness, often referred to as cancer stem cells (CSCs), can escape chemotherapy due to high expression levels of multidrug resistance proteins (ie, the adenosine triphosphate-binding cassette [ABC] transporters).[89,90] HCCs displaying biliary-HPC features or cholangiocellular carcinomas (thought to arise from HPCs) have been reported to exhibit increased expression of ABC transporters.[52,91,92] One approach to isolating CSCs is based on the functional ability of the ABC transporters to efflux xenobiotics across cell membranes against a concentration gradient.[93,94] Using the fluorescent dye Hoeschst33342, a side population (SP) can be cell sorted from the rest of the population. The SP was first reported by Goodell and colleagues[95] for the isolation of murine hematopoietic stem cells with long-term multilineage repopulating potential. By isolating the SP from different HCC cell lines, Chiba and colleagues,[96] in 2006, showed that this SP fraction expresses a high amount of K19 and harbors an enormous tumorigenic potential. In the same year, Haraguchi and colleagues[97] characterized the SP from the Huh7 HCC cell line using a microarray analysis approach and reported similar results: biliary-HPC markers (eg, *KRT19*, *KRT14*, *JAG1*), were up-regulated in the SP. JAG1 has been reported in a few bad prognosis gene signatures (see **Table 1**) and has been suggested to play a role in EMT in HCCs in vitro.[98] In 2012, Marquardt and colleagues[99] identified a 617-gene set that separated the SP from the non-SP in different HCC cell lines treated with zebularine, a DNA methyltransferase-1 inhibitor. The SP fractions of the zebularine-treated cell lines showed a higher expression of biliary-HPC cell markers (eg, *KRT19*, *SOX9*) but also differential expression of *PDGFRA*, *TWEAKR*, *laminin/integrin* subtypes, and *RICTOR*, a binding partner in the mechanistic target of rapamycin (mTOR) complex 2.[100] The mTOR complex 2 regulates processes such as cytoskeleton remodeling and survival, and has been reported to be activated in hypoxic conditions.[101–103] Inducing hypoxia in HepG2 HCC cells in vitro significantly induced the expression of ABC transporters.[104] Govaere and colleagues[44] showed a strong link between the cytoskeleton and chemoresistance in human HCCs because abolishing K19 expression induces chemosensitivity in HCC cells in vitro. Moreover, primary human K19-positive HCCs displayed a larger SP fraction, containing the K19-positive cells, compared with the K19-negative HCCs. mTOR could be the central player that ties up the links between biliary-HPC features, stemness, and the cytoskeleton.

## SUMMARY

Whether biliary-HPC features found in human HCCs arise due to mechanisms of dedifferentiation or reflect an HPC origin, they are generally linked with a worse prognosis, chemoresistance, and an aggressive behavior. In the future, the challenge will not only be to detect these HCCs correctly (because the tumor cells with biliary-HPC features might only be a minority of the entire tumor) but it will also be crucial to predict HCC behavior properly to adjust treatment accordingly. This would mean a huge step forward in personalized therapy design.

## REFERENCES

1. Jemal A, Bray F, Center MM, et al. Global cancer statistics. CA Cancer J Clin 2011;61(2):69–90.
2. McGlynn KA, London WT. The global epidemiology of hepatocellular carcinoma: present and future. Clin Liver Dis 2011;15(2):223–43 vii-x.
3. Roskams T, Kojiro M. Pathology of early hepatocellular carcinoma: conventional and molecular diagnosis. Semin Liver Dis 2010;30(1):17–25.
4. Sherman M. Hepatocellular carcinoma: epidemiology, surveillance, and diagnosis. Semin Liver Dis 2010;30(1):3–16.
5. Bruix J, Gores GJ, Mazzaferro V. Hepatocellular carcinoma: clinical frontiers and perspectives. Gut 2014;63(5):844–55.
6. Fausto N. Liver regeneration and repair: hepatocytes, progenitor cells, and stem cells. Hepatology 2004;39(6):1477–87.
7. Marshall A, Rushbrook S, Davies SE, et al. Relation between hepatocyte G1 arrest, impaired hepatic regeneration, and fibrosis in chronic hepatitis C virus infection. Gastroenterology 2005;128(1):33–42.
8. Roskams T. Liver stem cells and their implication in hepatocellular and cholangiocarcinoma. Oncogene 2006;25(27):3818–22.
9. Roskams TA, Theise ND, Balabaud C, et al. Nomenclature of the finer branches of the biliary tree: canals, ductules, and ductular reactions in human livers. Hepatology 2004;39(6):1739–45.
10. Gouw AS, Clouston AD, Theise ND. Ductular reactions in human liver: diversity at the interface. Hepatology 2011;54(5):1853–63.
11. Yoon SM, Gerasimidou D, Kuwahara R, et al. Epithelial cell adhesion molecule (EpCAM) marks hepatocytes newly derived from stem/progenitor cells in humans. Hepatology 2011;53(3):964–73.
12. van Eyken P, Sciot R, van Damme B, et al. Keratin immunohistochemistry in normal human liver. Cytokeratin pattern of hepatocytes, bile ducts and acinar gradient. Virchows Arch A Pathol Anat Histopathol 1987;412(1):63–72.
13. Boulter L, Govaere O, Bird TG, et al. Macrophage-derived Wnt opposes notch signaling to specify hepatic progenitor cell fate in chronic liver disease. Nat Med 2012;18(4):572–9.
14. Yimlamai D, Christodoulou C, Galli GG, et al. Hippo pathway activity influences liver cell fate. Cell 2014;157(6):1324–38.
15. Furuyama K, Kawaguchi Y, Akiyama H, et al. Continuous cell supply from a Sox9-expressing progenitor zone in adult liver, exocrine pancreas and intestine. Nat Genet 2011;43(1):34–41.
16. Pellicoro A, Ramachandran P, Iredale JP, et al. Liver fibrosis and repair: immune regulation of wound healing in a solid organ. Nat Rev Immunol 2014;14(3): 181–94.

17. Villanueva A. Rethinking future development of molecular therapies in hepato-cellular carcinoma: a bottom-up approach. J Hepatol 2013;59(2):392–5.
18. Moeini A, Cornellà H, Villanueva A. Emerging signaling pathways in hepatocel-lular carcinoma. Liver Cancer 2012;1(2):83–93.
19. Marquardt JU, Galle PR, Teufel A. Molecular diagnosis and therapy of hepato-cellular carcinoma (HCC): an emerging field for advanced technologies. J Hepatol 2012;56(1):267–75.
20. Lee JS, Chu IS, Heo J, et al. Classification and prediction of survival in hepato-cellular carcinoma by gene expression profiling. Hepatology 2004;40(3): 667–76.
21. Lee JS, Heo J, Libbrecht L, et al. A novel prognostic subtype of human hepato-cellular carcinoma derived from hepatic progenitor cells. Nat Med 2006;12(4): 410–6.
22. Boyault S, Rickman DS, de Reynies A, et al. Transcriptome classification of HCC is related to gene alterations and to new therapeutic targets. Hepatology 2007; 45(1):42–52.
23. Woo HG, Park ES, Cheon JH, et al. Gene expression-based recurrence predic-tion of hepatitis B virus-related human hepatocellular carcinoma. Clin Cancer Res 2008;14(7):2056–64.
24. Chiang DY, Villanueva A, Hoshida Y, et al. Focal gains of VEGFA and molec-ular classification of hepatocellular carcinoma. Cancer Res 2008;68(16): 6779–88.
25. Hoshida Y, Nijman SM, Kobayashi M, et al. Integrative transcriptome analysis re-veals common molecular subclasses of human hepatocellular carcinoma. Can-cer Res 2009;69(18):7385–92.
26. Villanueva A, Toffanin S, Llovet JM. Linking molecular classification of hepatocel-lular carcinoma and personalized medicine: preliminary steps. Curr Opin Oncol 2008;20(4):444–53.
27. Villanueva A, Minguez B, Forner A, et al. Hepatocellular carcinoma: novel mo-lecular approaches for diagnosis, prognosis, and therapy. Annu Rev Med 2010;61:317–28.
28. Villanueva A, Hoshida Y, Battiston C, et al. Combining clinical, pathology, and gene expression data to predict recurrence of hepatocellular carcinoma. Gastroenterology 2011;140:1501–12.e2.
29. Nault JC, De Reyniès A, Villanueva A, et al. A hepatocellular carcinoma 5-gene score associated with survival of patients after liver resection. Gastroenterology 2013;145(1):176–87.
30. Yamashita T, Forgues M, Wang W, et al. EpCAM and alpha-fetoprotein expres-sion defines novel prognostic subtypes of hepatocellular carcinoma. Cancer Res 2008;68(5):1451–61.
31. Villanueva A, Alsinet C, Yanger K, et al. Notch signaling is activated in human hepatocellular carcinoma and induces tumor formation in mice. Gastroenter-ology 2012;143(6):1660–9.e1667.
32. Van Eyken P, Sciot R, Paterson A, et al. Cytokeratin expression in hepatocellular carcinoma: an immunohistochemical study. Hum Pathol 1988;19(5):562–8.
33. Durnez A, Verslype C, Nevens F, et al. The clinicopathological and prognostic relevance of cytokeratin 7 and 19 expression in hepatocellular carcinoma. A possible progenitor cell origin. Histopathology 2006;49(2):138–51.
34. Uenishi T, Kubo S, Yamamoto T, et al. Cytokeratin 19 expression in hepatocellu-lar carcinoma predicts early postoperative recurrence. Cancer Sci 2003;94(10): 851–7.

35. Zhuang PY, Zhang JB, Zhu XD, et al. Two pathologic types of hepatocellular carcinoma with lymph node metastasis with distinct prognosis on the basis of CK19 expression in tumor. Cancer 2008;112(12):2740–8.

36. Yang XR, Xu Y, Shi GM, et al. Cytokeratin 10 and cytokeratin 19: predictive markers for poor prognosis in hepatocellular carcinoma patients after curative resection. Clin Cancer Res 2008;14(12):3850–9.

37. Ding SJ, Li Y, Tan YX, et al. From proteomic analysis to clinical significance: overexpression of cytokeratin 19 correlates with hepatocellular carcinoma metastasis. Mol Cell Proteomics 2004;3(1):73–81.

38. Wee A. Diagnostic utility of immunohistochemistry in hepatocellular carcinoma, its variants and their mimics. Appl Immunohistochem Mol Morphol 2006;14(3): 266–72.

39. Aishima S, Nishihara Y, Kuroda Y, et al. Histologic characteristics and prognostic significance in small hepatocellular carcinoma with biliary differentiation: subdivision and comparison with ordinary hepatocellular carcinoma. Am J Surg Pathol 2007;31(5):783–91.

40. Kim H, Choi GH, Na DC, et al. Human hepatocellular carcinomas with "Stemness"-related marker expression: keratin 19 expression and a poor prognosis. Hepatology 2011;54(5):1707–17.

41. Tsuchiya K, Komuta M, Yasui Y, et al. Expression of keratin 19 is related to high recurrence of hepatocellular carcinoma after radiofrequency ablation. Oncology 2011;80(3–4):278–88.

42. van Malenstein H, Komuta M, Verslype C, et al. Histology obtained by needle biopsy gives additional information on the prognosis of hepatocellular carcinoma. Hepatol Res 2012;42:990–8.

43. Andersen JB, Loi R, Perra A, et al. Progenitor-derived hepatocellular carcinoma model in the rat. Hepatology 2010;51(4):1401–9.

44. Govaere O, Komuta M, Berkers J, et al. Keratin 19: a key role player in the invasion of human hepatocellular carcinomas. Gut 2014;63(4):674–85.

45. Hirschfield GM. Genetic determinants of cholestasis. Clin Liver Dis 2013;17(2): 147–59.

46. Roskams T, Desmet V. Ductular reaction and its diagnostic significance. Semin Diagn Pathol 1998;15(4):259–69.

47. Desmet VJ. Ductal plates in hepatic ductular reactions. Hypothesis and implications. I. Types of ductular reaction reconsidered. Virchows Arch 2011;458(3): 251–9.

48. Desmet VJ. Ductal plates in hepatic ductular reactions. Hypothesis and implications. II. Ontogenic liver growth in childhood. Virchows Arch 2011;458(3): 261–70.

49. Desmet VJ. Ductal plates in hepatic ductular reactions. Hypothesis and implications. III. Implications for liver pathology. Virchows Arch 2011;458(3): 271–9.

50. Chen Y, Wong PP, Sjeklocha L, et al. Mature hepatocytes exhibit unexpected plasticity by direct dedifferentiation into liver progenitor cells in culture. Hepatology 2012;55(2):563–74.

51. Santos NP, Oliveira PA, Arantes-Rodrigues R, et al. Cytokeratin 7/19 expression in N-diethylnitrosamine-induced mouse hepatocellular lesions: implications for histogenesis. Int J Exp Pathol 2014;95(3):191–8.

52. Komuta M, Spee B, Vander Borght S, et al. Clinicopathological study on cholangiolocellular carcinoma suggesting hepatic progenitor cell origin. Hepatology 2008;47(5):1544–56.

53. Komuta M, Govaere O, Vandecaveye V, et al. Histological diversity in cholangio-cellular carcinoma reflects the different cholangiocyte phenotypes. Hepatology 2012;55:1876–88.
54. Spee B, Carpino G, Schotanus BA, et al. Characterisation of the liver progenitor cell niche in liver diseases: potential involvement of Wnt and Notch signalling. Gut 2010;59(2):247–57.
55. Alison M, Golding M, Lalani EN, et al. Wholesale hepatocytic differentiation in the rat from ductular oval cells, the progeny of biliary stem cells. J Hepatol 1997;26(2):343–52.
56. Zajicek G, Oren R, Weinreb M. The streaming liver. Liver 1985;5(6):293–300.
57. Boulter L, Lu WY, Forbes SJ. Differentiation of progenitors in the liver: a matter of local choice. J Clin Invest 2013;123(5):1867–73.
58. Giannelli G, Rani B, Dituri F, et al. Moving towards personalised therapy in patients with hepatocellular carcinoma: the role of the microenvironment. Gut 2014;63(10):1668–76.
59. Hoshida Y, Villanueva A, Kobayashi M, et al. Gene expression in fixed tissues and outcome in hepatocellular carcinoma. N Engl J Med 2008;359(19):1995–2004.
60. Givant-Horwitz V, Davidson B, Reich R. Laminin-induced signaling in tumor cells. Cancer Lett 2005;223(1):1–10.
61. Lorenzini S, Bird TG, Boulter L, et al. Characterisation of a stereotypical cellular and extracellular adult liver progenitor cell niche in rodents and diseased human liver. Gut 2010;59(5):645–54.
62. Español-Suñer R, Carpentier R, Van Hul N, et al. Liver progenitor cells yield functional hepatocytes in response to chronic liver injury in mice. Gastroenterology 2012;143(6):1564–75.e7.
63. Vestentoft PS, Jelnes P, Andersen JB, et al. Molecular constituents of the extracellular matrix in rat liver mounting a hepatic progenitor cell response for tissue repair. Fibrogenesis Tissue Repair 2013;6(1):21.
64. Petz M, Them N, Huber H, et al. La enhances IRES-mediated translation of laminin B1 during malignant epithelial to mesenchymal transition. Nucleic Acids Res 2012;40(1):290–302.
65. Gröger CJ, Grubinger M, Waldhör T, et al. Meta-analysis of gene expression signatures defining the epithelial to mesenchymal transition during cancer progression. PLoS One 2012;7(12):e51136.
66. Hashimoto K, Mori N, Tamesa T, et al. Analysis of DNA copy number aberrations in hepatitis C virus-associated hepatocellular carcinomas by conventional CGH and array CGH. Mod Pathol 2004;17(6):617–22.
67. Giannelli G, Fransvea E, Bergamini C, et al. Laminin-5 chains are expressed differentially in metastatic and nonmetastatic hepatocellular carcinoma. Clin Cancer Res 2003;9(10 Pt 1):3684–91.
68. Santamato A, Fransvea E, Dituri F, et al. Hepatic stellate cells stimulate HCC cell migration via laminin-5 production. Clin Sci (Lond) 2011;121(4):159–68.
69. Bergamini C, Sgarra C, Trerotoli P, et al. Laminin-5 stimulates hepatocellular carcinoma growth through a different function of alpha6beta4 and alpha3beta1 integrins. Hepatology 2007;46(6):1801–9.
70. Giannelli G, Azzariti A, Fransvea E, et al. Laminin-5 offsets the efficacy of gefitinib ('Iressa') in hepatocellular carcinoma cells. Br J Cancer 2004;91(11):1964–9.
71. Ke AW, Shi GM, Zhou J, et al. CD151 amplifies signaling by integrin $\alpha 6\beta 1$ to PI3K and induces the epithelial-mesenchymal transition in HCC cells. Gastroenterology 2011;140(5):1629–41.e5.

72. Fransvea E, Mazzocca A, Antonaci S, et al. Targeting transforming growth factor (TGF)-betaRI inhibits activation of beta1 integrin and blocks vascular invasion in hepatocellular carcinoma. Hepatology 2009;49(3):839–50.
73. Bedossa P, Peltier E, Terris B, et al. Transforming growth factor-beta 1 (TGF-beta 1) and TGF-beta 1 receptors in normal, cirrhotic, and neoplastic human livers. Hepatology 1995;21(3):760–6.
74. Mikula M, Proell V, Fischer AN, et al. Activated hepatic stellate cells induce tumor progression of neoplastic hepatocytes in a TGF-beta dependent fashion. J Cell Physiol 2006;209(2):560–7.
75. Reichl P, Dengler M, van Zijl F, et al. Signaling of Axl via 14-3-3zeta activates autocrine transforming growth factor-β signaling in hepatocellular carcinoma. Hepatology 2014. [Epub ahead of print].
76. Fan QM, Jing YY, Yu GF, et al. Tumor-associated macrophages promote cancer stem cell-like properties via transforming growth factor-beta1-induced epithelial-mesenchymal transition in hepatocellular carcinoma. Cancer Lett 2014;352(2): 160–8.
77. Dubois-Pot-Schneider H, Fekir K, Coulouarn C, et al. Inflammatory cytokines promote the retrodifferentiation of tumor-derived hepatocyte-like cells to progenitor cells. Hepatology 2014;60:2077–90.
78. van Zijl F, Mair M, Csiszar A, et al. Hepatic tumor-stroma crosstalk guides epithelial to mesenchymal transition at the tumor edge. Oncogene 2009;28(45): 4022–33.
79. Petz M, Them NC, Huber H, et al. PDGF enhances IRES-mediated translation of Laminin B1 by cytoplasmic accumulation of La during epithelial to mesenchymal transition. Nucleic Acids Res 2012;40(19):9738–49.
80. Stock P, Monga D, Tan X, et al. Platelet-derived growth factor receptor-alpha: a novel therapeutic target in human hepatocellular cancer. Mol Cancer Ther 2007; 6(7):1932–41.
81. Oseini AM, Roberts LR. PDGFRalpha: a new therapeutic target in the treatment of hepatocellular carcinoma? Expert Opin Ther Targets 2009;13(4):443–54.
82. Jakubowski A, Ambrose C, Parr M, et al. TWEAK induces liver progenitor cell proliferation. J Clin Invest 2005;115(9):2330–40.
83. Dwyer BJ, Olynyk JK, Ramm GA, et al. TWEAK and LTβ signaling during chronic liver disease. Front Immunol 2014;5:39.
84. Bird TG, Lu WY, Boulter L, et al. Bone marrow injection stimulates hepatic ductular reactions in the absence of injury via macrophage-mediated TWEAK signaling. Proc Natl Acad Sci U S A 2013;110(16):6542–7.
85. Kawakita T, Shiraki K, Yamanaka Y, et al. Functional expression of TWEAK in human hepatocellular carcinoma: possible implication in cell proliferation and tumor angiogenesis. Biochem Biophys Res Commun 2004;318(3):726–33.
86. Yin X, Luistro L, Zhong H, et al. RG7212 anti-TWEAK mAb inhibits tumor growth through inhibition of tumor cell proliferation and survival signaling and by enhancing the host antitumor immune response. Clin Cancer Res 2013; 19(20):5686–98.
87. Marquardt JU, Factor VM, Thorgeirsson SS. Epigenetic regulation of cancer stem cells in liver cancer: current concepts and clinical implications. J Hepatol 2010;53(3):568–77.
88. Marquardt JU, Thorgeirsson SS. Stem cells in hepatocarcinogenesis: evidence from genomic data. Semin Liver Dis 2010;30(1):26–34.
89. Reya T, Morrison SJ, Clarke MF, et al. Stem cells, cancer, and cancer stem cells. Nature 2001;414(6859):105–11.

90. Dean M, Fojo T, Bates S. Tumour stem cells and drug resistance. Nat Rev Cancer 2005;5(4):275–84.

91. Vander Borght S, Libbrecht L, Katoonizadeh A, et al. Breast cancer resistance protein (BCRP/ABCG2) is expressed by progenitor cells/reactive ductules and hepatocytes and its expression pattern is influenced by disease etiology and species type: possible functional consequences. J Histochem Cytochem 2006;54(9):1051–9.

92. Vander Borght S, Komuta M, Libbrecht L, et al. Expression of multidrug resistance-associated protein 1 in hepatocellular carcinoma is associated with a more aggressive tumour phenotype and may reflect a progenitor cell origin. Liver Int 2008;28(10):1370–80.

93. Alison MR, Guppy NJ, Lim SM, et al. Finding cancer stem cells: are aldehyde dehydrogenases fit for purpose? J Pathol 2010;222(4):335–44.

94. Golebiewska A, Brons NH, Bjerkvig R, et al. Critical appraisal of the side population assay in stem cell and cancer stem cell research. Cell Stem Cell 2011; 8(2):136–47.

95. Goodell MA, Brose K, Paradis G, et al. Isolation and functional properties of murine hematopoietic stem cells that are replicating in vivo. J Exp Med 1996; 183(4):1797–806.

96. Chiba T, Kita K, Zheng YW, et al. Side population purified from hepatocellular carcinoma cells harbors cancer stem cell-like properties. Hepatology 2006; 44(1):240–51.

97. Haraguchi N, Utsunomiya T, Inoue H, et al. Characterization of a side population of cancer cells from human gastrointestinal system. Stem Cells 2006;24(3): 506–13.

98. Tanaka S, Shiraha H, Nakanishi Y, et al. Runt-related transcription factor 3 reverses epithelial-mesenchymal transition in hepatocellular carcinoma. Int J Cancer 2012;131(11):2537–46.

99. Marquardt JU, Raggi C, Andersen JB, et al. Human hepatic cancer stem cells are characterized by common stemness traits and diverse oncogenic pathways. Hepatology 2012;54(3):1031–42.

100. Ma XM, Blenis J. Molecular mechanisms of mTOR-mediated translational control. Nat Rev Mol Cell Biol 2009;10(5):307–18.

101. Matter MS, Decaens T, Andersen JB, et al. Targeting the mTOR pathway in hepatocellular carcinoma: current state and future trends. J Hepatol 2014;60(4): 855–65.

102. Li W, Petrimpol M, Molle KD, et al. Hypoxia-induced endothelial proliferation requires both mTORC1 and mTORC2. Circ Res 2007;100(1):79–87.

103. Toschi A, Lee E, Gadir N, et al. Differential dependence of hypoxia-inducible factors 1 alpha and 2 alpha on mTORC1 and mTORC2. J Biol Chem 2008; 283(50):34495–9.

104. Vander Borght S, van Pelt J, van Malenstein H, et al. Up-regulation of breast cancer resistance protein expression in hepatoblastoma following chemotherapy: a study in patients and in vitro. Hepatol Res 2008;38(11):1112–21.

# Classification and Staging of Hepatocellular Carcinoma
## An Aid to Clinical Decision-Making

Benyam D. Addissie, MD, Lewis R. Roberts, MB ChB, PhD*

KEYWORDS

• Hepatocellular carcinoma • Tumor staging • Classification • Treatment selection

KEY POINTS

- Hepatocellular carcinoma is a heterogeneous malignancy and classification and staging methods help in stratifying patients for determining prognosis and planning treatments.
- Tumor characteristics, degree of liver dysfunction, and patient's performance status have been found to be key factors that determine prognosis and what treatment modalities are appropriate.
- There is no one classification method that is globally applicable in all populations.
- A multidisciplinary team approach is needed for planning individualized treatment for the best outcome.

## INTRODUCTION

Hepatocellular carcinoma (HCC) is a clinically and pathologically heterogeneous neoplasm. The outcomes of patients with HCC depend on the stage of disease at the time of diagnosis and the underlying biologic behavior of the tumor. HCCs fall along a broad spectrum of biologic behavior ranging from initiation as a single well-demarcated mass that progresses to a single large lesion to tumors that initiate as multifocal, infiltrative tumors with a high propensity to local, regional, or distant metastases. There seems to be a wide range of tumor phenotypes between these two extremes. A large subgroup of HCCs begin as single nodules that acquire more invasive characteristics as they grow, becoming multifocal with either local satellite lesions or more distant intrahepatic or extrahepatic metastases. Small unifocal HCCs are the

Disclosures: Dr Lewis Roberts receives grant support from ARIAD Pharmaceuticals, Gilead Sciences, Inova Diagnostics, and Wako Diagnostics. No disclosures for Dr Benyam Addissie.
Division of Gastroenterology and Hepatology, Mayo Clinic College of Medicine, 200 First Street Southwest, Rochester, MN 55905, USA
* Corresponding author.
E-mail address: roberts.lewis@mayo.edu

most easily treated, either by liver transplantation, surgical resection, or thermal ablation, with excellent long-term outcomes. As HCCs become larger and more invasive
and metastatic in their phenotypes, it becomes progressively more difficult to achieve
a radical cure. The effectiveness of local or locoregional therapies, surgical resection,
or liver transplantation for HCC depends on tumor size; unifocality or multifocality; the
presence, type, and extent of extrahepatic metastases; and the exact locations of tumor sites. Optimal treatment selection heavily depends on the tumor phenotype at the
time of diagnosis. There are also important patient characteristics that determine the
likely outcome in response to therapy. These characteristics are particularly important
in the case of patients with HCC because most of these cases worldwide occur in individuals with cirrhotic stage chronic liver disease. The presence of cirrhosis further
complicates the decision-making in patients with HCC because it substantially limits
the ability of patients to tolerate surgical resection or extensive ablative or embolic
therapy for HCC tumors, thus requiring careful evaluation of liver functional state in
relation to tumor burden. Classification and staging of HCC in a way that allows
optimal treatment selection is therefore challenging. There have been several advances in understanding the natural history and pathogenesis of HCC, and these advances have spurred changes in treatment that have improved the long-term
outcomes of patients with HCC. However, mortality from HCC is still rising worldwide,
indicating the need for further improvements in surveillance and early detection, access to care, and individualized selection of treatment options based on each patient's
unique clinical and molecular phenotype.

Over the past three decades, several classification and staging systems have been
used to stratify this heterogeneous malignancy and to aid providers in determining
prognosis and treatment. These systems use different variables to objectively score
tumor and patient characteristics. These factors have typically included tumor number, extent and location, severity of liver dysfunction, and performance status of the
patient (**Fig. 1**). Some classification schemes use a combination of these variables
for improved performance. The classification systems vary and do not necessarily
overlap. Some are used more frequently than others and there is notable geographic
variability in their use. This article summarizes some of these classification and staging
schemes and discusses the conceptual framework that guides optimal treatment
selection for each patient. The aim of this article is not to exhaustively discuss each
staging system proposed in the last three decades, but to review the most commonly
used staging systems, evaluate the rationale behind some of the newer staging
systems, and compare them focusing on their use in clinical decision-making, notably
choice of therapy.

## COMMON CLASSIFICATION AND STAGING METHODS
### Tumor-Node-Metastasis Classification

The TNM classification for solid tumors is a staging system that has been and is still a
method that is widely used for all solid tumors. It was first described in 1968 by the
French surgeon Pierre Denoix.[1] It is the accepted staging system by the International
Union Against Cancer and the American Joint Committee on Cancer for staging of solid
tumors in general, with amendments and modifications for different kinds of tumors.[2]
The TNM system is based on tumor size, extent of regional lymph node involvement,
and whether or not there is spread to distant structures. The staging may be based
on clinical or imaging findings (ie, clinical) or after open surgical resection or exploration
(ie, pathologic) (**Table 1**). The TNM classification method had been shown to have superior prognostic power in HCC when compared with three other commonly used

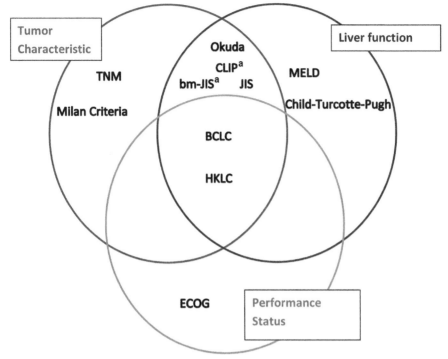

**Fig. 1.** Variables used in various HCC classification and staging methods. [a] Incorporated serum biomarkers, such as alpha fetoprotein. BCLC, Barcelona Clinic Liver Cancer staging; bm-JIS, biomarker combined JIS; CLIP, Cancer of the Liver Italian Program; ECOG, Eastern Cooperative Oncology Group; HKLC, Hong Kong Liver Cancer staging; JIS, Japanese Integrated Staging; MELD, Model for End-Stage Liver Disease; TNM, Tumor-Node-Metastasis staging. Performance Status score Milan criteria: single lesion ≤5 cm, or up to three lesions, each ≤3 cm.

classification methods in China, namely the Chinese University Prognostic Index, Okuda classification, or the Cancer of the Liver Italian Program (CLIP).[3] However, the outcome of patients with HCC varies greatly depending on the severity of their underlying liver disease, and because the TNM method does not account for this major prognostic variable, its use in determining management is limited.

### Okuda Classification

This method was the first to incorporate tumor characteristics and severity of liver dysfunction in a prognostic classification of HCC (**Table 2**). It was first published in 1985.[4] Okuda and colleagues stratified 850 Japanese patients with HCC into three groups based on tumor size (tumor involving either less than or greater than 50% of the liver) and liver function (presence of ascites, serum albumin, and serum bilirubin). This method was developed at a time when most patients were diagnosed at advanced stages of the malignancy. It now has lower predictive capacity because tumors are identified at much smaller sizes and local and potentially curative treatments are more commonly used.

### Cancer of the Liver Italian Program

This is a staging scheme developed by an Italian group in 1998 based on a retrospective study of 435 patients (**Table 3**).[5] The scheme incorporates tumor

**Table 1**
**Tumor-node-metastasis staging**

| Stage | Tumor | Node | Metastasis |
|---|---|---|---|
| Stage I | T1: solitary tumor without vascular invasion | N0: No regional node metastasis | M0: No distal metastasis |
| Stage II | T2: solitary tumor with vascular invasion or multiple tumors <5 cm | | |
| Stage IIIA | T3: multiple tumors >5 cm or tumor involving major branch of the portal vein | | |
| Stage IIIB | T4: tumor that invades adjacent organs other than gallbladder or perforates visceral peritoneum | | |
| Stage IIIC | Any T | N1: regional lymph node metastasis | |
| Stage IV | Any T | Any N | M1: distant metastasis |

*Adapted from* Edge SB, Byrd DR, Compton CC, eds. AJCC Cancer Staging Manual. 7th ed. New York, Springer; 2010. p. 222.

morphology, the presence or absence of portal vein thrombosis, and liver function. It has been validated in Western and Eastern populations.[6–8] The CLIP system has been shown to be a good indicator of long-term outcome after resection and other curative treatments. However, its accuracy would probably have been improved by the inclusion of performance status.

### Japan Integrated Staging

The Japan Integrated Staging (JIS) classification was introduced in 2003 by Kudo and colleagues[9] from Japan. It incorporated tumor characteristics using TNM staging and the severity of underlying liver disease using the Child-Turcotte-Pugh (CTP) score or class. TNM stages I to IV were assigned scores of 0 to 3, respectively, and CTP classes A to C were given scores of 0 to 2, respectively. The sum of the two scores was used to group tumors into total JIS scores of 0 to 5 (**Table 4**). This scoring system was modified in 2008 by Kitai and colleagues[10] with the addition of serum tumor biomarkers as variables, namely the serum alpha fetoprotein (AFP), lens culinaris

**Table 2**
**Okuda classification**

| | 0 Point | 1 Point |
|---|---|---|
| Tumor size | <50% of liver | >50% of liver |
| Ascites | No | Yes |
| Albumin | ≥3 g/dL | <3 g/dL |
| Total bilirubin | <3 mg/dL | ≥3 mg/dL |

Stage I, 0 points; Stage II, 1–2 points; Stage III, 3–4 points.
*Data from* Okuda K, Ohtsuki T, Obata H, et al. Natural history of hepatocellular carcinoma and prognosis in relation to treatment. Study of 850 patients. Cancer 1985;56(4):918–28.

**Table 3**
**Cancer of the Liver Italian Program**

|                        | 0 Point                          | 1 Point                                  | 2 Points          |
| ---------------------- | -------------------------------- | ---------------------------------------- | ----------------- |
| Child-Turcotte-Pugh class | A                             | B                                        | C                 |
| Tumor morphology       | Single tumor and <50% of liver   | Multiple tumors and <50% of liver        | >50% of liver     |
| Alpha fetoprotein      | <400 ng/mL                       | >400 ng/mL                               |                   |
| Portal vein thrombosis | No                               | Yes                                      |                   |

Early stage, 0 points; intermediate stage, 1–3 points; advanced stage, 4–6 points.

*Data from* A new prognostic system for hepatocellular carcinoma: a retrospective study of 435 patients: the Cancer of the Liver Italian Program (CLIP) investigators. Hepatology 1998; 28(3):751–5.

agglutinin reactive AFP (AFP-L3), and des-carboxyprothrombin, and was designated the biomarker-combined JIS. The biomarker-combined JIS was found to be superior to conventional JIS or CLIP, when evaluated in 1924 Asian patients with HCC. This method is yet to be validated in Western populations.

### Barcelona Clinic Liver Cancer Staging

The Barcelona Clinic Liver Cancer (BCLC) staging system was first proposed by the Barcelona Clinic group led by Bruix and Llovet and has had minor modifications.[11] The BCLC system was based on several studies that defined patient characteristics that resulted in the optimal outcomes for patients receiving different therapies for HCC. It incorporates a comprehensive group of predictive variables: size and extent of the primary lesion, macrovascular invasion and extrahepatic spread, liver function as assessed by CTP class, performance status, and the presence of cancer-related constitutional symptoms (**Fig. 2, Table 5**). This staging system is currently endorsed by the American Association for the Study of Liver Disease and the European Association for the Study of the Liver. The BCLC system was the first to link each stage to treatment recommendations for which there was a strong evidence-base of use. It has been externally validated in Western[12,13] and Eastern[14] populations and has excellent prognostic ability. Although the BCLC system has advantages over other systems, it has been recognized that the intermediate and advanced stages, BCLC-B and BCLC-C, can encompass relatively heterogeneous groups of patients with HCC and that the treatment proposed by the classification method may not be optimal for all patients in the group. Indeed, many experts recommend or implement alternative initial treatments for patients who initially present at these stages. Thus, the treatment recommendations need to be considered as guidelines and

**Table 4**
**Japanese Integrated Staging score**

|                        | 0 Point | 1 Point | 2 Points | 3 Points |
| ---------------------- | ------- | ------- | -------- | -------- |
| TNM                    | I       | II      | III      | IV       |
| Child-Turcotte-Pugh class | A    | B       | C        |          |

JIS score: Sum of points.

*Adapted from* Kudo M, Chung H, Osaki Y. Prognostic staging system for hepatocellular carcinoma (CLIP score): its value and limitations, and a proposal for a new staging system, the Japan Integrated Staging Score (JIS score). J Gastroenterol 2003;38(3):209; with permission.

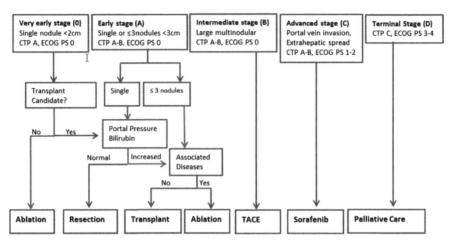

**Fig. 2.** Barcelona Clinic Liver Cancer staging and treatment strategy. TACE, transarterial chemoembolization. (*From* Forner A, Llovet JM, Bruix J. Hepatocellular carcinoma. Lancet 2012;379:1248; with permission.)

individualized for each patient based on their specific presentation. Additionally, most patients in the studies on which the BCLC system was based had hepatitis C virus–induced HCC and there may be differences in treatment outcomes in the predominantly hepatitis B virus–induced HCCs found in Eastern patient populations. Nevertheless, the BCLC system has stood the test of time as a prognostic tool and cemented

**Table 5**
**Barcelona Clinic Liver Cancer staging**

| BCLC Stage | Tumor Characteristics | Liver Function | Performance Status (ECOG) | Treatment Option |
|---|---|---|---|---|
| A 1 | Single tumor <5 cm | No portal hypertension | 0 | Surgery, RFA |
| A 2 | Single tumor <5 cm | Portal hypertension, normal bilirubin | 0 | Surgery, RFA, transplantation |
| A 3 | Single tumor <5 cm | Portal hypertension, abnormal bilirubin | 0 | RFA, transplantation |
| A 4 | 3 tumors <3 cm | | 0 | Transplant, TACE |
| B | Large multinodular | Child-Turcotte-Pugh A-B | 0 | TACE |
| C | Vascular invasion or metastasis | Child-Turcotte-Pugh A-B | 1–2 | Sorafenib |
| D | Any | Child-Turcotte-Pugh C | 3–4 | Supportive care |

ECOG, Eastern Cooperation Oncology Group; RFA, radiofrequency ablation; TACE, transarterial chemoembolization; TARE, transarterial radioembolization.
*Adapted from* Llovet JM, Bru C, Bruix J. Prognosis of hepatocellular carcinoma: the BCLC staging classification. Semin Liver Dis 1999;19(3):334; with permission.

the concept that the addition of patient performance status and constitutional symptoms enhances the discriminatory power of prognostic systems.

### Hong Kong Liver Cancer Prognostic Staging Scheme

Recently, a group of investigators from Hong Kong proposed another comprehensive staging and treatment system for HCC.[15] The Hong Kong Liver Cancer (HKLC) system was developed based on data from 3856 patients treated for HCC in the background of chronic liver disease, predominantly caused by hepatitis B, at the Queen Mary Hospital in Hong Kong between 1995 and 2008. The goal was to develop a prognostic classification scheme with treatment guidance for Asian patients with HCC. For the population studied, the HKLC group reported a significantly better prognostic ability when compared with BCLC. Particularly, the HKLC system identified patients in the intermediate and advanced BCLC stages who received more aggressive treatment than was recommended by the BCLC system, with improved survival outcomes (**Fig. 3**).[15] This classification and staging system is now being validated in Western populations and in populations with a different spectrum of causes of HCC. Potential arguments against the HKLC staging system may be that it was developed in a population of primarily hepatitis B–induced HCCs and may not be generalizable to regions with a high prevalence of hepatitis C virus or nonalcoholic steatohepatitis–induced HCCs.

### SELECTING TREATMENT MODALITIES BASED ON STAGE OF HEPATOCELLULAR CARCINOMA

The ultimate objective of all classification and staging methods is to guide providers in selecting the optimal treatment of patients with HCC. Currently available treatments include curative surgical procedures; percutaneous or intraoperative local ablation;

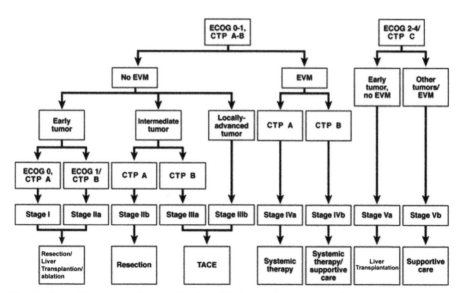

**Fig. 3.** Hong Kong Liver Cancer Staging. EVM, extrahepatic vascular invasion/metastasis. (*From* Yau T, Tang VY, Yao TJ, et al. Development of Hong Kong Liver Cancer staging system with treatment stratification for patients with hepatocellular carcinoma. Gastroenterology 2014;146(7):1696; with permission.)

external beam radiotherapy; catheter-based transarterial therapies; systemic chemotherapy; and best supportive care, including palliative measures.

It is important to recognize that the conceptual framework in which one selects treatment of individual patients with HCC is fundamentally different from the framework used to develop prognostic staging-treatment systems. Prognostic staging and treatment systems are often developed from the perspective of identifying the patient group that receives the optimal benefit from treatment with a particular modality; in contrast, treatment selection for individual patients ideally includes assessment by an experienced multidisciplinary group including radiologists, pathologists, transplant and hepatobiliary surgeons, medical oncologists, hepatologists, interventional radiologists, radiation oncologists, and palliative care specialists to determine the best evidence-based care for a patient at the point of clinical presentation. Fundamentally, the focus is on what treatment will result in optimal benefit for the individual patient, not necessarily whether the patient is the ideal candidate for the specific treatment under consideration. Social norms and ethical concepts, such as justice, equity, and harm, reach into the discussion, most notably as it relates to liver transplantation, where there is typically a limited supply of donor organs, but also importantly in resource-limited settings in low and middle income countries, where health system resources are often constrained.

At the time of initial presentation of a patient with chronic liver disease and a new HCC, the involvement of a hepatologist or primary care physician with experience in the care of patients with liver disease can be critical. If the chronic liver disease or cirrhosis has been previously unrecognized, the institution of standard care measures over the initial few weeks can often result in improvements in measures of liver function and patient performance status, thus potentially allowing revised classification of patients into earlier stages that are amenable to more aggressive therapies. This is particularly the case in reference to the performance status recommendations of the BCLC system, in which an Eastern Cooperative Oncology Group performance status of 1 (**Table 6**) shifts patients from the intermediate (BCLC-B) to advanced (BCLC-C) HCC stage regardless of tumor characteristics.

It may be that although overarching principles can be defined for HCC treatment, there will always be a need for regional guidelines because of the distinctive nature of the genetic, environmental, cultural, and health system factors that affect response to treatment and implementation of therapies. For example, the implementation of aggressive nationwide identification of those at risk for HCC and effective surveillance programs for at-risk individuals means that 70% of patients in Taiwan and Japan are diagnosed with HCC at the BCLC 0 and A stages; this is in marked contradistinction to

| Table 6 | |
|---|---|
| **Eastern Cooperation Oncology Group performance status** | |
| **Grade** | **Performance Status** |
| 0 | Able to perform at predisease level without limitations |
| 1 | Restricted in strenuous physical activities but able to do light activities, such as office work and light household work |
| 2 | Ambulatory and able to care for self, but not more work. Up and about more than 50% of the day |
| 3 | Limited to some self-care, confined to bed more than 50% of the day |
| 4 | Totally confined to bed or chair, cannot take care of self, completely disabled |
| 5 | Dead |

most other parts of the world, where at least 50% to 60% of cases are diagnosed at BCLC stages B and C. This results in fundamentally different responses to treatment and overall outcomes.

In practice, many experts approach the care of patients with HCC from the perspective of providing the most effective therapy that can be safely performed at each stage of management, from the initial presentation, through episodes of recurrence, progression, or metastasis as needed. When executed in concert with an experienced multidisciplinary team, this approach is more likely to achieve the best long-term outcomes for each patient. Because of the heterogeneity of presentations of HCC and the specific technical considerations involved in the selection of the main therapeutic options, including liver transplantation, surgical resection, local ablation, stereotactic or proton beam radiotherapy, and catheter-based therapies, comprehensive expertise and cross-disciplinary consultation is needed to achieve the best outcomes. Because of the high risk of tumor recurrence in patients who do not receive liver transplantation, it is also critical that patients have relatively close interval follow-up during therapy. This allows the identification of tumor recurrence at a relatively earlier stage when treatments are more effective and the amount of injury to benign liver tissue can also be minimized. Unfortunately, because of more aggressive biology, the tumors in some patients, even with the initial appearance of early stage disease, recur with multifocal or diffusely infiltrating disease that is difficult to treat.

## Liver Transplantation

Liver transplantation is the potentially curative treatment that achieves the best outcomes among the treatments offered to patients with HCC. This is not only because it achieves complete surgical removal of the cancer, but also because it removes the surrounding cirrhotic liver with its propensity to recurrent cancer and end-stage liver disease. Because liver transplantation involves allocation of a scarce resource, there are criteria to ensure that organs are allocated to those likely to experience the maximum benefit. In the pivotal study by Mazzaferro and colleagues[16] from Milan in 1996, it was shown that patients with a single tumor up to 5 cm or two or three tumors up to 3 cm in size without extrahepatic metastasis had the best 4-year overall and recurrence-free survival of 85% and 92%, respectively. These "Milan Criteria" are used as a selection criterion by organ allocation programs to identify the most appropriate liver transplant recipients. Adoption of these criteria has significantly improved the outcomes of those receiving liver transplantation for HCC.[17] Other criteria have also been proposed with the goal of expanding the availability of liver transplant to more patients with HCC. Yao and colleagues[18] from the University of California, San Francisco proposed expansion of the tumor size limitations to a solitary mass of less than or equal to 6.5 cm, or three or fewer masses of size less than or equal to 4.5 cm and total tumor diameter of less than or equal to 8 cm, and showed that the expanded criteria did not negatively impact survival. However, it should be noted that the study used posttransplantation pathologic data to determine eligibility for transplantation. To equalize the dropout rate between patients with HCC and those with nonmalignant chronic liver disease awaiting liver transplantation, the Model for End-Stage Liver score exception system was introduced. This system is designed to achieve approximately the same numbers of patients with HCC dropping off the list because of tumor progression as there are patients without HCC who die while waiting for a transplant. Even with these measures, wait time on the transplant list varies from months to years before transplantation, depending on the geographic region. Unlike noncancer transplant patients, however, a longer waiting time can paradoxically be associated with improved survival after liver transplant.[19] Patients commonly receive other modes of treatment while on the waiting list for transplantation, usually transarterial chemoembolization (TACE), radiofrequency ablation (RFA), or transarterial radioembolization (TARE). These treatments prevent tumor progression before transplantation and have been shown to lead to improved long-term posttransplant outcomes, particularly in those patients who are on the waiting list for several months before transplantation. Paradoxically, those patients with very short wait times do not benefit appreciably from treatment, because there is not sufficient time for progression to occur before transplant, and patients with very long wait times (>18 months) also have little benefit because of the propensity for the tumors to eventually recur before transplant. In a proportion of patients with disease that is beyond the transplant criteria, local or locoregional therapy is successful in downstaging the tumor to within criteria.[20,21]

### Surgical Resection

Surgical resection is another potentially curative mode of treatment of HCC. Resection is ideal for patients who have no cirrhosis and excellent liver function. In patients with cirrhosis, it is important to assess the patient's risk of liver decompensation after surgery. The risk is generally inferred from the baseline severity of liver disease, because one would need to consider the patient's CTP class, presence of portal hypertension (assessed clinically), and hepatic venous pressure gradient, because they have been found to independently affect postresection outcome.[22] In patients with normal liver function, the size of the tumor does not seem to affect the outcome of surgical resection as long as the surgery is technically feasible and the volume of remaining liver is sufficient to maintain liver function.[23] Results of several studies have defined the patients that are least likely to develop hepatic decompensation after surgical resection. One study, on which the BCLC recommendations are based, found that patients with CTP class A cirrhosis who had no evidence of clinically significant portal hypertension (defined as the presence of either hepatic vein pressure gradient >10 mm Hg, esophageal varices, or splenomegaly with a platelet count <100,000/mm$^3$) and normal serum bilirubin (<1 mg/dL) had a very low risk of hepatic decompensation after surgical resection.[22] In another study, patients with cirrhosis with a Model for End-stage Liver Disease score of 8 or less had a zero mortality after surgical resection of HCC, compared with a perioperative mortality of 29% in those with a Model for End-stage Liver Disease score of 9 or greater.[24] Some centers, particularly in Asia, use the indocyanine green retention at 15 minutes (ICG-R15) as a measure of clinically significant portal hypertension.[25] The ICG-R15 is a key component of the Makuuchi criteria that are used in Asia to determine eligibility of patients with cirrhosis for HCC resection. The criteria include the presence or absence of uncontrolled ascites, the serum bilirubin level, and the ICG-R15.[26]

One of the current areas of controversy is the selection of patients with HCC for surgical resection. The BCLC system recommends resection for those with Stage 0 disease, that is, CTP A, Eastern Cooperative Oncology Group of 0, and a single tumor of less than or equal to 2 cm, and also for patients with Stage A disease with single masses of any size without clinically significant portal hypertension or an elevated bilirubin.[11] In contrast, the HKLC classification expands these criteria, and recommends resection in patients with CTP A cirrhosis who have early stage tumors, which they define as a single tumor CTP less than or equal to 5 cm, or intermediate stage tumors, which they defined as a single tumor of size greater than or equal to 5 cm without intrahepatic vascular invasion or three or fewer tumors less than or equal to 5 cm.[15] Yet another recommendation is made by the recent Liver Cancer Study Group of Japan Consensus, which recommends consideration of resection for an even broader class of patients with HCC including patients with four or more lesions if there is no vascular invasion.[27] These more aggressive recommendations are based on data showing that in patients with preserved liver function, surgical resection achieved better overall survival than nonsurgical treatments even for patients with multiple tumors.[28,29]

### Local Ablation Methods

Local therapies include the use of thermal ablation methods, such as RFA, microwave ablation, and laser ablation, and chemical methods of tissue coagulation, such as alcohol injection. These therapies are generally most effective for tumors less than or equal to 3 cm in size, because the goal is usually to achieve a treatment volume that includes a surrounding margin of 1 cm of nontumorous tissue. Consequently, effective treatment of a 3-cm diameter tumor requires the ablation of a volumetric sphere of diameter 5 cm, approximately 65 cm$^3$. RFA is the most commonly used ablative modality and has been shown to be very effective for small tumors, with results rivaling those of surgical resection for tumors up to 2 cm in size. RFA involves the placement of a probe in the tumor by imaging guidance and the application of a rapidly alternating current to induce liquefactive necrosis. The main limitations of RFA are that it cannot be applied to subcapsular lesions that are adjacent to nearby organs because of the risk of heat injury, and that it is less effective when used on lesions adjacent to large blood vessels because of the heat sink effect of the vessels, which prevents adequate thermal injury to the tumor. The next most commonly used ablative therapy is percutaneous ethanol injection. RFA is more effective than percutaneous ethanol injection in inducing a complete response rate at 1 year.[30] However, percutaneous ethanol injection has the advantage of being inexpensive with comparable survival outcomes, which gives it high value in low resource settings.[30,31] Laser ablation and microwave ablation are other ablative therapies that are less commonly used.

Each ablative therapy has its own inherent nuances, strengths, and limitations. Because of this, although it is important to perform comparisons among the different techniques to establish their strengths and limitations, it is also important to develop an improved understanding of the biology of ablation and the potential adverse consequences of heat shock induced by thermal ablation, for example, which may be responsible for inducing a more aggressive biologic phenotype in any residual tumor cells at the ablation margin, potentially increasing the risk of postablation recurrence.[32] Different thermal and chemical ablation modalities, such as RFA, microwave ablation, and laser ablation, also have different characteristics as far as their sensitivity to the effects of heat shunting by large vessels, their propensity to induce biliary strictures when applied close to major bile ducts, the risk of local infection and abscess formation if there is any local or regional biliary obstruction, and the relative gradient/drop-off of thermal effect with distance from the point of ablation. The relative differences in the physical effects of the modalities and differences in the need for adjustments or accommodations, such as saline to separate the liver from adjacent bowel or the need to treat surface lesions with laparoscopically guided treatment, make it difficult to exactly compare these therapies. It is therefore important to have local practitioners with expertise in ideally several modalities so that the best modality can be selected for each individual patient.

### Radiotherapy: Stereotactic Body Radiation Therapy and Proton Beam Therapy

Although HCC is a radiosensitive tumor, radiation therapy is not as commonly used as the other local and locoregional therapies, primarily because of the radiosensitivity of the surrounding benign liver and propensity to development of radiation-induced liver injury with conventional radiation therapy. With the development of more precise targeting of tumors by stereotactic body radiation therapy and proton beam therapy, there is increasing use of these radiation therapies for the treatment of selected tumor nodules that are not as easily treated by other modalities. The development of respiratory gating has also made tumor targeting more precise. Key considerations in the use of stereotactic body radiation therapy and proton beam therapy include the avoidance of the large bile ducts in the hepatic hilum because of the risk of biliary strictures and the avoidance of difficulties in localizing the tumor and radiation toxicity to the liver and surrounding tissue. Radiation injury to surrounding bowel can be prevented by laparoscopic placement of AlloDerm spacers (LifeCell Corporation, Bridgewater, NJ, USA) to keep the bowel away from the liver during therapy. Retrospective studies have shown that stereotactic body radiation therapy and proton beam therapy can have a significant response rate and survival benefits in nonresectable tumors.[33,34] One of the largest recent studies was a retrospective review of clinical response to proton beam or carbon ion therapies by Komatsu and colleagues,[35] which reported 90.2% local control of the tumor after 5 years and a 5-year survival rate of 38.2%. The study included patients with CTP Class A and B cirrhosis (98%) and most patients had single tumor (86%), most (77%) of which were unresectable. Therefore, proton beam or carbon ion radiation therapies are to be considered as treatment options, although additional prospective and randomized studies need to be performed to compare these modalities with the other more commonly used and available treatments.

### Catheter-Based Treatments: Transarterial Chemoembolization, Transarterial Radioembolization, and Transarterial Chemoinfusion

Locoregional treatments also include catheter-based transarterial delivery of chemotherapeutic or radiation therapy with or without embolization. TACE involves injecting a combination of chemotherapy with polyvinyl alcohol particles with the goal of embolizing the branch of the hepatic artery that perfuses the tumor and achieving sustained release of chemotherapeutic agent (usually doxorubicin, cisplatin, and/or mitomycin C) to induce tumor ischemia and necrosis. This treatment is commonly used for unresectable tumors. BCLC classification identifies Class B patients with large multinodular tumors developing in the setting of CTP Class A or B cirrhosis to be the ideal patients for consideration of TACE.[11] The HKLC staging system also recommends TACE for patients with unresectable locally advanced tumors without extrahepatic spread or intermediate stage tumors.[15] The Japanese Society of Hepatology consensus-based guidelines recommend TACE for an even broader group of patients. In addition to the groups mentioned previously, others with CTP Class A and B cirrhosis but also vascular involvement of HCC and those with CTP Class C disease who are not transplant candidates despite being within the Milan Criteria should be considered for TACE.[27] The main contraindication to TACE in patients with HCC is the presence of complete portal vein thrombosis. Because TACE occludes the hepatic artery, in patients with portal vein thrombosis it results in ischemic necrosis of the liver. TACE is not contraindicated after placement of a transjugular intrahepatic portosystemic shunt (TIPS), although some studies suggest that it may be less effective after TIPS.[36,37]

TARE is another locoregional HCC treatment that uses injection of glass or resin microspheres impregnated with β-emitting yttrium-90 into the hepatic artery feeding the tumor. In several large cohort studies TARE has been shown to have similar efficacy and safety as TACE[38]; several prospective randomized trials of TARE are underway. TARE has a risk of radiation-induced pneumonitis; therefore, before therapy, a planning angiogram using technetium-macroaggregated albumin is performed to quantify the degree of vascular shunting through the tumor and estimate the lung dose that would result from the dose to the liver. Given the similarities with TACE in terms of efficacy and safety, it is considered for the same groups of patients to whom TACE would be offered. Because the yttrium-90 impregnated glass beads have high specific activity, the number of beads needed for a regional treatment is not sufficient to occlude the arterial vasculature; hence yttrium-90 microspheres can be used in patients with portal vein thrombosis. TARE seems to be safe in patients with a TIPS shunt, with one study suggesting that it may be associated with less toxicity than TACE.[39,40]

Transarterial chemoinfusion, typically of 5-fluorouracil, is used particularly in Japan and other Asian countries for treatment of intermediate and advanced stage HCC. The data supporting its use are mostly from large cohort studies and suggest that there is a degree of efficacy.

### Systemic Chemotherapy

The multikinase inhibitor sorafenib is the standard of care for patients with HCC for whom surgical and locoregional therapies are not feasible. It is the only agent that has been shown to have any survival benefit in advanced HCC, despite several randomized phase III clinical trials performed to test several new agents over the past 7 years.[41] Response treatment with sorafenib varies significantly. One factor that was found to predict improvement of survival after starting treatment with sorafenib is degree of liver dysfunction.[42] Patients with CTP Class A disease had significantly improved survival compared with those with CTP Class B or C disease. AFP was another factor that Kostner and colleagues[42] reported to predict overall outcome. Patients with AFP levels greater than 200 ng/mL seemed to have shorter survival. Unfortunately, no other chemotherapeutic agents have been approved as treatments outside of clinical trials. In a small proportion of patients sorafenib is profoundly effective, achieving partial or complete remissions of HCC. Several studies are beginning to characterize the molecular features of these highly sorafenib-responsive tumors, including the presence of genetic amplification of the fibroblast growth factor 3–4 locus at chromosome 11q13 and amplification of the vascular endothelial growth factor A locus.[43,44]

Another important consideration is the potential effect of pharmacogenetic differences between populations. For example, Asian physicians are convinced of the use of 5-fluorouracil–based regimens administered by different routes, including chemoinfusion, for treatment of advanced HCC, whereas most Western studies have been negative. Because there is a strong component of genetic determination of the pharmacokinetics and toxicity of 5-fluorouracil–based regimens, it may be that these factors are important in explaining this apparent discrepancy.[45,46]

### Palliative Care

When the stage of HCC is advanced and when performance status is poor, palliative care should be used. This primarily focuses on the patient's symptoms and uses various modalities of therapy to alleviate distress and provide best supportive care.

### DISCUSSION

The ultimate objective of these classification and staging methods is to be able to guide providers in selecting best treatments for patients with HCC. The current classification methods have been able to identify factors that significantly affect patient outcomes, namely tumor characteristics, severity of liver disease, and performance status, and in some cases serum tumor biomarkers. The systems allow providers to stratify patients based on these factors that alter prognosis. One of these methods, the BCLC staging system, has been incorporated into the HCC treatment guidelines of the American Association for the Study of Liver Disease and European Association for the Study of the Liver. Similarly, there are Asian, Japanese, Korean,[47] and Hong Kong guidelines for use in these respective regions. However, these classifications are often geared toward identifying which patients would be ideal candidates for a

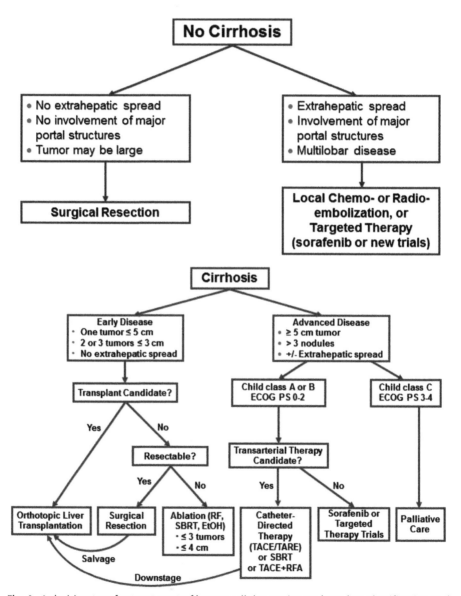

**Fig. 4.** A decision tree for treatment of hepatocellular carcinoma based on classification and staging variables. EtOH, ethanol; RF, radiofrequency ablation.

particular treatment modality, and not necessarily to help identify which treatment modality would give the best outcome for a particular patient. Despite advancements made in these classifications and staging methods, selection of best treatments for patients can be challenging in practice. In fact, results of multicenter studies have shown that a large proportion of patients with HCC are not being treated strictly according to these guidelines.[48,49] This implies that more needs to be done to devise practical decision trees to aid clinicians in selecting the best treatment of patients based on the known factors that alter prognosis. **Fig. 4** is a proposed decision tree that incorporates the major factors that are known to impact prognosis and treatment planning.

## SUMMARY

HCC is a heterogeneous malignancy and patients present with different combinations of severity of liver disease, variable performance status, and tumor characteristics, all of which affect treatment options and prognosis. A simplified approach to treatment, therefore, is not always feasible. Various classification and staging methods have been proposed over the past three decades, and the ones that incorporate tumor characteristics, degree of liver dysfunction, and patient performance status tend to be more useful in identifying which patient would best benefit from a particular treatment modality. Ideally, a strategy that enables providers to select the best treatment for a particular patient needs to be taken. This will require a multidisciplinary team approach involving hepatologists, oncologists, liver surgeons, and interventional radiologists for the best outcome to the patient. Of importance, the difference in treatment approaches according to staging classification in different regions of the world, particularly East versus West, also has important implications for the design and conduct of international multicenter clinical trials.

## REFERENCES

1. Denoix P. The treatment of tumors as a function of our knowledge concerning the role of the host. Rev Fr Etud Clin Biol 1965;10(6):583–6 [in French].
2. Greene FL, Sobin LH. The staging of cancer: a retrospective and prospective appraisal. CA Cancer J Clin 2008;58(3):180–90.
3. Lu W, Dong J, Huang Z, et al. Comparison of four current staging systems for Chinese patients with hepatocellular carcinoma undergoing curative resection: Okuda, CLIP, TNM and CUPI. J Gastroenterol Hepatol 2008;23(12):1874–8.
4. Okuda K, Ohtsuki T, Obata H, et al. Natural history of hepatocellular carcinoma and prognosis in relation to treatment. Study of 850 patients. Cancer 1985; 56(4):918–28.
5. A new prognostic system for hepatocellular carcinoma: a retrospective study of 435 patients: the Cancer of the Liver Italian Program (CLIP) investigators. Hepatology 1998;28(3):751–5.
6. Ueno S, Tanabe G, Sako K, et al. Discrimination value of the new western prognostic system (CLIP score) for hepatocellular carcinoma in 662 Japanese patients. Cancer of the Liver Italian Program. Hepatology 2001;34(3):529–34.
7. Levy I, Sherman M. Staging of hepatocellular carcinoma: assessment of the CLIP, Okuda, and Child-Pugh staging systems in a cohort of 257 patients in Toronto. Gut 2002;50(6):881–5.
8. Zhao WH, Ma ZM, Zhou XR, et al. Prediction of recurrence and prognosis in patients with hepatocellular carcinoma after resection by use of CLIP score. World J Gastroenterol 2002;8(2):237–42.

9. Kudo M, Chung H, Osaki Y. Prognostic staging system for hepatocellular carcinoma (CLIP score): its value and limitations, and a proposal for a new staging system, the Japan Integrated Staging score (JIS score). J Gastroenterol 2003; 38(3):207–15.

10. Kitai S, Kudo M, Minami Y, et al. A new prognostic staging system for hepatocellular carcinoma: value of the biomarker combined Japan Integrated Staging score. Intervirology 2008;51(Suppl 1):86–94.

11. Llovet JM, Bru C, Bruix J. Prognosis of hepatocellular carcinoma: the BCLC staging classification. Semin Liver Dis 1999;19(3):329–38.

12. Marrero JA, Fontana RJ, Barrat A, et al. Prognosis of hepatocellular carcinoma: comparison of 7 staging systems in an American cohort. Hepatology 2005; 41(4):707–16.

13. Cillo U, Vitale A, Grigoletto F, et al. Prospective validation of the Barcelona Clinic Liver Cancer staging system. J Hepatol 2006;44(4):723–31.

14. Wang JH, Changchien CS, Hu TH, et al. The efficacy of treatment schedules according to Barcelona Clinic Liver Cancer staging for hepatocellular carcinoma: survival analysis of 3892 patients. Eur J Cancer 2008;44(7):1000–6.

15. Yau T, Tang VY, Yao TJ, et al. Development of Hong Kong Liver Cancer staging system with treatment stratification for patients with hepatocellular carcinoma. Gastroenterology 2014;146(7):1691–700.e3.

16. Mazzaferro V, Regalia E, Doci R, et al. Liver transplantation for the treatment of small hepatocellular carcinomas in patients with cirrhosis. N Engl J Med 1996; 334(11):693–9.

17. Yoo HY, Patt CH, Geschwind JF, et al. The outcome of liver transplantation in patients with hepatocellular carcinoma in the United States between 1988 and 2001: 5-year survival has improved significantly with time. J Clin Oncol 2003;21(23):4329–35.

18. Yao FY, Ferrell L, Bass NM, et al. Liver transplantation for hepatocellular carcinoma: expansion of the tumor size limits does not adversely impact survival. Hepatology 2001;33(6):1394–403.

19. Schlansky B, Chen Y, Scott DL, et al. Waiting time predicts survival after liver transplantation for hepatocellular carcinoma: a cohort study using the United Network for Organ Sharing registry. Liver Transpl 2014;20(9):1045–56.

20. Graziadei IW, Sandmueller H, Waldenberger P, et al. Chemoembolization followed by liver transplantation for hepatocellular carcinoma impedes tumor progression while on the waiting list and leads to excellent outcome. Liver Transpl 2003;9(6):557–63.

21. Mazzaferro V, Battiston C, Perrone S, et al. Radiofrequency ablation of small hepatocellular carcinoma in cirrhotic patients awaiting liver transplantation: a prospective study. Ann Surg 2004;240(5):900–9.

22. Bruix J, Castells A, Bosch J, et al. Surgical resection of hepatocellular carcinoma in cirrhotic patients: prognostic value of preoperative portal pressure. Gastroenterology 1996;111(4):1018–22.

23. Roayaie S, Haim MB, Emre S, et al. Comparison of surgical outcomes for hepatocellular carcinoma in patients with hepatitis B versus hepatitis C: a western experience. Ann Surg Oncol 2000;7(10):764–70.

24. Teh SH, Christein J, Donohue J, et al. Hepatic resection of hepatocellular carcinoma in patients with cirrhosis: Model of End-Stage Liver Disease (MELD) score predicts perioperative mortality. J Gastrointest Surg 2005;9(9):1207–15 [discussion: 1215].

25. Lisotti A, Azzaroli F, Buonfiglioli F, et al. Indocyanine green retention test as a noninvasive marker of portal hypertension and esophageal varices in compensated liver cirrhosis. Hepatology 2014;59(2):643–50.

26. Makuuchi M, Kosuge T, Takayama T, et al. Surgery for small liver cancers. Semin Surg Oncol 1993;9(4):298–304.
27. Kudo M, Matsui O, Izumi N, et al. JSH consensus-based clinical practice guidelines for the management of hepatocellular carcinoma: 2014 update by the liver cancer study group of Japan. Liver Cancer 2014;3(3–4):458–68.
28. Ishizawa T, Hasegawa K, Aoki T, et al. Neither multiple tumors nor portal hypertension are surgical contraindications for hepatocellular carcinoma. Gastroenterology 2008;134(7):1908–16.
29. Ho MC, Huang GT, Tsang YM, et al. Liver resection improves the survival of patients with multiple hepatocellular carcinomas. Ann Surg Oncol 2009;16(4):848–55.
30. Brunello F, Veltri A, Carucci P, et al. Radiofrequency ablation versus ethanol injection for early hepatocellular carcinoma: a randomized controlled trial. Scand J Gastroenterol 2008;43(6):727–35.
31. Shiina S, Tateishi R, Imamura M, et al. Percutaneous ethanol injection for hepatocellular carcinoma: 20-year outcome and prognostic factors. Liver Int 2012;32(9): 1434–42.
32. Thompson SM, Callstrom MR, Butters KA, et al. Role for putative hepatocellular carcinoma stem cell subpopulations in biological response to incomplete thermal ablation: in vitro and in vivo pilot study. Cardiovasc Intervent Radiol 2014;37(5): 1343–51.
33. Seong J, Park HC, Han KH, et al. Clinical results and prognostic factors in radiotherapy for unresectable hepatocellular carcinoma: a retrospective study of 158 patients. Int J Radiat Oncol Biol Phys 2003;55(2):329–36.
34. Mornex F, Girard N, Beziat C, et al. Feasibility and efficacy of high-dose three-dimensional-conformal radiotherapy in cirrhotic patients with small-size hepatocellular carcinoma non-eligible for curative therapies: mature results of the French Phase II RTF-1 trial. Int J Radiat Oncol Biol Phys 2006;66(4):1152–8.
35. Komatsu S, Fukumoto T, Demizu Y, et al. Clinical results and risk factors of proton and carbon ion therapy for hepatocellular carcinoma. Cancer 2011;117(21): 4890–904.
36. Kang JW, Kim JH, Ko GY, et al. Transarterial chemoembolization for hepatocellular carcinoma after transjugular intrahepatic portosystemic shunt. Acta Radiol 2012;53(5):545–50.
37. Kuo YC, Kohi MP, Naeger DM, et al. Efficacy of TACE in TIPS patients: comparison of treatment response to chemoembolization for hepatocellular carcinoma in patients with and without a transjugular intrahepatic portosystemic shunt. Cardiovasc Intervent Radiol 2013;36(5):1336–43.
38. Moreno-Luna LE, Yang JD, Sanchez W, et al. Efficacy and safety of transarterial radioembolization versus chemoembolization in patients with hepatocellular carcinoma. Cardiovasc Intervent Radiol 2013;36(3):714–23.
39. Donahue LA, Kulik L, Baker T, et al. Yttrium-90 radioembolization for the treatment of unresectable hepatocellular carcinoma in patients with transjugular intrahepatic portosystemic shunts. J Vasc Interv Radiol 2013;24(1):74–80.
40. Padia SA, Chewning RH, Kogut MJ, et al. Outcomes of locoregional tumor therapy for patients with hepatocellular carcinoma and transjugular intrahepatic portosystemic shunts. Cardiovasc Intervent Radiol 2014. [Epub ahead of print].
41. Llovet JM, Ricci S, Mazzaferro V, et al. Sorafenib in advanced hepatocellular carcinoma. N Engl J Med 2008;359(4):378–90.
42. Kostner AH, Sorensen M, Olesen RK, et al. Sorafenib in advanced hepatocellular carcinoma: a nationwide retrospective study of efficacy and tolerability. ScientificWorldJournal 2013;2013:931972.

43. Arao T, Ueshima K, Matsumoto K, et al. FGF3/FGF4 amplification and multiple lung metastases in responders to sorafenib in hepatocellular carcinoma. Hepatology 2013;57(4):1407–15.
44. Horwitz E, Stein I, Andreozzi M, et al. Human and mouse VEGFA-amplified hepatocellular carcinomas are highly sensitive to sorafenib treatment. Cancer Discov 2014;4(6):730–43.
45. Oie S, Ono M, Fukushima H, et al. Alteration of dihydropyrimidine dehydrogenase expression by IFN-alpha affects the antiproliferative effects of 5-fluorouracil in human hepatocellular carcinoma cells. Mol Cancer Ther 2007;6(8):2310–8.
46. Qin S, Bai Y, Lim HY, et al. Randomized, multicenter, open-label study of oxaliplatin plus fluorouracil/leucovorin versus doxorubicin as palliative chemotherapy in patients with advanced hepatocellular carcinoma from Asia. J Clin Oncol 2013; 31(28):3501–8.
47. Choi JY. Treatment algorithm for intermediate and advanced stage hepatocellular carcinoma: Korea. Oncology 2011;81(Suppl 1):141–7.
48. Borzio M, Fornari F, De Sio I, et al. Adherence to American association for the study of liver diseases guidelines for the management of hepatocellular carcinoma: results of an Italian field practice multicenter study. Future Oncol 2013; 9(2):283–94.
49. Torzilli G, Belghiti J, Kokudo N, et al. A snapshot of the effective indications and results of surgery for hepatocellular carcinoma in tertiary referral centers: is it adherent to the EASL/AASLD recommendations? An observational study of the HCC East-West study group. Ann Surg 2013;257(5):929–37.

# Screening and Detection of Hepatocellular Carcinoma

Heather N. Simpson, MD, Brendan M. McGuire, MD*

## KEYWORDS

- Hepatocellular carcinoma • Tumors • Screening • Treatment

## KEY POINTS

- The increasing incidence of hepatocellular carcinoma (HCC) has led to the need to identify patients at risk for HCC so that a program of screening can be undertaken.
- Screening for HCC has led to earlier diagnosis of tumors and thus has aided in initiating optimal medical treatment earlier in the disease course.
- Advances in radiological techniques and the identification of more accurate serum tests to diagnose HCC continue to be important areas of study and exploration.
- As advances in the diagnosis and treatment of HCC continue to be achieved, it is hoped that morbidity and mortality related to HCC can be decreased.

## ROLE OF SCREENING FOR HEPATOCELLULAR CARCINOMA

The incidence of hepatocellular carcinoma (HCC) continues to increase worldwide, and especially in westernized countries due to a rising incidence of nonalcoholic fatty liver disease (NAFLD) and a peak in the number of patients with hepatitis C-induced cirrhosis. In contrast to other malignancies, the prevalence of HCC is predicted to continue to escalate over the next 20 to 30 years. The increasing burden of HCC has led to the need to develop a screening system that will help identify tumors when they are small, and thus more likely to be amenable to treatment and optimally to cure. The role of screening for any malignancy is to reduce mortality related to the disease. In order to be successful in this goal, there must be proper identification of the at-risk population, and the most sensitive and specific tests should be applied to this population at the appropriate time intervals (surveillance intervals). There must also be a validated system in place to determine appropriate follow-up of abnormal findings that maximizes the likelihood of detecting false-positive results and minimizes the number of tests needed to confirm the diagnosis of HCC.

The authors have nothing to disclose.
The University of Alabama School of Medicine, Department of Medicine, Division of Gastroenterology & Hepatology, Boshell Diabetes Building, 1808 7th Avenue South, Birmingham, AL 35233, USA
* Corresponding author.
*E-mail address:* bmcguire@uab.edu

## DEFINITION OF THE AT-RISK POPULATION

The population of patients who are at the highest risk of developing HCC are those who benefit most from being entered into a screening program. This population includes those people that have the highest incidence of HCC. It is well known that advanced fibrosis and in particular, cirrhosis of the liver, predisposes to the development of primary liver cancer. The primary question is what is the level of incidence at which screening becomes effective? An intervention is considered effective if it increases life in the population by at least 3 months.[1] Interventions that can be achieved at a cost of less than $50,000/year of life gained are considered cost-effective.[2] There have been several cost-effective analyses for HCC surveillance that have been published.[3–12] These models have varied in regards to the population being studied, the intervention that has been applied for screening, and differences among the sensitivity and specificity of the surveillance tests. The conclusion among these studies has found that surveillance for HCC is cost-effective using ultrasonography[5] among those who have the highest risk of HCC. The at-risk population identified to have the highest risk of development of HCC includes those patients who have cirrhosis of any etiology, as these patients have a 1.5% to 2% incidence per year of developing HCC. Therefore, among patients with cirrhosis of various etiologies, surveillance should be undertaken when the risk of developing HCC is 1.5% per year or greater (**Table 1**).

Patients who have chronic hepatitis B represent a unique population that remains at higher risk of developing HCC without cirrhosis compared with other populations with chronic liver disease. A prospective controlled study by Beasley and colleagues[13,14] showed that the annual incidence of hepatocellular cancer in hepatitis B carriers was 0.5%. The annual incidence increases with age greater than 70 years, with the chance of developing HCC rising to 1%. The incidence of HCC development among hepatitis B carriers with known cirrhosis increased to 2.5%/year. Uncontrolled prospective cohort studies in North America have suggested that the incidence of HCC in chronic hepatitis B carriers varies significantly.[15–17] Non-Asian chronic carriers with long-term inactive disease (anti-HBe positive with low viral loads) who are not cirrhotic appear to have a very low risk of developing HCC.[18–21] Thus, this population may not be worthy of screening for HCC. However, results of many studies have shown that Asian carriers of chronic hepatitis B without cirrhosis remain at increased risk for HCC regardless of their replication status.[18,22–24] Risk of HCC appears to persist also in Asian HBV carriers who lose surface antigen positivity (HBsAg), and thus this population should continue to be screened for HCC.[25] Overall, the annual incidence of HCC in male hepatitis B carriers from South East Asia starts to exceed 0.2% around age 40,[14] and this is unrelated to whether cirrhosis is present or disease activity is high. This is in contrast to Caucasians with chronic hepatitis B, in whom the risk of development of HCC appears to be increased with presence of cirrhosis and greater inflammatory activity. Unlike Asians who lose surface antigen and are at risk of developing HCC, Caucasian HBV carriers who lose surface antigen appear to have a decline in their risk of HCC development.[26,27] In general, recommendations are for Asian men with HBV to begin receiving screening at age 40, and Asian women with HBV to initiate screening at age 50. All hepatitis B carriers with cirrhosis should be screened for HCC regardless of age.

## SURVEILLANCE TESTS

There are 2 types of screening tests used to detect HCC: radiological and serologic. Radiological tests include ultrasonography, dynamic contrast computed tomography (CT), and dynamic contrast magnetic resonance imaging (MRI). The most widely used

**Table 1**
**Groups for whom HCC surveillance is recommended or in whom the risk of HCC is increased, but in whom efficacy of surveillance has not been demonstrated**

| Surveillance Recommended | Threshold Incidence for Efficacy of Surveillance (>.25 life year gained) (%/y) | Incidence of HCC |
|---|---|---|
| **Population group** | | |
| Asian male hepatitis B carriers over age 40 | 0.2 | 0.4%–0.6%/y |
| Asian female hepatitis B carriers over age 50 | 0.2 | 0.3%–0.6%/y |
| Hepatitis B carrier with family history of HCC | 0.2 | Incidence higher than without family history |
| African/North American Blacks with hepatitis B | 0.2 | HCC occurs at a younger age |
| Cirrhotic hepatitis B carriers | 0.2–1.5 | 3%–8%/y |
| Hepatitis C cirrhosis | 1.5 | 3%–5%/y |
| Stage 4 primary biliary cirrhosis | 1.5 | 3%–5%/y |
| Genetic hemochromatosis and cirrhosis | 1.5 | Unknown, but probably >1.5%/y |
| Alpha 1-antitrypsin deficiency and cirrhosis | 1.5 | Unknown, but probably >1.5%/y |
| Other cirrhosis | 1.5 | Unknown |
| **Surveillance benefit uncertain** | | |
| Hepatitis B carriers younger than 40 (males) or 50 (females) | 0.2 | <0.2%/y |
| Hepatitis C and stage 3 fibrosis | 1.5 | <1.5%/y |
| Noncirrhotic NAFLD | 1.5 | <1.5%/y |

*From* Bruix J, Sherman M. Management of hepatocellular carcinoma: an update. In: American Association for the Study of Liver Diseases practice guidelines. Hepatology 2011;53:1020–1022.

imaging test for surveillance is ultrasonography. Ultrasound has been reported to have a sensitivity of between 65% and 80% and specificity greater than 90% when used as a screening test.[28] The appearance of HCC on ultrasound can vary from an echogenic to a hypoechoic lesion. A further challenge in using ultrasonography is the difficulty of identifying a lesion given the background of a nodular cirrhotic liver. In addition, obesity poses another obstacle in the performance of ultrasound for HCC screening. There have been a number of studies of CT scans as screening tests for HCC.[29–31] There are no data available on the use of CT for HCC as a screening rather than a diagnostic test. The performance characteristics of CT scanning in HCC surveillance are unknown. In order to increase sensitivity, multiphase (triple-phase or four-phase) CT is necessary to more accurately identify tumors as arterial phase only CT results in a large number of false-positive results. In addition, because of radiation exposure, CT scanning may carry an increased risk of carcinogenesis when used regularly over a period of many years.[32] Furthermore, the use of multiphase CT for screening would not be cost-effective. Estimates have indicated that using CT or MRI for HCC screening would increase cost by $100,000 to $300,000 per quality-adjusted life year.[7] Thus, for these reasons, CT scanning is not endorsed as a screening test for

HCC. Ultrasound remains the test of choice for HCC screening. CT or MRI with contrast can attain a higher diagnostic accuracy than ultrasound, but these tests are not cost-effective for screening purposes in all populations. However, in clinical practice, a high-quality ultrasound may not be possible to obtain. This may be due to deficiencies in operator expertise, or suboptimal quality of the equipment used to perform the ultrasound. In addition, obesity, which has become increasingly common, has posed another significant challenge in achieving an adequate ultrasound assessment. Thus, CT or MRI should be considered in these cases, although there are currently no guidelines to support this practice.

## SCREENING INTERVAL

There has been some debate as to the optimal surveillance interval in HCC screening. The only randomized controlled trial of HCC screening was performed in China and used a 6-month interval, and this was associated with increased survival compared with no screening intervention.[33] Results of a retrospective study, however, suggested that survival was not different in patients screened at 6- versus 12-month intervals.[34] Current American Association for the Study of Liver Diseases (AASLD) guidelines recommend a screening interval of 6 months. There is no rationale for shortening the surveillance interval for patients who are felt to be a higher risk of developing HCC, as the frequency of screening is based on the average tumor doubling time.

## ROLE OF ALPHA FETOPROTEIN IN SCREENING

Alpha fetoprotein (AFP) is a glycoprotein that is typically produced during embryologic development by the fetal liver and yolk sac. In adults, elevations in AFP can be seen in the setting of multiple malignancies, including HCC, germ cell tumors, gastric cancer, and intrahepatic cholangiocarcinoma.[35–37] In addition, elevation of serum AFP levels can occur in cirrhotic patients in the absence of malignancy. The elevation may be related to the grade of fibrosis and inflammatory activity on liver biopsy or may correlate with elevations of aminotransferase levels.[38] AFP used alone as a screening test for HCC appears to be inadequate.[39–41] Receiver operating characteristic analysis of AFP as a diagnostic test suggests that a value of 20 ng/mL provides an optimal balance of sensitivity and specificity.[39] However, at this level, the sensitivity is only 60%, and thus a large number of HCCs would be missed. If the cut off value were reduced, then a much higher false-positive result would occur. This would then increase cost overall by leading to additional and ultimately unnecessary tests being ordered. AFP appears to lack the necessary specificity and sensitivity to make it a good screening test. The lack of efficacy of AFP as a surveillance test was confirmed recently as part of the Hepatitis C Antiviral Long-term Treatment against Cirrhosis (HALT-C) study.[42] Although AASLD and European Association for the Study of the Liver (EASL) practice guidelines do not endorse the use of AFP in conjunction with ultrasound for HCC screening, other guidelines from Asia and the National Comprehensive Cancer network in the United States continue to support use of both tests for HCC screening. Thus, surveillance recommendations for HCC screening include obtaining high-quality ultrasound every 6 months with or without measurement of serum AFP. The use of AFP as a diagnostic test for HCC will be discussed later in this article.

## DIAGNOSIS OF HEPATOCELLULAR CARCINOMA

The tests used to diagnose HCC include radiological tests, liver biopsy, and serum AFP. Each of these will be discussed separately.

## IMAGING MODALITIES

The diagnosis of HCC has typically been able to be made on a radiologic basis alone, without the need for biopsy as long as typical imaging characteristics for HCC are present.[43–50] This does require a contrast-enhanced study such as multiphasic computed tomography (CT) scanning or MRI. HCC becomes hyperintense compared with the surrounding liver in the arterial phase. The hyperintensity is due to the fact that the HCC only contains arterial blood that retains contrast, whereas the rest of the liver maintains its dual blood supply from both the hepatic artery and portal vein, and the venous blood does not contain contrast. Thus, the rest of the liver outside the tumor appears hypointense. In the venous phase, the HCC enhances less than the surrounding liver (ie, there is washout of contrast). The presence of arterial uptake followed by washout is highly specific for HCC.[48,49,51]

## NEED FOR NEEDLE BIOPSY/LIMITATIONS

If atypical features are seen on 1 imaging modality such as CT or MRI, then typically an alternative imaging test is obtained to see if typical features are present. Liver biopsy of suspected small HCCs between 1 and 2 cm has become an accepted alternative strategy for diagnosis of lesions with atypical features on imaging (**Fig. 1**). Indeed, biopsy may significantly improve the likelihood of obtaining the correct diagnosis in small nodules. A false-negative rate of 20% to 38% has been reported in use of MRI for diagnosis of small HCC lesions between 1 and 2 cm with atypical features.[52,53]

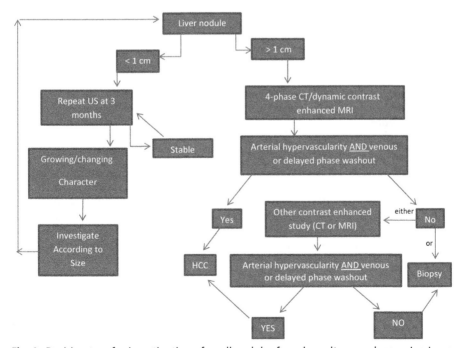

**Fig. 1.** Decision tree for investigation of small nodules found on ultrasound screening in patients at risk for HCC. (*From* Bruix J, Sherman M. Management of hepatocellular carcinoma: an update. In: American Association for the Study of Liver Diseases practice guidelines. Hepatology 2011;53:1020–1022).

In addition, earlier diagnosis of HCC improves the chances of obtaining the best outcome, as earlier treatment can be initiated. Ideally, this would mean that a lesion should be diagnosed when it is less than 2 cm.[54] Biopsy thus remains an important tool in the diagnosis of HCC.

Biopsy is overall well-tolerated and generally safe. Biopsy can also provide important information regarding the tumor grade that cannot be determined otherwise.[55] Biopsy does have its limitations, however, in particular, regarding small lesions. Obtaining a reliable specimen becomes challenging when nodules are less than 2 cm in size, and there is a significant chance of a false-negative result due to sampling error. In 1 prospective study evaluating patients with cirrhosis who had a biopsy of a single nodule smaller than 2 cm, false-negative rates up to 30% were reported.[51] In over half of the patients who initially had a negative result, a second biopsy performed during an additional session resulted in a diagnosis of HCC. Although the overall sensitivity, specificity, and positive predictive value of biopsy for the diagnosis of HCC have been reported to be as high as 90% to 100%, the negative predictive value has been found to be extremely low, at 14%.[56–58] Thus, in a suspected small HCC, if biopsy is negative, this does not definitively rule out the presence of HCC, and a negative result should not preclude a second attempt to biopsy the lesion if suspicion remains high for HCC.

## SAFETY OF BIOPSY/RISK OF SEEDING

Several studies have looked at the risk of needle tract seeding. This has been proven to happen, but overall it appears to be a rare phenomenon. One series, the largest to date, reviewed over 1000 patients with HCC who underwent percutaneous biopsy by means of ultrasound guidance and found that the frequency of tumor seeding was 0.76%.[59] Another much smaller study of approximately 100 patients reported the prevalence of tumor seeding following biopsy to be 1.6% to 3.4%.[58] Bleeding risk with needle biopsy appears to be no different than for routine liver biopsy.[60,61]

## ROLE OF CURRENTLY USED TUMOR MARKERS IN HEPATOCELLULAR CARCINOMA DIAGNOSIS
### Alpha Fetoprotein

Historically, serum AFP was a useful biomarker in the diagnosis of HCC when it was used along with imaging. However, as imaging modalities improve in their accuracy in identifying HCC, the role of AFP as a diagnostic test will likely continue to decline. As previously discussed, at lower levels AFP is less sensitive and thus tumors may be missed. This may be particularly true for smaller tumors. A retrospective series of patients diagnosed with a single HCC less than 2 cm reported low sensitivities associated with serum AFP. Indeed, only 20% of patients had an AFP level greater than 100 ng/mL, and only 11% had a level greater than 200 ng/mL.[62] A large prospective study of more than 1000 patients diagnosed with HCC revealed that 46% of patients had normal AFP levels (<20 ng/mL).[63] As AFP levels increase to more than 200 ng/mL, the specificity approaches 100%; however, the sensitivity is reduced to as low as 20%.[64,65] AFP levels of greater than 400 ng/mL have been virtually diagnostic of HCC, but sensitivity is then decreased further to less than 20%.[65,66] As mentioned previously, AFP lacks the necessary specificity and sensitivity to make it a good screening test, and the use of AFP has been mostly tested in its use as a diagnostic test for HCC. One area where AFP continues to have some utility is in regards to prognosis. Elevations in AFP are associated with increased tumor size, tumor stage, vascular invasion, portal vein thrombosis, extrahepatic metastases, and decreased survival.[63] Progression of AFP levels may be particularly helpful when used to follow patients who are listed for liver transplantation, as a significant rise in levels is associated with tumor recurrence and decreased survival following transplantation.[67]

### Les Culinaris Agglutinin-Reactive Alpha Fetoprotein

Les culinaris agglutinin-reactive alpha fetoprotein (AFP-L3) is an isoform of AFP that has been found to be significantly increased when expressed as a percent of the total serum AFP in patients who have HCC, but elevated levels of AFP-L3 have not been seen in patients who have high total serum AFP levels but who do not have HCC.[68] This is of value in distinguishing AFP elevation caused by diseases other than HCC. There have been several prospective studies, results of which have shown a higher sensitivity and specificity associated with AFP-L3 in the diagnosis of HCC (relative to total serum AFP) in patients with elevated baseline AFP levels.[68–71] However, it has not been shown that AFP-L3 has a distinct advantage over AFP. It may be more likely that AFP-L3 plays an important role as a secondary test when it is used along with total AFP. It has also been shown that both the sensitivity and specificity of AFP-L3 improved as AFP level increased, when the negative predictive value of AFP-L3 was greater than 80%.[71]

### Des-Gamma Carboxy Prothrombin

Des-gamma carboxy prothrombin (DCP) is also known as protein induced by vitamin K absence-II (PIVKA-II). DCP is an abnormal prothrombin produced as a result of defective post-translational carboxylation of the precursor protein to prothrombin. In 1 study, Marrero and colleagues[72] found that DCP at a cut-off of 125 mAU/mL had a higher sensitivity and specificity than AFP at a cut-off of 11 ng/mL, with sensitivities of 89% versus 77% and specificities of 95% versus 73%, in distinguishing HCC from chronic liver diseases. DCP will be elevated in patients who are taking vitamin K antagonists such as warfarin or in patients who are vitamin K deficient.

How does AFP compare with DCP and AFP-L3? It has a higher sensitivity than AFP-L3% and DCP for detecting early stage HCC, with a sensitivity of 65% and a specificity of 82% at the cut off of 10.9 ng/mL.[73] As discussed previously, used alone AFP remains an insufficient test for screening purposes, due to its lack of sensitivity and specificity. The combination of using AFP along with AFP-L3 or DCP may be better than using AFP alone as a biomarker for HCC diagnosis.

### Newer Tumor Markers

Much emphasis has been placed on finding new biomarkers that can help with not only the diagnosis of HCC, but also for guiding targeted therapies for HCC. In addition, novel biomarkers may be able to help predict response to current therapies and also help to predict likelihood of disease recurrence and patient survival. Cancer biomarkers either indicate the presence of cancer, or are predictors for the future development of cancer in the body. They can be in the form of DNAs, RNAs, proteins, metabolites, or antibodies. Biomarkers can be detected in the serum, or measured from other sources such as cancer tissue. There are several difficult challenges that come with the attempted development of new biomarkers. The unique molecular heterogeneity of both people and cancers makes it nearly impossible to find a perfect biomarker.

Several newer biomarkers have shown promise in aiding with the diagnosis of HCC. These include: Osteopontin, Golgi protein 73 (GP73), squamous cell carcinoma antigen (SCCA), sulfite oxidase (SUOX), aldo-ketoreductase family member B10 (AKR1B10), and hematopoietic progenitor cell antigen (CD34) expression.

Osteopontin is an extracellular matrix protein that is a member of the small integrin-binding ligand N-linked glycoprotein (SIBLING) protein family. It has important roles in cell signaling pathways that control inflammation, tumorigenesis, invasion, and metastasis of multiple cancers, including HCC.[74] One trial studying Osteopontin showed that at a cut-off of 91 ng/mL, it had a better performance for early diagnosis of HCC than AFP at a cut-off of 20 ng/mL.[75] The sensitivity and specificity for early HCC diagnosis were 74% and 66% for Osteopontin versus 53% and 93% for AFP, respectively. Thus it is possible that Osteopontin could be used along with AFP to aid with diagnosis of HCC. GP73 is an integral membrane protein located in the Golgi of normal epithelial cells. It has been found in high levels only in the presence of HCC.[76] Two recent meta-analyses studied the performance of GP73 compared with AFP. In 1 study, GP73 was comparable to AFP, while in another, GP73 outperformed AFP as a diagnostic marker.[77,78] SCCA is a serine protease inhibitor found in the squamous epithelium that has been shown to be expressed in high quantities in epithelial neoplasms including HCC.[79] A recent meta-analysis reported that SCCA was inferior to AFP in the diagnosis of HCC.[78] SUOX protein expression increases greatly in hepatocytes during the process of tumor development, whereas AKR1B10 protein and CD34 expression levels decrease during the process of tumor development. These biomarkers have been used to help separate well differentiated small HCCs from premalignant high-grade dysplastic nodules with a sensitivity of 94% and specificity of 95%.[80]

In addition, several single nucleotide polymorphisms (SNPs) have been identified as susceptibility gene loci for HCC development. Thus far, no single SNP has performed well enough to be clinically meaningful. This is likely because of the underlying heterogeneity of HCC. However, it is possible that in the future that a panel of susceptibility SNPs could be used along with other biomarkers to help improve the performance of these tests in predicting the risk of HCC development.

## SUMMARY

The increasing incidence of HCC has led to the need to identify patients at risk for HCC so that a program of screening can be undertaken. Screening for HCC has led to earlier diagnosis of tumors and thus has aided in initiating optimal medical treatment earlier in the disease course. Advances in radiological techniques and the identification of more accurate serum tests to diagnose HCC continue to be important areas of study and exploration. In particular, there have been efforts to develop new tumor markers to aid in the diagnosis of HCC and guide therapy of tumors based on novel genetic make-up. As advances in the diagnosis and treatment of HCC continue to be achieved, it is hoped that morbidity and mortality related to HCC can be decreased.

## REFERENCES

1. Naimark D, Naglie G, Detsky A. The meaning of life expectancy: what is a clinically significant gain? J Gen Intern Med 1994;9:702–7.
2. Laupacis A, Feeny D, Detsky A, et al. How attractive does a new technology have to be to warrant adoption and utilization? Tentative guidelines for using clinical and economic evaluations. CMAJ 1992;146:473–81.
3. Arguedas M, Chen VK, Eloubeidi M, et al. Screening for hepatocellular carcinoma in patients with hepatitis C cirrhosis: a cost-utility analysis. Am J Gastroenterol 2003;98:679–90.

4. Nouso K, Tanaka H, Uematsu S, et al. Cost-effectiveness of the surveillance program of hepatocellular carcinoma depends on the medical circumstances. J Gastroenterol Hepatol 2008;23:437–44.

5. Lin OS, Keeffe EB, Sanders GD, et al. Cost-effectiveness of screening for hepatocellular carcinoma in patients with cirrhosis due to chronic hepatitis C. Aliment Pharmacol Ther 2004;19:1159–72.

6. Thompson Coon J, Rogers G, Hewson P, et al. Surveillance of cirrhosis for hepatocellular carcinoma: systematic review and economic analysis. Health Technol Assess 2007;11:1–206.

7. Andersson K, Salomon J, Goldie S, et al. Cost effectiveness of alternative surveillance strategies for hepatocellular carcinoma in patients with cirrhosis. Clin Gastroenterol Hepatol 2008;6:1418–24.

8. Patel D, Terrault N, Yao F, et al. Cost-effectiveness of hepatocellular carcinoma surveillance in patients with hepatitis C virus-related cirrhosis. Clin Gastroenterol Hepatol 2005;3:75–84.

9. Sarasin F, Giostra E, Hadengue A. Cost-effectiveness of screening for detection of small hepatocellular carcinoma in western patients with Child-Pugh class A cirrhosis. Am J Med 1996;101:422–34.

10. Saab S, Ly D, Nieto J, et al. Hepatocellular carcinoma screening in patients waiting for liver transplantation: a decision analytic model. Liver Transpl 2003;9:672–81.

11. Shih ST, Crowley S, Sheu J. Cost-effectiveness analysis of a two-stage screening intervention for hepatocellular carcinoma in Taiwan. J Formos Med Assoc 2010; 109:39–55.

12. Collier J, Krahn M, Sherman M. A cost-benefit analysis of the benefit of screening for hepatocellular carcinoma. Hepatology 1999;30:481A.

13. Beasley RP, Hwant LY, Lin C, et al. Hepatocellular carcinoma and hepatitis B virus. A prospective study of 22707 men in Taiwan. Lancet 1981;2:1129–33.

14. Beasley R. Hepatitis B virus as the etiologic agent in hepatocellular carcinoma. Hepatology 1982;2:21S–6S.

15. Villeneuve JP, Desrochers M, Infante-Rivard C, et al. A long-term follow-up study of asymptomatic hepatitis B surface antigen-positive carriers in Montreal. Gastroenterology 1994;106:1000–5.

16. McMahon BJ, Alberts SR, Wainwright R, et al. Hepatitis B-related sequelae. Prospective study in 1400 hepatitis B surface antigen-positive Alaska native carriers. Arch Intern Med 1990;150:1051–4.

17. Sherman M, Peltekian K, Lee C. Screening for hepatocellular carcinoma in chronic carriers of hepatitis B virus: incidence and prevalence of hepatocellular carcinoma in a North American urban population. Hepatology 1995;22:432–8.

18. Hsu YS, Chien R, Yeh CT, et al. Long-term outcome after spontaneous HBeAg seroconversion in patients with chronic hepatitis B. Hepatology 2002;35:1522–7.

19. de Franchis R, Meucii G, Vecchi M, et al. The natural history of asymptomatic hepatitis B surface antigen carriers. Ann Intern Med 1993;118:191–4.

20. Sanchez-Tapias JM, Costa J, Mas A, et al. Influence of hepatitis B virus genotype on the long-term outcome of chronic hepatitis B in western patients. Gastroenterology 2002;123:1848–56.

21. Fattovich G. Natural history of hepatitis B. J Hepatol 2003;39(Suppl 1):S50–8.

22. Yang HI, Lu SN, Liaw YF, et al. Hepatitis B e antigen and the risk of hepatocellular carcinoma. N Engl J Med 2002;347:168–74.

23. Evans A, Chen G, Ross E, et al. Eight-year follow-up of the 90,000-person Haimen City cohort: I. Hepatocellular carcinoma mortality, risk factors, and gender differences. Cancer Epidemiol Biomarkers Prev 2002;11:369–76.

24. Huo TI, Wu JC, Lee PC, et al. Sero-clearance of hepatitis B surface antigen in chronic carriers does not necessarily imply a good prognosis. Hepatology 1998;28:231–6.
25. Yuen MF, Wong DK, Sablon E, et al. HBsAg seroclearance in chronic hepatitis B in the Chinese: virological, histological, and clinical aspects. Hepatology 2004; 39:1694–701.
26. Fattovich G, Giustina G, Realdi G, et al. Long-term outcome of hepatitis B e antigen-positive patients with compensated cirrhosis treated with interferon alfa. European Concerted Action on Viral Hepatitis (EUROHEP). Hepatology 1997;26:1338–42.
27. Fattovich G, Giustina G, Sanchez-Tapias J, et al. Delayed clearance of serum HBsAg in compensated cirrhosis B: relation to interferon alpha therapy and disease prognosis. European Concerted Action on Viral Hepatitis (EUROHEP). Am J Gastroenterol 1998;93:896–900.
28. Bolondi L, Sofia S, Siringo S, et al. Surveillance programme of cirrhotic patients for early diagnosis and treatment of hepatocellular carcinoma: a cost-effectiveness analysis. Gut 2001;48:251–9.
29. Di Tommaso L, Franchi G, Park YN, et al. Diagnostic value of HSP70, glypican 3, and glutamine synthetase in hepatocellular nodules in cirrhosis. Hepatology 2007;45:725–34.
30. Paradis V, Degos F, Dargere D, et al. Identification of a new marker of hepatocellular carcinoma by serum protein profiling of patients with chronic liver diseases. Hepatology 2005;41:40–7.
31. Sherman M. Screening for hepatocellular carcinoma. Baillieres Best Pract Res Clin Gastroenterol 1999;13:623–35.
32. Brenner DJ, Hall EJ. Computed tomography—an increasing source of radiation exposure. N Engl J Med 2007;357:2277–84.
33. Zhang BH, Yang BH, Tang ZY. Randomized controlled trial of screening for hepatocellular carcinoma. J Cancer Res Clin Oncol 2004;130:417–22.
34. Trevisani F, De NS, Rapaccini G, et al. Semiannual and annual surveillance of cirrhotic patients for hepatocellular carcinoma: effects on cancer stage and patient survival (Italian experience). Am J Gastroenterol 2002;97:734–44.
35. Terentiev AA, Moldogazieva NT. Structural and functional mapping of alpha-fetoprotein. Biochemistry (Mosc) 2006;71:120–32.
36. Adachi Y, Tsuchihashi J, Shiraishi N, et al. AFP-producing gastric carcinoma: multivariate analysis of prognostic factors in 270 patients. Oncology 2003;65: 95–101.
37. Shen WF, Zhong W, Xu F, et al. Clinicopathological and prognostic analysis of 429 patients with intrahepatic cholangiocarcinoma. World J Gastroenterol 2009;15: 5976–82.
38. Di Bisceglie AM, Sterling RK, Chung RT, et al. Serum alpha-fetoprotein levels in patients with advanced hepatitis C: results from the HALT-C Trial. J Hepatol 2005;43:434–41.
39. Trevisani F, D'Intino PE, Morselli-Labate AM, et al. Serum alpha-fetoprotein for diagnosis of hepatocellular carcinoma in patients with chronic liver disease: influence of HBsAg and anti-HCV status. J Hepatol 2001;34:570–5.
40. Sherman M. Alphafetoprotein: an obituary. J Hepatol 2001;34:603–5.
41. Forner A, Reig M, Bruix J. Alpha-fetoprotein for hepatocellular carcinoma diagnosis: the demise of a brilliant star. Gastroenterology 2009;137:26–9.
42. Lok AS, Sterling RK, Everhart JE, et al. Des-gamma-carboxy prothrombin and alpha-fetoprotein as biomarkers for the early detection of hepatocellular carcinoma. Gastroenterology 2010;138:493–502.

43. Forns X, Ampurdanes S, Llovet JM, et al. Identification of chronic hepatitis C patients without hepatic fibrosis by a simple predictive model. Hepatology 2002;36:986–92.
44. Moriyama M, Matsumura H, Aoki H, et al. Long-term outcome, with monitoring of platelet counts, in patients with chronic hepatitis C and liver cirrhosis after interferon therapy. Intervirology 2003;46:296–307.
45. Kojiro M. Focus on dysplastic nodules and early hepatocellular carcinoma: an eastern point of view. Liver Transpl 2004;10:S3–8.
46. Levy I, Greig PD, Gallinger S, et al. Resection of hepatocellular carcinoma without preoperative tumor biopsy. Ann Surg 2001;234:206–9.
47. Torzilli G, Makuuchi M, Inoue K, et al. No-mortality liver resection for hepatocellular carcinoma in cirrhotic and noncirrhotic patients: is there a way? A prospective analysis of our approach. Arch Surg 1999;134:984–92.
48. Burrel M, Llovet JM, Ayuso C, et al. MRI angiography is superior to helical CT for detection of HCC prior to liver transplantation: an explant correlation. Hepatology 2003;38:1034–42.
49. Yu JS, Kim KW, Kim EK, et al. Contrast enhancement of small hepatocellular carcinoma: usefulness of three successive early image acquisitions during multiphase dynamic MR imaging. AJR Am J Roentgenol 1999;173:597–604.
50. Mueller GC, Hussain HK, Carlos RC, et al. Effectiveness of MR imaging in characterizing small hepatic lesions: routine versus expert interpretation. AJR Am J Roentgenol 2003;180:673–80.
51. Forner A, Vilana R, Ayuso C, et al. Diagnosis of hepatic nodules 20 mm or smaller in cirrhosis: prospective validation of the noninvasive diagnostic criteria for hepatocellular carcinoma. Hepatology 2008;47:97–104.
52. Leoni S, Piscaglia F, Golfieri R, et al. The impact of vascular and nonvascular findings on the noninvasive diagnosis of small hepatocellular carcinoma based on the EASL and AASLD criteria. Am J Gastroenterol 2010;105:599–609.
53. Bolondi L, Gaiani S, Celli N, et al. Characterization of small nodules in cirrhosis by assessment of vascularity: the problem of hypovascular hepatocellular carcinoma. Hepatology 2005;42:27–34.
54. Bremner KE, Bayoumi AM, Sherman M, et al. Management of solitary 1 cm to 2 cm liver nodules in patients with compensated cirrhosis: a decision analysis. Can J Gastroenterol 2007;21:491–500.
55. Colecchia A, Scaioli E, Montrone L, et al. Pre-operative liver biopsy in cirrhotic patients with early hepatocellular carcinoma represents a safe and accurate diagnostic tool for tumour grading assessment. J Hepatol 2011;54(2):300–5.
56. Durand F, Regimbeau JM, Belghiti J, et al. Assessment of the benefits and risks of percutaneous biopsy before surgical resection of hepatocellular carcinoma. J Hepatol 2001;35:254–8.
57. Caturelli E, Solmi L, Anti M, et al. Ultrasound guided fine needle biopsy of early hepatocellular carcinoma complicating liver cirrhosis: a multicenter study. Gut 2004;53:1356–62.
58. Durand F, Belghiti J, Paradis V. Liver transplantation for hepatocellular carcinoma: role of biopsy. Liver Transpl 2007;13:S17–23.
59. Chang S, Kim SH, Lim HK, et al. Needle tract implantation after sonographically guided percutaneous biopsy of hepatocellular carcinoma: evaluation of doubling time, frequency, and features on CT. AJR Am J Roentgenol 2005;185:400–5.
60. Silva MA, Hegab B, Hyde C, et al. Needle track seeding following biopsy of liver lesions in the diagnosis of hepatocellular cancer: a systematic review and meta-analysis. Gut 2008;57:1592–6.

61. Stigliano R, Marelli L, Yu D, et al. Seeding following percutaneous diagnostic and therapeutic approaches for hepatocellular carcinoma. What is the risk and the outcome? Seeding risk for percutaneous approach of HCC. Cancer Treat Rev 2007;33:437–47.

62. Rapaccini GL, Pompili M, Caturelli E, et al. Hepatocellular carcinoma <2 cm in diameter complicating cirrhosis: ultrasound and clinical features in 153 consecutive patients. Liver Int 2004;24:124–30.

63. Farinati F, Marino D, De Giorgio M, et al. Diagnostic and prognostic role of alpha-fetoprotein in hepatocellular carcinoma: both or neither? Am J Gastroenterol 2006;101:524–32.

64. Gupta S, Bent S, Kohlwes J. Test characteristics of alpha-fetoprotein for detecting hepatocellular carcinoma in patients with hepatitis C. A systematic review and critical analysis. Ann Intern Med 2003;139:46–50.

65. Daniele B, Bencivenga A, Megna AS, et al. Alpha-fetoprotein and ultrasonography screening for hepatocellular carcinoma. Gastroenterology 2004;127: S108–12.

66. Gebo KA, Chander G, Jenckes MW, et al. Screening tests for hepatocellular carcinoma in patients with chronic Hepatitis C: a systematic review. Hepatology 2002;36:S84–92.

67. Vibert E, Azoulay D, Hoti E, et al. Progression of alpha-fetoprotein before liver transplantation for hepatocellular carcinoma in cirrhotic patients: a critical factor. Am J Transplant 2010;10:129–37.

68. Sato Y, Nakata K, Kato Y, et al. Early recognition of hepatocellular carcinoma based on altered profiles of alpha-fetoprotein. N Engl J Med 1993;328:1802–6.

69. Shiraki K, Takase K, Tameda Y, et al. A clinical study of lectin-reactive alpha-fetoprotein as an early indicator of hepatocellular carcinoma in the follow-up of cirrhotic patients. Hepatology 1995;22:802–7.

70. Wang SS, Lu RH, Lee FY, et al. Utility of lentil lectin affinity of alpha-fetoprotein in the diagnosis of hepatocellular carcinoma. J Hepatol 1996;25:166–71.

71. Sterling RK, Jeffers L, Gordon F, et al. Clinical utility of AFP-L3% measurement in North American patients with HCV-related cirrhosis. Am J Gastroenterol 2007; 102:2196–205.

72. Marrero JA, Su GL, Wei W, et al. Des-gamma carboxyprothrombin can differentiate hepatocellular carcinoma from nonmalignant chronic liver disease in American patients. Hepatology 2003;37:1114–21.

73. Marrero JA, Feng Z, Wang Y, et al. Alpha-fetoprotein, des-gamma carboxyprothrombin, and lectin-bound alpha-fetoprotein in early hepatocellular carcinoma. Gastroenterology 2009;137:110–8.

74. McAllister SS, Gifford AM, Greiner AL, et al. Systemic endocrine instigation of indolent tumor growth requires osteopontin. Cell 2008;133:994–1005.

75. Shang S, Plymoth A, Ge S, et al. Identification of osteopontin as a novel marker for early hepatocellular carcinoma. Hepatology 2012;55:483–90.

76. Marrero JA, Romano PR, Nikolaeva O, et al. GP73, a resident golgi glycoprotein, is a novel serum marker for hepatocellular carcinoma. J Hepatol 2005;43: 1007–12.

77. Zhou Y, Yin X, Ying J, et al. Golgi protein 73 versus alpha-fetoprotein as a biomarker for hepatocellular carcinoma: a diagnostic meta-analysis. BMC Cancer 2012;12:17.

78. Witjes CD, van Aalten SM, Steyerberg EW, et al. Recently introduced biomarkers for screening of hepatocellular carcinoma: a systematic review and meta-analysis. Hepatol Int 2013;7:59–64.

79. Beneduce L, Castaldi F, Marino M, et al. Squamous cell carcinoma antigen-immunoglobulin M complexes as novel biomarkers for hepatocellular carcinoma. Cancer 2005;103:2558–65.
80. Jin GZ, Yu WL, Dong H, et al. SUOX is a promising diagnostic and prognostic biomarker for hepatocellular carcinoma. J Hepatol 2013;59:510–7.

# Elevated Alpha-Fetoprotein

## Differential Diagnosis - Hepatocellular Carcinoma and Other Disorders

Robert J. Wong, MD, MS[a], Aijaz Ahmed, MD[b,c],
Robert G. Gish, MD[c,d],*

### KEYWORDS

- Hepatocellular carcinoma • Alpha-fetoprotein • Chronic hepatitis C virus infection
- Chronic hepatitis B virus infection
- *Lens culinaris* agglutinin-reactive fraction of alpha-fetoprotein
- Des-gamma-carboxy prothrombin

### KEY POINTS

- The incidence of cirrhosis-related hepatocellular carcinoma (HCC) is rising in the United States, with the associated disease burden expected to grow through 2020.
- Surveillance with alpha-fetoprotein (AFP) in combination with abdominal ultrasonography every 6 months was once widely recommended for HCC surveillance.
- Increased AFP is seen in chronic liver disease without HCC, nonhepatic malignancies, and normal pregnancy; thus, AFP levels must be interpreted within the context of the clinical presentation.
- Results of cross-sectional HCC screening studies show the benefit of diagnosing additional cases of HCC with AFP, but highlight the lack of cost-effectiveness owing to the increased false-positive results.
- US Food and Drug Administration guidelines for HCC risk assessment include using *Lens culinaris* agglutinin-reactive fraction of alpha-fetoprotein (AFP-L3) with des-gamma-carboxy prothrombin (DCP), or the combination of AFP-L3 with AFP and DCP.

The authors have nothing to disclose.
[a] Division of Gastroenterology and Hepatology, Alameda Health System-Highland Hospital, Highland Care Pavilion, 5th floor, 1411 East 31st Street, Oakland, CA 94602, USA; [b] Division of Gastroenterology and Hepatology, Stanford University School of Medicine, 750 Welch Road, Suite# 210, Palo Alto, CA 94304, USA; [c] Liver Transplant Program, Stanford University Medical Center, 750 Welch Road, Suite# 210, Palo Alto, CA 94304, USA; [d] Hepatitis B Foundation, 3805 Old Easton Road, Doylestown, PA 18902, USA
* Corresponding author. Robert G. Gish Consultants LLC, 6022 La Jolla Mesa Drive, San Diego, CA 92037.
*E-mail address:* rgish@robertgish.com

Clin Liver Dis 19 (2015) 309–323
http://dx.doi.org/10.1016/j.cld.2015.01.005
1089-3261/15/$ – see front matter © 2015 Elsevier Inc. All rights reserved.

liver.theclinics.com

## INTRODUCTION

Globally, up to approximately 800,000 new cases of hepatocellular carcinoma (HCC) are diagnosed annually.[1,2] The incidence of cirrhosis-related HCC is rising in the United States, with approximately 34,000 cases diagnosed each year as of 2014. The disease burden associated with HCC is expected to grow through 2020. The incremental increase in the incidence of HCC in the United States is largely a reflection of the natural history of chronic infection with hepatitis C virus (HCV) and the emerging epidemic of nonalcoholic steatohepatitis.[3,4] It is estimated that as many as 1 to 2 million patients with chronic HCV infection in the United States will develop cirrhosis and related complications in the near future.[3,4] Currently, HCV-related HCC is the leading indication for liver transplantation in patients with HCC in the United States.[4] Recent data have demonstrated that nonalcoholic steatohepatitis is the fastest growing etiology of chronic liver disease among HCC-related liver transplantations in the United States.[5] It is estimated that nonalcoholic steatohepatitis–related cirrhosis and its complications will peak in the United States in the next 10 to 15 years.[5] Chronic infection with hepatitis B virus (HBV) is the most common cause of HCC worldwide; it contributes to HCC prevalence in the United States as a result of increasing immigration from high-prevalence regions of the world.[1] Curative surgical options, including hepatic resection and liver transplantation, are available, with acceptable outcomes if HCC is diagnosed at an early stage. The 5-year tumor-free survival is 15% to 40% with resection and up to 80% with liver transplantation.[6–10] Therefore, it is important to establish screening and surveillance protocols for HCC with a focus on diagnosing HCC at an early stage.

In this review, we discuss the differential diagnosis of increased serum biomarker levels and the role of these markers in the early diagnosis of HCC and in HCC surveillance programs. The impact of newly cleared risk biomarkers for HCC and their use in conjunction with serum alpha-fetoprotein (AFP) is reviewed.

## SURVEILLANCE FOR HEPATOCELLULAR CARCINOMA

The goal of any screening and surveillance program is to effectively identify disease at an early stage such that potentially curative treatment options can be offered, and this principle is true for HCC screening and surveillance. Surveillance strategies with the goal of increasing the rate of early detection of HCC are needed to optimize the management of these patients by providing them with potentially curative surgical options, including hepatic resection and liver transplantation, as well as locoregional therapies, including ablation therapy, that can include thermal and transarterial ablation, and a reliable mechanism to follow the response to therapy.[6–10]

### Evolution of Surveillance Guidelines

In the past, the combination of serum AFP level and an abdominal imaging study was recommended for HCC surveillance.[11] However, recent data have shown conclusively that the low sensitivity of serum AFP and its high false-negative rate and suboptimal discriminatory impact impair the diagnosis of HCC.[12] The low sensitivity and specificity of AFP for HCC diagnosis is complicated additionally by variations in tumor-specific and patient-specific heterogeneity, which further reduces its positive and negative predictive values.

The sensitivity of combined serum AFP level and abdominal ultrasonography to detect early stage HCC varies from 40% to 65%.[12–15] Owing to the lack of sensitivity and specificity of serum AFP, its use was withdrawn from the American Association for the Study of Liver Diseases (AASLD) guidelines for HCC surveillance.[16] However, the Asian Pacific Association for the Study of the Liver (APASL) and the National

Comprehensive Cancer Network (NCCN) continue to recommend inclusion of AFP in HCC screening and surveillance decision trees.

Abdominal ultrasonography is recommended by AASLD as the preferred abdominal imaging modality for HCC surveillance. Abdominal ultrasonography performed every 6 months is cost effective for HCC surveillance despite its low and variable sensitivity as a diagnostic test[15,17] and the observation that the sensitivity of abdominal ultrasonography is further compromised in obese patients. Triphasic CT and MRI of the abdomen have become the gold standard to diagnose HCC in the setting of cirrhosis.[17–19] However, owing to high cost, radiation exposure, and the risks associated with intravenous contrast media, the routine use of a CT scan or MRI of the abdomen as the primary modality for HCC surveillance is not recommended.[16,17] AFP use remains the standard of care in the community as part of surveillance regimens owing to the low quality of ultrasonography in many centers and problems with image quality in patients with obesity.

The US Food and Drug Administration (FDA)-cleared tests *Lens culinaris* agglutinin-reactive fraction of AFP (AFP-L3) and des-gamma-carboxy prothrombin (DCP), which are discussed fully elsewhere in this article, are being recognized in the global peer-reviewed medical literature[20–25] and may become standard components of the HCC surveillance armamentarium.

### Worldwide Variation in Hepatocellular Carcinoma Surveillance Guidelines

Serum AFP measurement is recommended for HCC surveillance by APASL and the NCCN.[26,27] These guidelines stipulate that patients with increased risk of developing HCC undergo surveillance with an ultrasound of the abdomen and serum AFP level measurements every 6 to 12 months. In Japan, the national health practice guidelines allow for the testing of tumor markers that include AFP-L3 and DCP, in conjunction with abdominal ultrasonography for HCC surveillance.[28] In contrast, the AASLD,[16] the European Association for the Study of the Liver (EASL) and the European Organization for Research and Treatment of Cancer (EORTC)[29] all recommend against the use of serum AFP levels in combination with abdominal ultrasonography in HCC surveillance schema.

## SERUM ALPHA-FETOPROTEIN

AFP is a glycoprotein molecule with structural features similar to albumin.[30] Serum AFP is synthesized by the fetal liver and yolk sac during embryogenesis.[30]

### Causes of Elevation in Serum Alpha-Fetoprotein Level

In addition to low sensitivity, the poor specificity of solely using AFP as a screening diagnostic tool for HCC is reflected in the many other medical conditions that can lead to serum AFP elevations, contributing to high rates of false positivity. Elevations in serum AFP levels can be seen in patients with acute hepatitis, chronic liver diseases, cirrhosis, HCC, intrahepatic cholangiocarcinoma, colitis, ataxia telangiectasia, gastric cancer, germ cell tumors, and fetal disorders, and at the onset of normal pregnancy with steady decline as the gestation progresses (**Box 1**).[31–33] In patients with chronic liver disorders, the elevation in serum AFP level can be a reflection of histologic necroinflammatory activity within the liver and may be associated with elevation in serum aminotransferase levels.[33] For example, Di Bisceglie and colleagues[33] observed AFP levels greater than 20 ng/mL in 16.6% of chronic HCV patients without HCC in the Hepatitis Antiviral Long-term Treatment against Cirrhosis (HALT-C) trial in which the cohort with cirrhosis had significantly higher levels of serum AFP compared with noncirrhotics; female gender, black race, and platelet count were independently

---

**Box 1**
**Causes of elevation in serum alfa-fetoprotein level**

Hepatocellular carcinoma

Acute hepatitis

Chronic liver diseases

Cirrhosis

Intrahepatic cholangiocarcinoma

Colitis

Ataxia telangiectasia

Gastric cancer

Germ cell tumors

Fetal disorders

Normal pregnancy with steady decline as the gestation progresses

---

associated with higher AFP levels. In a prospective study of 432 chronic HBV patients without HCC, Liaw and colleagues[34] observed elevated AFP levels of greater than 20 ng/mL in 45.6% of patients, with 19.4% of patients demonstrating AFP levels of greater than 100 ng/mL and a highest recorded AFP level of 2520 ng/mL.

### Factors Impacting Serum Alpha-Fetoprotein Level as a Tumor Marker

The cause of underlying liver disease, the ethnicity of the population undergoing surveillance, the prevalence of HCC within a region, and the tumor size of HCC may impact the accuracy of serum AFP level as a tumor marker (**Box 2**).[35–38] In a prospective cohort study with more than 1000 HCC patients, it was demonstrated that 46% of cases had normal (<20 ng/mL) serum AFP levels.[12] Evidence from case control and prospective cohort studies in the setting of chronic HCV-related cirrhosis have demonstrated sensitivities of 41% to 65% and specificities of 80% to 94% for elevated serum AFP levels of greater than 20 ng/mL in diagnosing HCC.[12–15] The specificity of serum AFP level can increase to 100% at serum AFP levels of greater than 200 ng/mL, but the sensitivity is reduced to 20%.[13,14] **Fig. 1** shows the change in sensitivity and sensitivity of AFP in detecting HCC with increasing AFP. In a multi-center, retrospective, case control study of chronic HCV patients with and without HCC, Nguyen and colleagues[37] demonstrated significant racial disparities in the sensitivity of serum AFP in diagnosis of HCC. When using an AFP cutoff of greater than 20 ng/mL, the sensitivity for detecting HCC was 42.9% among blacks and 66.0% among nonblacks. Implementing AFP for the detection of HCC yielded an area under the receiver operating curve of 0.56 for blacks and 0.81 for nonblacks.

---

**Box 2**
**Factors impacting the accuracy of serum alpha-fetoprotein level as a tumor marker**

Etiology of underlying liver disease

Ethnicity of patient population

Prevalence of hepatocellular carcinoma within a region

Tumor burden of hepatocellular carcinoma

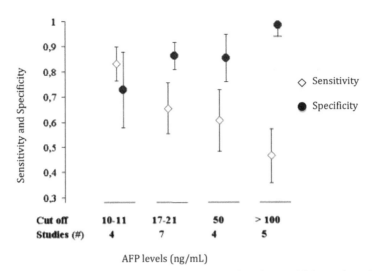

AFP levels (ng/mL)

**Fig. 1.** Pooled estimates from a systematic review assessing the sensitivity and specificity of different cutoff thresholds of alpha-fetoprotein (AFP) for detection of hepatocellular carcinoma (HCC). The x-axis presents the different thresholds of AFP cutoff values and the numbers of studies included for each threshold. The y-axis presents the pooled sensitivity and specificity for each group of studies. White diamonds refer to sensitivity and black circles refer to specificity. Bars represent 95% CIs. (*From* Colli A, Fraquelli M, Casazza G, et al. Accuracy of ultrasonography, spiral CT, magnetic resonance, and alpha-fetoprotein in diagnosing hepatocellular carcinoma: a systematic review. Am J Gastroenterol 2006;101:518; with permission.)

The sensitivity of serum AFP level is lower in the setting of a solitary HCC lesion measuring less than 2 cm in size compared with larger lesions; this was demonstrated in a retrospective study in which fewer than 20% of patients were noted to have a serum AFP level of greater than 100 ng/mL and only 11% a level of greater than 200 ng/mL.[38] Of additional diagnostic value is the observation that an increase in serum AFP level can provide prognostic information and is predictive of large tumor size, advanced stage, extrahepatic metastases, portal vein thrombosis, and posttransplant HCC recurrence, leading to poor survival outcome (**Box 3**).[12]

### The Role of Serum Alpha-Fetoprotein in Hepatocellular Carcinoma Surveillance

In a cross-sectional HCC screening study by Zhang and Yang[39] in Shanghai, China, AFP gave a benefit by diagnosing an additional 6% to 8% of cases, but lacked cost effectiveness owing to the concomitant increased false-positive rate that resulted

| Box 3 |
|---|
| **Prognostic value: increase in serum alpha-fetoprotein level predicts** |
| Large tumor size |
| Advanced stage |
| Extrahepatic metastases |
| Portal vein thrombosis |
| Posttransplant hepatocellular carcinoma recurrence leading to poor survival outcome |

with the addition of AFP testing to screening with abdominal ultrasonography alone. The cost for each case of HCC detected with abdominal ultrasonography alone nearly doubled with the addition of serum AFP level, increasing from $1982 to $3639.[39] In another surveillance strategy study by the same group utilizing combined serum AFP level and abdominal ultrasonography performed every 6 months (compared with no routine surveillance), 17,920 patients with chronic HBV infection were randomized to either surveillance (n = 8109) or no surveillance (n = 9711) with a mean follow-up of 14.4 months.[40] A total of 38 HCC cases were detected in the surveillance group and 18 in the control, no surveillance group. None of the 18 patients with HCC in the no surveillance group met the criteria for hepatic surgical resection and demonstrated 1-year mortality of 100%. However, 24 of the 29 patients in the surveillance group underwent hepatic resection with a 2-year survival rate of 77.5%. These observations are further supported by results from a randomized, controlled trial, also from Shanghai, in which 18,816 patients with chronic HBV infection were assigned either to a control group (n = 9443) or screening group (n = 9373) with serum AFP level being checked with abdominal ultrasonography every 6 months.[41] In the group undergoing HCC screening, early stage HCC was diagnosed in 60.5% of patients versus 0% in the unscreened group; 46.5% in the screened group were able to undergo curative hepatic resection versus only 7.5% in the unscreened group. In short, HCC screening demonstrated a 37% reduction in mortality (83.2 vs 131.5 per 100,000 individuals; $P<.01$). Because HCC surveillance with serum AFP level and abdominal ultrasonography every 6 months in HBV-infected patients demonstrated a survival benefit, this provides support for serum AFP level to be included in HCC surveillance programs in this Asian population, as still recommended by APASL.[26]

HCV-related cirrhosis is a leading risk factor for HCC in Western nations and Japan. Unfortunately, comparably large randomized trials for HCC surveillance are lacking in these populations and observations are limited to small, prospective studies. For example, data derived from the prospective HALT-C trial showed that abdominal ultrasonography diagnosed 14 of 24 early stage HCC cases (60%), doubling of serum AFP level identified 5 (20%), and a combination of other tests diagnosed the remaining 5 (20%) patients.[42] Results of studies evaluating the role of abdominal ultrasonography alone in HCC surveillance demonstrated a sensitivity of 32% for detecting early, small HCC. Serum AFP level combined with abdominal ultrasonography increased the sensitivity to 63.4% ($P<.001$) with minimal compromise in specificity.[18] Given the low sensitivity and specificity of AFP, the utilization of this test for routine HCC screening has been abandoned in some regions.[16,29] In addition to sensitivity and specificity, the utility of a screening test also depends on the disease prevalence in the population. Thus, despite lower sensitivity and specificity, serum AFP may still be useful in high prevalence regions where a positive test will lead to a higher positive predictive value. In the United States, the AASLD guideline recommendation for not routinely incorporating AFP into HCC screening reflects the consensus for using a threshold of 1.5% annual HCC incidence to determine cost effectiveness of screening modalities.[11] Therefore, combined use of serum AFP level and abdominal ultrasonography every 6 months seems to be the most pragmatic approach for HCC surveillance in the setting of cirrhosis and, as allowed in Japan, the inclusion of testing of other tumor markers.[29]

### The Role of Alpha-Fetoprotein in Predicting Hepatic Fibrosis

In addition to the role of AFP in HCC diagnosis, studies have evaluated the potential role of AFP in predicting advanced fibrosis in patients with chronic HCV. In a recent study of 541 chronic HCV patients with confirmed positive RNA, Bruce and colleagues[43] evaluated the sensitivity and specificity of serum AFP in predicting Ishak stage 3 fibrosis, at least, on liver biopsy. Utilizing an AFP level of 8 µg/L or greater yielded sensitivity of 39% and specificity of 95% in predicting Ishak stages 3 to 6 fibrosis. Thus, although AFP may not be an adequate screening test for fibrosis, given the low sensitivity, it may have diagnostic value as a confirmatory test when other clinical or laboratory markers are suggestive of advanced fibrosis.

### The Role of Alpha-Fetoprotein in Modeling to Predict Hepatocellular Carcinoma

In addition to patient-specific and tumor-specific heterogeneity that can further impact the positive and negative predictive values of serum AFP for HCC screening, the underlying severity and acuity of liver disease and liver inflammation can also impact the accuracy of this test. In a recent study utilizing the Department of Veterans Affairs Hepatitis C Virus Clinical Case Registry, El-Serag et al[44] developed a predictive model that includes serum AFP, alanine aminotransferase (ALT), and platelets, to distinguish between chronic HCV cirrhosis patients with and without HCC. To account for the effect of degree of liver inflammation and disease acuity on serum AFP levels, potential interactions between AFP and ALT, and between AFP and platelets were incorporated into the prediction model. The authors noted that, regardless of AFP level, low platelets and serum ALT levels and older age were associated with greater HCC risk. In addition, patients with high levels of ALT and normal to high levels of platelets had significantly lesser risk for HCC.[44]

### Serum Alpha-Fetoprotein Level and Liver Transplantation

Strategies can be developed to identify patients with increased AFP and other risk biomarkers to expedite their liver transplant evaluation or prioritize the status if a patient is already listed for liver transplantation.[45] On the other hand, guidelines can be formulated with a cutoff threshold of elevated serum AFP level and other risk biomarkers that will make liver transplantation prohibitive owing to a greater risk of HCC recurrence after liver transplantation. Currently, these discussions are limited by the lack of prospective clinical data despite the fact that these policies will optimize organ utilization in the era of major donor shortage. At the conclusion of a US national conference of transplant physicians, surgeons, and other medical specialists, held under the auspices of the Organ Procurement and Transplantation Network (OPTN)/United Network for Organ Sharing (UNOS), the American Society of Transplant Surgeons, the American Society of Transplantation, and the International Liver Transplantation Society that was convened to address liver transplantation for HCC, an allocation policy was proposed that states that the elevated serum AFP level should not exceed 500 ng/mL because it predicts a high risk of posttransplant HCC recurrence leading to graft loss and mortality.[46] Patients with tumors that may qualify them as liver transplant candidates should be considered for aggressive locoregional therapies by interventional radiology in an effort to slow the progression of HCC. Current best practices dictate that these patients be managed by a multidisciplinary liver tumor board. A decrease in serum AFP levels may be an indication of response to therapy correlating with tumor regression or stability. Serum AFP level and other biomarkers can play a central role in assessing the impact of these bridging locoregional therapies. Patients who respond to these locoregional therapies may demonstrate a decline in serum AFP levels, with a goal of reduction to less than 500 ng/mL. In this context, the previous UNOS policy of awarding Model for End-Stage Liver Disease (MELD) exception points to prioritize patients with elevated serum AFP level has been withdrawn owing to the concern that patients with advanced HCC may undergo liver transplantation with high risk of HCC recurrence posttransplant, resulting in poor organ utilization.[47]

## RISK BIOMARKERS FOR HEPATOCELLULAR CARCINOMA

FDA cleared as risk biomarkers for HCC, AFP-L3 and DCP are used in conjunction with abdominal ultrasonography for HCC surveillance. The combination of these serum biomarkers with abdominal ultrasonography achieves a sensitivity of 85% and a specificity of 95% in HCC diagnosis.[20–25,36,48–55] Of note, these biomarkers represent the only FDA-cleared use of AFP as a combination test for HCC diagnosis. Furthermore, recent improvements in the laboratory methods for testing AFP-L3 and DCP have contributed additionally to better consistency and applicability of these tools for HCC screening.[55] Recent studies demonstrate that AFP-L3 had a sensitivity of 37% to 60% and a specificity of 85% to 92% for HCC detection, whereas DCP had a sensitivity of 39% to 89% and a specificity of 90% to 95%.[56]

### Lens culinaris Agglutinin-Reactive Alpha-Fetoprotein

Serum AFP can be differentiated into 3 major isoforms by electrophoresis-based reactivity to certain lectins.[30] One of these isoforms, a fucosylated variant reactive to AFP-L3, has been associated with HCC.[30,48] The relative increase in AFP-L3 compared with total serum AFP level improves the accuracy of risk assessment in patients with HCC.[48] Serum AFP-L3 level of 10% or greater identifies patients with increased risk for development of HCC. The AFP-L3 fraction is elevated in patients with HCC and improves the sensitivity and specificity of serum AFP level. Prospective data are available, demonstrating greater sensitivity and specificity associated with AFP-L3 in the diagnosis of HCC relative to total serum AFP level.[20–25,48–55]

### Des-Y-Carboxyprothrombin

DCP, also known as prothrombin-induced by vitamin K absence II (PIVKA II), is a defective prothrombin protein formed as result of absent vitamin K-dependent activity of y-glutamyl carboxylase on the pre-prothrombin protein. DCP is a prothrombin precursor that undergoes carboxylation in hepatocytes before secretion. HCC cells lack carboxylation ability and secrete DCP, a noncarboxylated prothrombin precursor. Thus, serum DCP levels are increased in patients with HCC secondary to defective vitamin K carboxylation.[51–55] The detection of DCP in serum reflects underlying HCC activity, and thus DCP has been labeled as a risk biomarker for HCC. Limited prospective data have demonstrated that DCP has a greater specificity of 91% compared with 78% for serum AFP, but that the sensitivity of DCP is low at 41%.[53] Thus, DCP measurement is not superior to serum AFP as a screening test. The low sensitivity associated with DCP can be negated by simultaneous measurement of serum AFP levels. Another caveat is that elevated DCP levels can be seen in patients taking warfarin and other 4-hydroxycoumarin-containing anticoagulants[51] that owe their anticoagulant action to interference with vitamin K carboxylation. **Fig. 2** presents the performance characteristics of AFP, DCP, and AFP-L3 in the detection of HCC.[57,58] The box and whisker plots compare the median values (with 25th and 75th percentile with the whiskers) of AFP, DCP, and AFP-L3 among patients with HCC, non-HCC chronic liver disease, and healthy controls, demonstrating the discriminatory value of these diagnostic tools in differentiating between HCC and non-HCC patients.

### Improved Risk Assessment with an Expanded Biomarker Panel with Alpha-Fetoprotein

An increase in serum biomarker levels is an indication of higher risk for HCC. Therefore, the FDA cleared AFP-L3 (with AFP) and DCP to assess the risk of HCC but not necessarily to diagnose HCC. Thus, although not approved directly for

**Log AFP, log AFP-L3, and log DCP values in the hepatocellular carcinoma, CLD, and healthy control patient cohorts, showing the median value and 25th and 75th percentiles.**

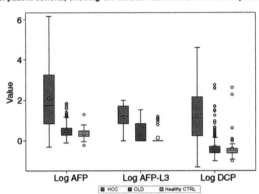

**Fig. 2.** Box and whisker plot demonstrating the distribution of alpha-fetoprotein (AFP), des-gamma-carboxy prothrombin (DCP), and AFP-L3 among patients with hepatocellular carcinoma (HCC) compared with controls with chronic liver disease. CTRL, control. (*From* Johnson PJ, Pirrie SJ, Cox TF, et al. The detection of hepatocellular carcinoma using a prospectively developed and validated model based on serologic biomarkers. Cancer Epidemiol Biomarkers Prev 2014;23:147; with permission.)

diagnosis, the implementation of these tests in patients at risk for HCC can help to further risk stratify the need for further noninvasive or invasive testing. Applying results from these tests to an at-risk population can help to modify an individual's pretest probability of HCC such that the posttest probability can provide enough certainty to forego further testing and proceed to treatment or not. Furthermore, the utility of these tests can be especially helpful in situations where traditional, noninvasive diagnostic testing is equivocal for HCC diagnosis. Although serum AFP level has never been evaluated by the FDA for approval as an independent test for HCC surveillance, it is now FDA cleared in combination with AFP-L3. Based on new FDA guidelines, clinicians could use either the combination of AFP-L3 with DCP, or the combination of AFP-L3 with AFP and DCP to help risk stratify the probability of HCC in at-risk populations to guide further diagnostic and treatment decisions.

Increased biomarkers are also useful indicators of a high risk of metastatic disease, vascular invasion, and the presence of poorly differentiated HCC; poorly differentiated HCC has been associated with high elevations in several biomarker levels. For example, a systematic review by Hakeem and colleagues[59] included 13 studies that evaluated the prognostic role of AFP in predicting post liver transplantation outcomes. Despite the poor quality of studies identified for inclusion in this systematic review, increased levels of AFP before transplantation were associated consistently with higher rates of vascular invasion, poor HCC differentiation and post liver transplant HCC recurrence, with lesser overall survival after liver transplantation. This is of interest because patients with poorly differentiated HCC are more likely to develop recurrence, metastases, and vascular invasion, with or without treatment, making them poor liver transplant candidates.

It is important to understand that biomarkers should guide the diagnostic workup within the matrix of HCC risk or HCC management and not be used as independently operating diagnostic tests. Results from biomarker testing can help to improve the posttest probability of HCC such that patients at very a high probability of having HCC may not require extensive and costly imaging to confirm an HCC diagnosis. In addition, patients with very low posttest probability of having HCC based on biomarker testing may be able to forego additional testing, thereby reducing the amount of resources needed for serial imaging modalities. However, bearing in mind the well-known patient-specific and tumor-specific heterogeneity of HCC, the use of biomarkers needs to be individualized; prospective data are lacking to develop concrete guidelines. For example, in a patient with cirrhosis and body mass index of 35 to 40 kg/m$^2$ with all 3 biomarkers in the normal range and a good quality negative abdominal ultrasonography, an MRI or CT scan for further evaluation may not be necessary. On the other hand, if the same obese patient was noted to have increasing DCP and AFP-L3 levels, an MRI or CT scan to rule out an early stage HCC would be a prudent step, despite a good quality negative abdominal ultrasonography. The latter patient has a higher risk of underlying HCC than the former, which may be missed on ultrasonography alone. Finally, patients with chronic HCV infection and compensated cirrhosis who have achieved a sustained virologic response to antiviral therapy should continue to undergo HCC surveillance. Similar to the previous clinical scenario, the imaging modality should be selected based on the entire clinical presentation, including trends in biomarkers.

## INVESTIGATIONAL TUMOR MARKERS

Several additional serum biomarkers have been identified and are being studied for their role in early diagnosis of HCC, including glypican-3 (GPC-3), α-L-fucosidase A1, human telomerase reverse transcriptase, squamous cell carcinoma antigen, Golgi protein 73, and transforming growth factor B1.[60–63]

### Glypican-3

GPC-3 is a cell-surface heparin sulfate proteoglycan.[64–70] GPC-3 is overexpressed in HCC and may be a marker of tumor growth. GPC-3 can be identified histologically through immunohistochemistry and in the serum of patients with underlying HCC. Tissue GPC-3 has demonstrated high specificity, ranging from 90% to 100% in patients with HCC. However, the sensitivity of serum GPC-3 in patients with HCC remains low. Improvement in sensitivity is reported when GPC-3 is measured in conjunction with serum AFP level.

## SUMMARY

- The utilization of combined serum AFP levels and abdominal ultrasonography every 6 months for HCC screening and surveillance demonstrates significantly improved early detection of HCC, leading to improved treatment options and improved overall survival. This approach is supported by guidelines from APASL and the NCCN, but not the AASLD, EASL, or EORTC.
- Increased AFP levels can be seen in the absence of HCC, including chronic liver disease without HCC, nonhepatic malignancies, and normal pregnancy, and thus AFP levels must be interpreted within the context of the entire clinical presentation.
- Increases in serum AFP level can provide prognostic value and are predictive of large tumor size, advanced stage, extrahepatic metastases, portal vein thrombosis, and posttransplant HCC recurrence leading to poor survival outcome.
- The improved detection of HCC is balanced by the increased costs associated with a combined modality approach, because patient-specific heterogeneity and tumor-specific heterogeneity contribute to false-positive rates, which subsequently affect the cost effectiveness of HCC screening and surveillance programs.

- The emergence of serum biomarkers AFP-L3 and DCP with significantly improved sensitivity and specificity for HCC facilitated FDA clearance of these biomarkers in combination with AFP as risk markers for HCC.
- Based on FDA guidelines for HCC risk assessment, clinicians could use either the combination of AFP-L3 with DCP, or the combination of AFP-L3 with AFP and DCP.
- An update in AASLD practice guidelines is warranted to redefine the role of serum AFP level in conjunction with risk biomarkers.

## REFERENCES

1. Bosetti C, Turati F, La Vecchia C. Hepatocellular carcinoma epidemiology. Best Pract Res Clin Gastroenterol 2014;28(5):753–70.
2. Flores A, Marrero JA. Emerging trends in hepatocellular carcinoma: focus on diagnosis and therapeutics. Clin Med Insights Oncol 2014;8:71–6.
3. Kabiri M, Jazwinski AB, Roberts MS, et al. The changing burden of hepatitis C virus infection in the United States: model –based predictions. Ann Intern Med 2014;161(3):170–80.
4. Biggins SW, Bambha KM, Terrault NA, et al. Projected future increase in aging hepatitis C virus-infected liver transplant candidates: a potential effect of hepatocellular carcinoma. Liver Transpl 2012;18(12):1471–8.
5. Wong RJ, Cheung R, Ahmed A. Nonalcoholic steatohepatitis is the most rapidly growing indication for liver transplantation in patients with hepatocellular carcinoma in the US. Hepatology 2014;59(6):2188–95.
6. Choe WH, Kim YJ, Parks HS, et al. Short-term interval chemoembolization and radiofrequency ablation for hepatocellular carcinoma. World J Gastroenterol 2014;20(35):12588–94.
7. Dong W, Zhang T, Wang ZG, et al. Clinical outcome of small hepatocellular carcinoma after different treatments: a meta-analysis. World J Gastroenterol 2014;20(29):10174–82.
8. Xu XS, Liu C, Qu K, et al. Liver transplantation versus liver resection for hepatocellular carcinoma: a meta-analysis. Hepatobiliary Pancreat Dis Int 2014;13(3):234–41.
9. Earl TM, Chapman WC. Hepatocellular carcinoma: resection versus transplantation. Semin Liver Dis 2013;33(3):282–92.
10. Earl TM, Chapman WC. Conventional surgical treatment of hepatocellular carcinoma. Clin Liver Dis 2011;15(2):353–70.
11. Bruix J, Sherman M. Management of hepatocellular carcinoma. Hepatology 2005;42:1208–36.
12. Farinati F, Marino D, De Giorgio M, et al. Diagnostic and prognostic role of alpha-fetoprotein in hepatocellular carcinoma: both or neither? Am J Gastroenterol 2006;101:524–32.
13. Gebo KA, Chander G, Jenckes MW, et al. Screening tests for hepatocellular carcinoma in patients with chronic hepatitis C: a systemic review. Hepatology 2002;36:S84–92.
14. Gupta S, Bent S, Kohlwes J. Test characteristics of alpha-fetoprotein for detecting hepatocellular carcinoma in patients with hepatitis C. A systemic review and critical analysis. Ann Intern Med 2003;139:46–50.
15. Daniele B, Bencivenga A, Megna AS, et al. Alpha-fetoprotein and ultrasonography screening for hepatocellular carcinoma. Gastroenterology 2004;127:S108–12.

16. Bruix J, Sherman M. Management of hepatocellular carcinoma: an update. Hepatology 2011;53:1020–2.
17. Singal A, Volk ML, Waljee A, et al. Meta-analysis: surveillance with ultrasound for early stage hepatocellular carcinoma in patients with cirrhosis. Aliment Pharmacol Ther 2009;30:37–47.
18. Singal AG, Conjeevaram HS, Volk ML, et al. Effectiveness of hepatocellular carcinoma surveillance in patients with cirrhosis. Cancer Epidemiol Biomarkers Prev 2012;21:793–9.
19. Teefey SA, Hildeboldt CC, Dehdashti F, et al. Detection of primary hepatic malignancy in liver transplant candidates: prospective comparison of CT, MR imaging, US, and PET. Radiology 2003;226:533–42.
20. Kumada T, Nakano S, Takeda I, et al. Clinical utility of Lens culinaris agglutinin-reactive alpha-fetoprotein in small hepatocellular carcinoma: special reference to imaging diagnosis. J Hepatol 1999;30(1):125–30.
21. Makuuchi M, Kokudo N, Arii S, et al. Development of evidence-based clinical guidelines for the diagnosis and treatment of hepatocellular carcinoma in Japan. Hepatol Res 2008;38(1):37–51.
22. Koike Y, Shiratori Y, Sato S, et al. Des-gamma-carboxy prothrombin as a useful predisposing factor for the development of portal venous invasion in patients with hepatocellular carcinoma: a prospective analysis of 227 patients. Cancer 2001;91(3):561–9.
23. Shimauchi Y, Tanaka M, Kuromatsu R, et al. A simultaneous monitoring of Lens culinaris agglutinin A-reactive alpha-fetoprotein and des-gamma-carboxy prothrombin as an early diagnosis of hepatocellular carcinoma in the follow-up of cirrhotic patients. Oncol Rep 2000;7(2):249–56.
24. Toyoda H, Kumada T, Kiriyama S, et al. Prognostic significance of simultaneous measurement of three tumor markers in patients with hepatocellular carcinoma. Clin Gastroenterol Hepatol 2006;4(1):111–7.
25. Volk ML, Hernandez JC, Su GL, et al. Risk factors for hepatocellular carcinoma may impair the performance of biomarkers: a comparison of AFP, DCP, and AFP-L3. Cancer Biomark 2007;3(2):79–87.
26. Omata M, Lesmana LA, Tateishi R, et al. Asian Pacific Association for the study of the liver consensus recommendations on hepatocellular carcinoma. Hepatol Int 2010;4(2):439–74.
27. National Comprehensive Cancer Network (NCCN). NCCN clinical practice guidelines in oncology: hepatobiliary cancers. Version 2013. Fort Washington (PA): NCCN; 2013.
28. Kudo M, Izumi N, Kokudo N, et al. Management of hepatocellular carcinoma in Japan: consensus-based clinical practice guidelines proposed by the Japan Society of Hepatology (JSH) 2010 updated version. Dig Dis 2011;29: 339–64.
29. European Association for the Study of the Liver, European Organization for Research and Treatment of Cancer. EASL-EORTC clinical practice guidelines: management of hepatocellular carcinoma. J Hepatol 2012;56:908–43.
30. Mizejewski GJ. Alpha-fetoprotein structure and function: relevance to isoforms, epitopes, and conformational variants. Exp Biol Med (Maywood) 2001;226: 377–408.
31. Adachi Y, Tsuchihashi J, Shiraishi N, et al. AFP-producing gastric carcinoma: multivariate analysis of prognostic factors in 270 patients. Oncology 2003;65: 95–101.

32. Shen WF, Zhong W, Xu F, et al. Clinicopathological and prognostic analysis of 429 patients with intrahepatic cholangiocarcinoma. World J Gastroenterol 2009;15: 5976–82.

33. Di Bisceglie AM, Sterling RK, Chung RT, et al. Serum alpha-fetoprotein levels in patients with advanced hepatitis C: results from the HALT-C Trial. J Hepatol 2005;43:434–41.

34. Liaw YF, Tai DI, Chen TJ, et al. Alpha-fetoprotein changes in the course of chronic hepatitis: relation to bridging hepatic necrosis and hepatocellular carcinoma. Liver 1986;6(3):133–7.

35. McMahon BJ, Bulkow L, Harpster A, et al. Screening for hepatocellular carcinoma in Alaska natives infected with chronic hepatitis B: a 16-year population-based study. Hepatology 2000;32:842–6.

36. Trevisani F, D'Intino PE, Morselli-Labate AM, et al. Serum alpha-fetoprotein for diagnosis of hepatocellular carcinoma in patients with chronic liver disease: influence of HBsAg and anti-HCV status. J Hepatol 2001;34:570–5.

37. Nguyen MH, Garcia RT, Simpson PW, et al. Racial differences in effectiveness of alpha-fetoprotein for diagnosis of hepatocellular carcinoma in hepatitis C virus cirrhosis. Hepatology 2002;36:410–7.

38. Rapaccini GL, Pompili M, Caturelli E, et al. Hepatocellular carcinomas <2 cm in diameter complicating cirrhosis: ultrasound and clinical features in 153 consec- utive patients. Liver Int 2004;24:124–30.

39. Zhang B, Yang B. Combined alpha fetoprotein testing and ultrasonography as a screening test for primary liver cancer. J Med Screen 1999;6:108–10.

40. Yang B, Zhang B, Xu Y, et al. Prospective study of early detection for primary liver cancer. J Cancer Res Clin Oncol 1997;123:357–60.

41. Zhang BH, Yang BH, Tang ZY. Randomized controlled trial of screening for hepatocellular carcinoma. J Cancer Res Clin Oncol 2004;130:417–22.

42. Lok AS, Sterling RK, Everhart JE, et al. Des-gamma-carboxy prothrombin and alpha-fetoprotein as biomarkers for early detection of hepatocellular carcinoma. Gastroenterology 2010;138:493–502.

43. Bruce MG, Bruden D, McMahon BJ, et al. Clinical significance of elevated alpha- fetoprotein in Alaskan Native patients with chronic hepatitis C. J Viral Hepat 2008; 15(3):179–87.

44. El-Serag HB, Kanwal F, Davila JA, et al. A new laboratory-based algorithm to pre- dict development of hepatocellular carcinoma in patients with hepatitis C and cirrhosis. Gastroenterology 2014;146(5):1249–55.

45. Vibert E, Azoulay D, Hoti E, et al. Progression of alpha-fetoprotein before liver transplantation for hepatocellular carcinoma in cirrhotic patients: a critical factor. Am J Transplant 2010;10:129–37.

46. Pomfret EA, Washburn K, Wald C, et al. Report of a national conference on liver allocation in patients with hepatocellular carcinoma in the United States. Liver Transpl 2010;16:262–78.

47. Toso C, Asthana S, Bigam DL, et al. Reassessing selection criteria prior to liver transplantation for hepatocellular carcinoma utilizing the scientific registry of transplant recipients database. Hepatology 2009;49:832–8.

48. Sato Y, Nakata K, Kato Y, et al. Early recognition of hepatocellular carcinoma based on altered profiles of alpha-fetoprotein. N Engl J Med 1993;328:1802–6.

49. Shiraki K, Takase K, Tameda Y, et al. A clinical study of lectin-reactive alpha-feto- protein as an early indicator of hepatocellular carcinoma in the follow-up of cirrhotic patients. Hepatology 1995;22:802–7.

50. Wang SS, Lu RH, Lee FY, et al. Utility of lentil lectin affinity of alpha-fetoprotein in the diagnosis of hepatocellular carcinoma. J Hepatol 1996;25:166–71.

51. Sterling RK, Jeffers L, Gordon F, et al. Clinical utility of AFP-L3% measurement in North American patients with HCV-related cirrhosis. Am J Gastroenterol 2007; 102:2196–205.

52. Inagaki Y, Tang W, Makuuchi M, et al. Clinical and molecular insights into the hepatocellular carcinoma tumour marker des-gamma-carboxyprothrombin. Liver Int 2011;31(1):22–35.

53. Ishii M, Gama H, Chida N, et al. Simultaneous measurements of serum alpha-fetoprotein and protein induced by vitamin K absence for detecting hepatocellular carcinoma. South Tohoku District Study Group. Am J Gastroenterol 2000;95: 1036–40.

54. Marrero JA, Feng Z, Wang Y, et al. Alpha-fetoprotein, des-gamma carboxyprothrombin, and lectin-bound alpha-fetoprotein in early hepatocellular carcinoma. Gastroenterology 2009;137:110–8.

55. Nakamura S, Nouso K, Sakaguchi K, et al. Sensitivity and specificity of des-gamma-carboxy prothrombin for diagnosis of patients with hepatocellular carcinoma varies according to tumor size. Am J Gastroenterol 2006;101: 2038–43.

56. Rich N, Singal AG. Hepatocellular carcinoma tumour markers: current role and expectations. Best Pract Res Clin Gastroenterol 2014;28(5):843–53.

57. Colli A, Fraquelli M, Casazza G, et al. Accuracy of ultrasonography, spiral CT, magnetic resonance, and alpha-fetoprotein in diagnosing hepatocellular carcinoma: a systematic review. Am J Gastroenterol 2006;101(3):513–23.

58. Johnson PJ, Pirrie SJ, Cox TF, et al. The detection of hepatocellular carcinoma using a prospectively developed and validated model based on serological biomarkers. Cancer Epidemiol Biomarkers Prev 2014;23(1):144–53.

59. Hakeem AR, Young RS, Marangoni G, et al. Systematic review: the prognostic role of alpha-fetoprotein following liver transplantation for hepatocellular carcinoma. Aliment Pharmacol Ther 2012;35(9):987–99.

60. Poon TC, Yip TT, Chan AT, et al. Comprehensive proteomic profiling identifies serum proteomic signatures for detection of hepatocellular carcinoma and its subtypes. Clin Chem 2003;49:752–60.

61. Paradis V, Degos F, Dargere D, et al. Identification of a new marker of hepatocellular carcinoma by serum protein profiling of patients with chronic liver diseases. Hepatology 2005;41:40–7.

62. Schwegler EE, Cazares L, Steel LF, et al. SELDI-TOF MS profiling of serum for detection in the progression of chronic hepatitis C to hepatocellular carcinoma. Hepatology 2005;41:634–42.

63. Zinkin NT, Grall F, Bhasker K, et al. Serum proteomics and biomarkers in hepatocellular carcinoma and chronic liver disease. Clin Cancer Res 2008;14: 470–7.

64. Sung YK, Hwang SY, Park MK, et al. Glypican-3 is overexpressed in human hepatocellular carcinoma. Cancer Sci 2003;94:259–62.

65. Zhu ZW, Friess H, Wang L, et al. Enhanced glypican-3 expression differentiates the majority of hepatocellular carcinomas from benign hepatic disorders. Gut 2001;48:558–64.

66. Capurro MI, Xiang YY, Lobe C, et al. Glypican-3 promotes the growth of hepatocellular carcinoma by stimulating canonical Wnt signaling. Cancer Res 2005;65: 6245–54.

67. Hippo Y, Watanabe K, Watanabe A, et al. Identification of soluble NH2-terminal fragment of glypican-3 as a serological marker for early-stage hepatocellular carcinoma. Cancer Res 2004;64:2418–23.
68. Nakatsura T, Yoshitake Y, Senju S, et al. Glypican-3, overexpressed specifically in human hepatocellular carcinoma, is a novel tumor marker. Biochem Biophys Res Commun 2003;306:16–25.
69. Capurro M, Wanless IR, Sherman M, et al. Glypican-3: a novel serum and histochemical marker for hepatocellular carcinoma. Gastroenterology 2003;125:89–97.
70. Liu H, Li P, Zhai Y, et al. Diagnostic value of glypican-3 in serum and liver for primary hepatocellular carcinoma. World J Gastroenterol 2010;16:4410–5.

# Imaging of Hepatocellular Carcinoma

## New Approaches to Diagnosis

Munazza Anis, MD

## KEYWORDS

- Liver • Imaging • HCC • LI-RADS • MRI

## KEY POINTS

- The liver imaging reporting and data system (LI-RADS) is a form of structured reporting that is being made congruent with the US Organ Procurement and Transplant Network (OPTN) classification of liver nodules in cirrhotic patients.
- Major diagnostic imaging features for hepatocellular carcinoma (HCC) are arterial phase hyperenhancement, tumor size (diameter), washout, capsule presence and appearance, and interval threshold tumor growth.
- LI-RADS and OPTN class 5 are essentially equivalent, conveying almost 100% certainty for HCC using imaging features for lesions greater than 10 mm in size.

## INTRODUCTION

Hepatocellular carcinoma (HCC) is the sixth most frequent tumor and second leading cause of cancer death worldwide.[1] A variety of treatment options are available for HCC,[2,3] such as surgical resection for an early-stage tumor with normal portal pressures and serum bilirubin and liver transplantation (LT) in patients with early-stage cancer and without prohibitive comorbid disease. Locoregional therapy, such as transarterial chemoembolization, radiofrequency ablation, and other destructive techniques, might be appropriate for patients who are poor surgical candidates. The multikinase inhibitor, sorafenib, has been recently approved for systemic therapy for the treatment of advanced disease HCC patients.

In clinical practice, the appropriate management of a given specific stage of HCC depends on the accuracy of the imaging diagnosis of HCC, because negative outcome risk factors are usually not known unless a biopsy of the tumor is obtained, and this is becoming increasingly uncommon. Abdominal ultrasound is the initial imaging test suggested in all guidelines for screening and surveillance of HCC in

The author has nothing to disclose.
Hunter Holmes McGuire VAMC, 1201 Broad Rock Boulevard, Richmond, VA 23249, USA
*E-mail address:* Munazza.Anis@va.gov

Clin Liver Dis 19 (2015) 325–340
http://dx.doi.org/10.1016/j.cld.2015.01.013
1089-3261/15/$ – see front matter **liver.theclinics.com**

high-risk individuals,[2,3] followed generally by contrast-enhanced computed tomography (CT) or MRI. The American Association for the Study of Liver Diseases (AASLD), the European Association for the Study of the Liver, the Organ Procurement and Transplantation Network (OPTN) in the United States (which is administered by the United Network for Organ Sharing), the Japan Society of Hepatology, and several other organizations have published guidelines for the imaging diagnosis of HCC,[4–12] such as "arterial phase hyperenhancement" and "washout," after intravenous contrast administration; some also incorporate an evaluation of nodule growth on serial examinations. Heretofore, the AASLD and other organizations generally stratified imaging diagnoses simply as positive, negative, or indeterminate for HCC,[2,3] but there is now a move toward greater precision and expression of degree of certainty.

### American Association for the Study of Liver Diseases-Organ Procurement and Transplant Network Criteria for Hepatocellular Carcinoma Diagnosis

According to the latest AASLD guidelines,[13] imaging surveillance for HCC should be based on serial ultrasound. However, in practice, surveillance is often performed with serial dynamic multiphasic CT or MRI (**Table 1**). Also, a 10- to 20-mm nodule initially detected by ultrasound, according to the AASLD guidelines, can be definitively diagnosed as HCC with arterial phase hyperenhancement and washout on CT or MRI.[2,14,15] Diagnosis of HCCs between 10 and 20 mm is particularly important, because these tumors can be cured by LT, although they do not get priority points on the transplant wait list according OPTN criteria until the size exceeds 2 cm. The finding of "arterial phase enhancement and washout" provides only 87% to 95% specificity for diagnosis of HCC.[5,8,14] However, the visualization of a liver nodule on surveillance ultrasound raises the probability of HCC in an at-risk population with a positive predictive value of approximately 100%.[2,3,14]

The OPTN[14,15] updated its liver imaging policy in October 2013 by requiring minimum technical specifications on CT and MRI, a structured reporting (the Liver Imaging Reporting and Data System [LI-RADS]), and for the scan to be interpreted by a

---

**Table 1**
**US Organ Procurement and Transplant Network classification of cirrhotic nodules**

| Class | Description |
|-------|-------------|
| 0 | Incomplete or inadequate study (repeat) |
| 1 | No evidence of HCC (normal follow-up) |
| 2 | Benign lesion or diffuse disease; no focal mass (transplant center discretion for further imaging) |
| 3 | Abnormal scan; indeterminate lesion not meeting criteria for HCC (follow-up imaging 6–12 mo) |
| 4 | Abnormal scan; intermediate suspicion for HCC (3 mo imaging follow-up) |
| 5 | Meets criteria for HCC<br>5A: Greater than or equal to 1 cm and <2 cm (potentially eligible for automatic exception)<br>5A-G: Lesion that has demonstrated threshold growth (potentially eligible for automatic exception)<br>5B: Maximum diameter greater than or equal to 2 cm and less than or equal to 5 cm (potentially eligible for automatic exception)<br>5T: Prior local regional treatment of HCC (potentially eligible for automatic exception)<br>5X: Maximum diameter greater than or equal to 5 cm (not eligible for automatic exception) |

radiologist at a transplant center. The classification of OPTN nodules is shown in **Table 1**. A candidate with a stage 2 HCC tumor by TNM classification is considered eligible for LT if the patient has undergone a thorough assessment to evaluate the number and size of tumors, as classified by the Milan[16] or University of California at San Francisco criteria.[17] The patients must have undergone dynamic contrast-enhanced CT or MRI imaging to rule out any extrahepatic spread (ie, lymph node involvement) and/or macrovascular involvement (ie, tumor thrombus in a portal or hepatic vein). Any imaging examination performed for the purpose of obtaining or updating priority points on the transplant wait list should meet minimum recommended technical and imaging protocol requirements for CT and MRI (**Boxes 1** and **2**). In addition, a radiologist at an OPTN-approved transplant center must interpret the scans. Technically inadequate or incomplete imaging examinations must be classified as OPTN class 0 and be repeated or completed to be considered for priority point allocation. All nodules in cirrhotic patients are to be categorized according to the OPTN classification (see **Table 1**), which refers to LI-RADS for nodule designation (**Table 2**). Several classification systems have been put forth in radiology literature[18,19]; detailed descriptions of the radiological appearances can be found in the earlier article by Anis and Irshad[20] and 2 recent reviews[21,22]; however, the focus of this article is LI-RADS,[23,24] which is later discussed in detail.

*Summary*

1. Numerous organizations have proposed guidelines for the imaging diagnosis of HCC,[2,13,14] such as "arterial phase hyperenhancement" and "washout"; some also incorporate an evaluation of nodule growth on serial examinations.
2. AASLD guidelines outline serial ultrasound as the modality of choice for HCC surveillance.
3. According to AASLD guidelines, a 10- to 20-mm lesion in high-risk patients with cirrhosis can be definitively diagnosed as HCC with imaging features of arterial phase hyperenhancement and washout appearance on CT or MRI.
4. OPTN class 5 nodules are equivalent to LI-RADS 5 lesions; OPTN class 5 nodules greater than 2 cm in diameter receive added priority model of end-stage liver disease (MELD) points on the transplant wait list. The OPTN classification now refers to LI-RADS for nodule classes 1 to 4.

## LIVER IMAGING REPORTING AND DATA SYSTEM

LI-RADS is a form of structured reporting that has been devised to standardize the reporting and data collection of CT and MR imaging for HCC in cirrhotic patients. This method of categorizing liver findings for patients with cirrhosis allows the radiology community to apply consistent terminology, reduce imaging interpretation variability and errors, enhance communication with referring clinicians, and facilitate

---

**Box 1**
**Technical requirements for computed tomography**

1. Multirow multidetector CT with thin slice reconstruction (5 mm or thinner)
2. Dual-chamber, power injector with saline push
3. 4–6 mL/s (minimum 3 mL/s) for a minimum of 300 mg of Iodine/mL for a dose of 1.5 mg Iodine/kg of body weight; bolus tracking or timing bolus
4. Three phases of contrast are mandatory: late arterial, portal venous, and delayed phase

---

**Box 2**
**Technical requirements for MRI**

1. 1.5 T or higher strength MRI with phased array multichannel torso coil

2. Precontrast and postgadolinium 3D gradient-echo T1 sequences, in-phase and out-of-phase T1 sequences and T2 with and without fat saturation sequences

3. 2–3 mL/s of extracellular contrast with a dual chamber power injector

4. Precontrast, late arterial (bolus tracking), portal venous (35–55 s), and delayed phases (120–180 s) are mandatory; 5 mm or less slice thickness

---

quality assurance and research. LI-RADS is devised only for individuals at increased risk for HCC and should not be applied to the general population. There are 5 categories of liver observations that are referred to as LR 1-5 (see **Table 2**). Other categories include other malignancy (OM); LR-5t that describes a definite HCC that has received locoregional treatment for downgrading; and LR-5V that indicates an advanced HCC with tumor extension (invasion) into the hepatic or portal veins.

### Major Features Described in Liver Imaging Reporting and Data System

Major features included in the diagnostic criteria include arterial phase enhancement, tumor size (diameter), washout appearance, the presence and nature of a capsule, and threshold growth.

#### Arterial phase enhancement

The hepatic arterial phase may be subdivided into early and late hepatic arterial phases, when the portal vein is either not yet enhanced or is enhanced, respectively (portal vein is enhanced) (**Fig. 1**). The late hepatic arterial phase is needed for the diagnosis of HCC.

- Isoenhancement or hypoenhancement: In this circumstance, lesion enhancement is less than the surrounding liver. These findings may be categorized as LR-3 or LR-4, depending on the diameter of the mass and other features. Subtraction images are helpful if these lesions demonstrate a T1 hyperintense signal on MRI, keeping in mind that the precontrast and postcontrast images need to be coregistered (ie, overlayed exactly at the same position precontrast and postcontrast, which requires the same breath intake at all slice positions).

---

**Table 2**
**Liver imaging reporting and data system classification 1–5**

| | Arterial Hypoenhancement or Isoenhancement | | Arterial Phase Hyperenhancement | | |
|---|---|---|---|---|---|
| | <20 mm | ≥20 mm | <10 mm | 10–19 mm | ≥20 mm |
| No associated features (WO, C, G) | LR-3 | LR-3 | LR-3 | LR-3 | LR-4 |
| One associated feature (WO, C, G) | LR-3 | LR-4 | LR-4 | LR-4 LR-5 | LR-5 |
| Two or more of associated features (WO, C, G) | LR-4 | LR-4 | LR-4 | LR-5 | LR-5 |

Observations in the liver in high-risk patient: definitely benign = LR-1, probably benign = LR-2.
   *Abbreviations:* C, capsule; G, growth; WO, washout.
   *Adapted from* LIRAD-ACR Web site. Available at: http://nrdr.acr.org/lirads/. Accessed November 20, 2014.

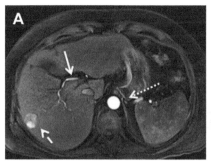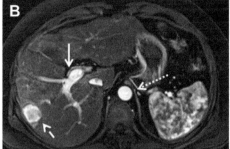

Fig. 1. MRI axial postcontrast images in early (*A*) and late (*B*) arterial phases. Early phase (*A*) demonstrates nonopacification of the portal vein (*arrow center liver*), whereas the portal vein is enhancing in the late arterial phase with marked conspicuity of the HCC (*small arrow right liver*). Aorta, dotted arrow.

- Hyperenhancement: Here the lesion enhancement is unequivocally greater than that of surrounding liver, and this is the hallmark of an HCC.

### Diameter

For masses with arterial phase hyperenhancement, the key diameter threshold is less than 10 mm versus 10 to 19 mm. Masses less than 10 mm cannot be categorized as LR-5, regardless of other major features, which maintains congruency with the OPTN classification that does not allow less than 10-mm lesions to be classified as OPTN 5. Masses of 10 to 19 mm with arterial phase hyperenhancement can be categorized LR-5A if the major criteria are met. For arterial phase hypoenhancing or isoenhancing masses, lesions, which are less than 2 cm with one other major feature such as washout, capsule presence, or growth, are categorized as LR-3, whereas lesions greater than 2 cm are categorized LR-3 if none of the associated major features are present.

### Washout

Washout is determined visually by the radiologist, on the portal venous (immediately following the arterial phase) or delayed phases (ie, the last phase of contrast administration) (**Fig. 2**). Delayed phase may be superior to the portal venous phase

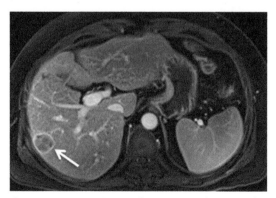

Fig. 2. Axial delayed postcontrast MRI image demonstrates lesion washout with progressive enhancement of the rim compatible with a capsule appearance (*arrow*).

for depicting washout appearance because some HCCs may show a washout appearance only in the delayed phase. Region of interest measurements, time-enhancement curves, or, at MRI, subtraction images and other techniques can also be used as needed.

### Capsule

A capsule is described if there is a thick peripheral rim of smooth hyperenhancement in the portal venous phase or delayed phase that is more conspicuous than the rims surrounding background nodules (see **Fig. 2**). Such capsule appearance has a high positive predictive value for HCC in at-risk patients. There is some overlap between these findings of a capsule and "corona enhancement." If rim enhancement increases in the portal venous or delayed phases, then it likely represents a "capsule," whereas if the rim enhancement occurs only in the arterial phase and then fades, it represents "corona enhancement" that is considered an ancillary feature (see later discussion), aiding the diagnosis of HCC.

### Threshold growth

A diameter increase 50% or more over a period of 6 months or shorter, or greater than 100% over a period of 6 months, is considered *threshold growth*, which is a major feature of HCC (**Fig. 3**).

### Ancillary features

Features that may favor HCC include mild to moderate T2 hyperintensity, restricted diffusion (ie, the restricted diffusion of water molecules seen in cancer cells), corona enhancement (as explained above), mosaic architecture, nodule-in-nodule architecture, intralesional fat, lesional iron-sparing (**Figs. 4** and **5**), blood products from bleeding within the lesion, and diameter increase less than threshold growth.

Features that may favor benignity include homogeneous marked T2 hyperintensity, homogeneous marked T2 or T2* hypointensity, undistorted vessels, parallels blood pool enhancement, diameter reduction, and diameter stability for more than or equal to 2 years.

These features are used to upgrade or downgrade a lesion and are used as tie-breaking rules, keeping in mind that a lesion cannot be upgraded to beyond LR 4.

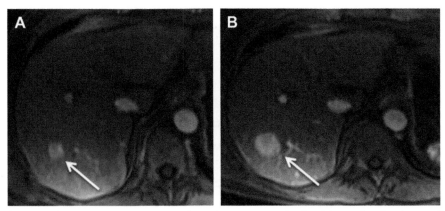

**Fig. 3.** Axial postcontrast MRI images (*A, B*; image B was obtained 6 months after image A) demonstrating interval doubling of right hepatic lobe HCC in 6 months (*arrows*).

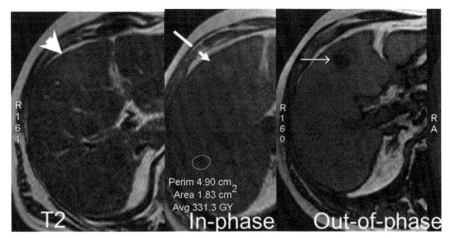

**Fig. 4.** Two ancillary features described for HCC, including T2 hyperintense signal (*arrowhead*), and in-phase and out-of-phase signal dropout (*arrow*).

## LIVER IMAGING REPORTING AND DATA SYSTEM 1

Category LR-1 refers to observations that have typical characteristics for a benign diagnosis (**Fig. 6**) and include cysts, hemangiomas, vascular anomalies, perfusion alteration, hepatic fat deposition or sparing, hypertrophic pseudomass (ie, an area of hepatic hypertrophy giving a false appearance of a mass), confluent fibrosis, and focal scar. Observations that spontaneously disappear are also classified as LI-RADS category 1 lesions. The 2 most common cysts in the liver are hepatic cysts and cystic biliary hamartomas. Peribiliary cysts are rare cysts associated with advanced cirrhosis that represent cystic dilatation of the extramural glands in the periductal connective tissue. They parallel the bile ducts in distribution and may be misinterpreted as dilated bile ducts. Hepatic cysts, cystic biliary hamartomas, and peribiliary cysts do not communicate with the bile ducts.

### Summary

1. LI-RADS is only to be used in individuals at increased risk for HCC.
2. LR-1 refers to features that are diagnostic of benign entities.
3. These do not need to be reported as LI-RADS lesions.

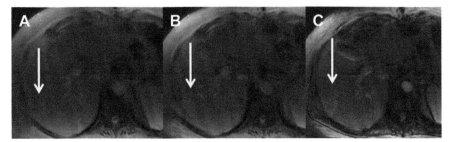

**Fig. 5.** Multiecho T2* images (A-C) demonstrating darkening of the background liver due to iron deposition in cirrhosis with increasing time to echo but the HCC demonstrates intralesional iron sparing appearing increasingly brighter (*arrow*).

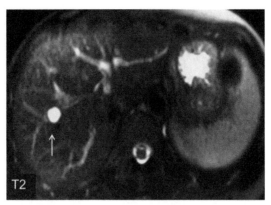

**Fig. 6.** T2 hyperintense homogenous lesion in the right lobe (*arrow*) compatible with a cyst: definitely benign: LI-RADS 1.

## LIVER IMAGING REPORTING AND DATA SYSTEM 2

LR-2 observations include findings with features suggestive of but not diagnostic of a benign entity (eg, cysts with mildly atypical features or low-density lesions that are too small to accurately characterize at CT) (**Fig. 7**). These LR-2 findings also include hemangiomas, vascular anomalies, perfusion alteration, hepatic fat deposition or sparing, confluent fibrosis, and focal scars without typical findings. The updated LI-RADS 2013 version does not include focal nodular hyperplasia or adenoma in this category, because these lesions are rare and difficult to diagnose reliably by noninvasive imaging. Cirrhosis-associated nodules are categorized as LR-2 if the diameter is less than 2 cm and the lesion is homogeneous with isoenhancement compared with background cirrhotic nodules. These lesions may differ from the background nodules by being distinctly larger, having mild to moderate T2 hypointensity, having mild to moderate T1 hyperintensity, or having mild to moderate CT hyperattenuation. LI-2 nodules do not require reporting as LI-RADS observations. Continued surveillance is generally recommended for LR-2 lesions.

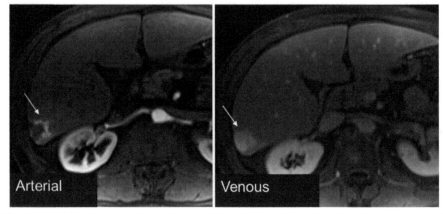

**Fig. 7.** Arterial and venous phases demonstrate a focal peripherally enhancing mass (*arrows*) with centripetal filling on delayed images compatible with a hemangioma: probably benign: LI-RADS 2.

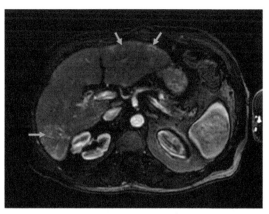

**Fig. 5.** Multifocal, bilobar HCC (*arrows*).

cirrhosis often have multicentric tumors and typically do not tolerate major hepatic lobar resections. Segmental or nonanatomic resections to preserve hepatic parenchyma can be considered in patients with single tumors and well-compensated cirrhosis. Occasionally a large encapsulated, exophytic tumor can be safely resected with minimal parenchymal loss in patients with cirrhosis (**Fig. 6**).

The cause of cirrhosis plays a significant role in selecting patients for hepatic resection. Patients with chronic hepatitis B often have softer, less fibrotic livers; although most of these patients have cirrhosis, they typically have less portal hypertension

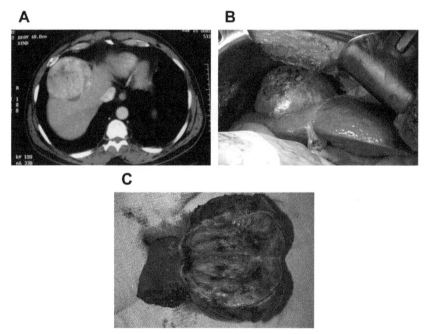

**Fig. 6.** A large exophytic encapsulated HCC in a patient with underlying cirrhosis. (*A*) CT scan image, (*B*) at operation, (*C*) the resected specimen.

and are likely to tolerate partial hepatectomy.[11] In contrast, virtually all patients with hepatitis C have cirrhosis with significant hepatic inflammation and portal hypertension making surgical resection prohibitively hazardous. In this population, hepatic resection may be considered for small tumors measuring less than 2 cm and in a peripheral location allowing resection of the least possible hepatic parenchyma with minimum blood loss (**Fig. 7**). Larger tumors and tumors located deep within the liver that would require a major hepatic resection should be considered for other therapeutic modalities (**Fig. 8**).

### Outcome of Hepatic Resection

The reported outcome of hepatic resection for HCC varies widely as a result of significant geographic variations in population characteristics, cause of the underlying liver disease, presentation, and tumor features. Refinements in patient selection, anesthetic methods, surgical techniques, and postoperative care have reduced the operative mortality after partial hepatectomy to less than 5% in patients with normal livers and 5% to 10% in patients with cirrhosis.[4,12–15] **Table 1** lists some of the largest series of partial hepatic resection for patients with HCC. These series include a wide spectrum of patients ranging from those with small tumors who underwent minor resections to patients with large (>10 cm) and/or multifocal tumors, including those with major vascular invasion. Most reports included patients with and without cirrhosis, although 2 reports (Chen and colleagues[19] and Laurent and colleagues[20]) focused their analysis exclusively on noncirrhotic patients. The overall 5-year survival ranges from 29% to 81%, and recurrence rates range from 51% to 69%. In these reports, the presence of cirrhosis negatively impacted hospital mortality and long-term survival. The report by Taura and colleagues[22] demonstrates the impact of underlying liver disease on outcomes after hepatic resection. They analyzed the outcome of 293 patients with either a single tumor less than 5 cm or up to 3 tumors each measuring less than 3 cm (similar to the Milan criteria[25] that are used to select a patient for liver transplantation). The 5-year patient survival was 81% in patients without cirrhosis, 54% in patients with CTP A, and 28% in patients with CTP B cirrhosis. The annual recurrence rate in the first 3 years was 22% and 15% in cirrhotic and

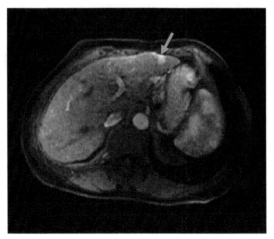

**Fig. 7.** HCC at the edge of segment II (*arrow*) in a patient with cirrhosis can be resected with a small wedge resection.

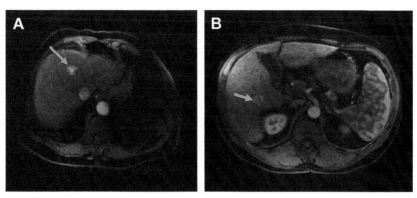

**Fig. 8.** HCC (*arrows*) in patients with cirrhosis and portal hypertension located deep in the hepatic parenchyma (*A*) segment IV and (*B*) segment VI.

noncirrhotic patients, respectively. Similar studies have compared the outcome of hepatic resection in patients with cirrhosis with that of liver transplantation. Although a 5-year survival equivalent to that of transplantation can be achieved in select patients, the rate of recurrence remains significantly higher after hepatic resection.[4,17,23]

The cause of the underlying chronic liver disease also affects the outcome after hepatic resection. Better long-term survival is achieved after partial hepatectomy for patients with hepatitis B as compared with those with hepatitis C or alcohol-related cirrhosis.[11,26,27] This improved survival has been attributed to patients' demographics as well as tumor characteristics. HCCs in patients with HCV are often multifocal, more likely to have microvascular invasion, and occur in an older age group.[26,27]

The heterogeneity of the various patient populations with HCC and the varied tumor characteristics have made it difficult to identify reliable prognostic factors associated with improved survival after hepatic resection. Prognostic factors that have consistently been associated with improved survival include CTP stage, preoperative AFP levels, size and number of tumor nodules, absence of satellite nodules, size of resection margins, and absence of vascular invasion.[28]

| Table 1 | | | |
|---|---|---|---|
| **Results of some of the published series of hepatic resection for HCC** | | | |
| **Author, Year** | **No. of Patients** | **5-y Survival (%)** | **Recurrence Rate (%)** |
| Bismuth et al,[3] 1995 | 68 | 40 | 59 |
| Nagasue et al,[16] 2001 | 100 | 50 | 51 |
| Poon et al,[17] 2002 | 135 | 70 | 51 |
| Belghiti et al,[18] 2002 | 328 | 37 | — |
| Chen et al,[19] 2003 | 254 | 36 | 57 |
| Laurent et al,[20] 2005 | 108 | 29 | 52 |
| Bège et al,[21] 2007 | 116 | 40 | 69 |
| Taura et al,[22] 2007 | 127 | 81 | 54 |
| Cherqui et al,[23] 2009 | 67 | 72 | 54 |
| Lee et al,[24] 2010 | 130 | 52 | 51.5 |

*Data from* Refs.[3,16–24]

### Management of Tumor Recurrence

Chronic inflammation with ongoing necrosis, hepatocyte cell division, and regeneration in patients with cirrhosis creates a favorable environment for the development of cellular mutations that could lead to overt malignancy.

Recurrence is usually highest in the first 2 years after resection but has been reported to occur up to 10 years after resection.[17] Using genomic data to characterize a recurrence as either metastatic or de novo has clearly shown that a recurrence of HCC in the liver appearing more than 2 years after resection is nearly always a de novo tumor.[29] Recurrence caused by metastatic spread from the primary tumor is usually seen within the first 2 years and is typically multinodular and carries a poor prognosis.

Because the most common site of recurrence is the remaining liver, patients undergoing hepatic resection should be followed with serial imaging studies to detect recurrence early. It is recommended that patients undergo imaging every 3 months for the first year then every 6 months thereafter. Recurrent tumors detected early (within 2 years) can be considered for additional surgical resection or LRT. Salvage transplantation is considered for a recurrence occurring more than 2 years from resection because this likely represents a de novo tumor. These procedures are often associated with excessive blood loss and higher morbidity. The long-term results of salvage transplantation vary widely, with some groups reporting comparable outcomes with primary transplantation for HCC,[23,30–32] whereas others report high operative mortality and poor long-term outcomes.[33] Currently there are no agreed on selection criteria for determining patient eligibility for salvage liver transplantation for recurrent HCC. Some regions in the United States give priority for liver transplantation to patients within 2 years of surgical resection for an HCC that was within listing criteria who develop a recurrence of tumor that remains within the listing criteria.

### Surgical Techniques

Most hepatic resections for HCC are performed with a standard open technique. Minimizing blood loss and transfusion are essential in performing a hepatic resection in patients with HCC, especially those with underlying cirrhosis. Several devices are available to divide the liver with minimal blood loss; their use depends on the surgeon's preference. These devices include the ultrasonic harmonic scalpel (Ethicon, Cincinnati, OH), advanced bipolar devices (Enseal, Ethicon, Cincinnati, OH), radiofrequency monopolar devices (TissueLink, Medtronic, Minneapolis, MN), and electrothermal vessel sealer (LigaSure Covidien, Dublin, Ireland). The use of intraoperative ultrasound allows precise localization of the tumor in relation to vascular structures and affords detection of other lesions that may not have been seen on preoperative imaging studies. The authors perform formal lobar hepatic resections using a standardized approach of ligating the inflow and outflow vessels followed by parenchymal transection. The authors occasionally use intermittent inflow occlusion (Pringle maneuver) during hepatic resections to minimize blood loss.

Recent advances in minimally invasive surgery and wide acceptance of using the laparoscopic approach for the treatment of malignancy have encouraged hepatobiliary surgeons to consider laparoscopy for hepatic resection for HCC. Equivalent long-term outcomes have been reported with a laparoscopic approach as compared with an open technique. The laparoscopic technique has the advantage of less postoperative pain, shorter hospital stay, and earlier return to functional status. Currently most laparoscopic resections are performed for small tumors in favorable locations that can be resected with minimal blood loss. Although a few groups have performed major lobar hepatic resections for HCC using the laparoscopic approach,[23,34–36] these are techniques that should be reserved for surgeons and centers with extensive expertise in laparoscopic surgery and complex hepatobiliary resections.

## LIVER TRANSPLANTATION FOR HEPATOCELLULAR CARCINOMA

HCC was among the earliest indications for liver transplantation, as logic suggests that transplantation would provide the most effective cure for HCC in patients with underlying cirrhosis by completely removing the tumor and restoring normal hepatic function. Yet, the initial experience with liver transplantation for HCC in the 1980s was plagued by high recurrence rates and poor outcomes. As a result, HCC became a contraindication to liver transplantation, as the consensus was to offer the limited supply of donor organs to patients who would gain the most benefit. It was later observed that patients with incidental HCC, too small to be detected by preoperative imaging studies that were found in the explanted liver, had outcomes equivalent to transplantation for non-HCC patients. These early observations showed that the tumor burden is crucial to the success of liver transplantation for HCC. Over the ensuing decades, reports of good long-term survival for patients with early HCC led to the development of acceptable criteria to ensure optimal outcome for patients with HCC and avoid wasting the scarce donor organs in patients expected to do poorly. Therefore, it was agreed on to offer liver transplantation to patients with early stage HCC who have predicted 5-year survival comparable with non-HCC patients.

### The Milan Criteria

The prospective landmark study by Mazzaferro and colleagues[25] in 1996 reported excellent long-term outcomes when restrictive criteria were applied in selecting patients with HCC for liver transplantation. The Milan criteria are defined as one lesion less than 5 cm or 3 lesions each measuring less than 3 cm with no evidence of macrovascular invasion. In that seminal study, the 5-year survival in patients transplanted within the Milan criteria was 70%, which was equivalent to liver transplantation for other indications. The development of the Milan criteria set the stage for orthotopic liver transplantation to be widely accepted as a curative treatment of patients with early stage HCC. As a result, the Milan criteria were adopted worldwide as the basis for selecting appropriate patients with HCC for liver transplantation and have served as the gold standard comparison for all other suggested criteria. Many groups around the world independently validated these results. Recently Mazzaferro and colleagues[37] reported an analysis of 190 studies over a 15-year period and found the Milan criteria to be an independent prognostic factor, impacting outcomes after liver transplantation for HCC.

Intent-to-treat studies have demonstrated that the risk of removal caused by HCC progression beyond the Milan criteria (dropout rate) is greater than the risk of death while patients are awaiting transplantation.[5] For these reasons, in the United States, the Organ Procurement and Transplantation Network (OPTN) has developed an organ allocation policy for deceased donor liver transplantation that allows for increased priority for liver transplant candidates with stage II HCC.[38]

### The University of California at San Francisco Criteria

Concerns began to be raised regarding whether the Milan criteria may be too restrictive, thus, excluding patients who would have otherwise done well after liver transplantation. The University of California at San Francisco (UCSF) group reported the outcome of 70 consecutive patients over a 12-year period who had tumors exceeding the Milan criteria on explant liver pathology and yet achieved a 5-year survival of

75%.[39] Their results suggested that patients with 4 or more lesions or gross vascular invasion had poor survival after liver transplant. They also demonstrated the importance of total tumor burden (ie, the sum of the diameter of all tumor nodules being <8 cm) as a significant predictor of survival. Based on this analysis, they proposed a modified pathologic HCC staging criteria for liver transplantation known as the UCSF criteria: a solitary tumor less than or equal to 6.5 cm or up to 3 nodules with the largest lesion measuring less than 4.5 cm and total tumor diameter of 8 cm or less. These results were subsequently validated prospectively by the same group in patients prospectively selected based on pretransplant imaging.[40]

In contrast, other single-center studies have shown that selecting patients exceeding the Milan criteria but within the UCSF criteria was associated with reduced survival but still achieved a 5-year survival of 50%.[41,42]

The effect of incrementally expanding the Milan criteria for patients awaiting liver transplantation may negatively impact the wait-list mortality for non-HCC patients because transplanting a patient with HCC results in a patient without a tumor possibly missing a chance for liver transplant. Volk and colleagues[43] examined the posttransplant survival that would justify expansion of the Milan criteria for liver transplantation using a Markov model. They found that 5-year survival following liver transplantation for the expanded-criteria patients had to exceed 61% before expansion of the Milan criteria resulted in an improvement in overall survival and did not harm patients without HCC.

When compared with standard MELD patients, HCC candidates seem to have increased access to deceased donor transplantation despite having inferior adjusted 3-year posttransplant patient survival.[44] This disparity is exacerbated depending on the availability of deceased donors in a particular region or country; therefore, the expansion of the Milan criteria should remain conservative when considering the allocation of deceased donor organs. Some regions in the United States with shorter waiting times and lower mortality on the waiting list have adopted modest expansions of the Milan criteria, whereas other regions with longer waiting times and higher waiting-list mortality have not. In regions that do not offer any priority for patients beyond the Milan criteria, transplantation from living donors offers the only realistic hope.

Despite the resulting controversies sparked by concerns over how expansion of the criteria would disadvantage non-HCC candidates, there is acceptance among the transplant community that modest expansion of the Milan criteria can be considered using the UCSF criteria as a benchmark.

### Beyond the University of California at San Francisco Criteria

Several other single-center criteria have been proposed (**Box 1**) that represent progressive expansion beyond both the Milan and UCSF criteria, with 5-year survival exceeding 70%. These criteria, however, have not been prospectively validated and are not widely used.

The concept of the Metro Ticket was introduced by Mazzaferro and colleagues[49] to demonstrate that the expansion of these criteria can have a price in terms of patient survival after liver transplantation (**Fig. 9**). The authors showed that survival was correlated with the tumor size, number of tumors, and the presence of microvascular invasion in explanted liver. The concept explains that the further the distance from the conventional limits (the higher the number and size of the tumors), the higher the price paid (high recurrence and reduced survival).

### Priority Allocation for Hepatocellular Carcinoma Candidates

Assigning organ allocation priority to patients with HCC has been an ongoing topic of debate. The MELD allocation scheme allowing for increased priority for liver transplant

---

**Box 1**
**History of MELD exception points for patients with HCC within Milan criteria**

Asan Medical Center[45]

    Tumor size less than or equal to 5 cm and number less than or equal to 6 without gross vascular invasion

University of Toronto[46]

    Any size, any number; biopsy showing no poorly differentiated tumors

    Aggressive bridging therapy

University of Tokyo[47]

    Tumor size less than or equal to 5 cm and number less than or equal to 5 nodules

The Hangzhou Criteria[48]

    Size less than 8 cm in total, with no restriction in number of nodules

    If greater than 8 cm, then biopsy grade I/II differentiation and AFP less than 400 ng/mL

---

candidates with HCC was instituted in the United States in 2002. The score assigned to patients with HCC within the Milan criteria has undergone multiple revisions, as the number of patients transplanted for HCC has increased dramatically and was clearly shown to disadvantage those patients without tumor undergoing liver transplantation (**Table 2**). Additional MELD exception points equivalent to a 10% increase in mortality is allowed every 3 months provided the patients remain within the Milan criteria. Currently, HCC is the primary indication in 10% to 20% of deceased donor liver transplants performed in the United States under the MELD organ allocation scheme.

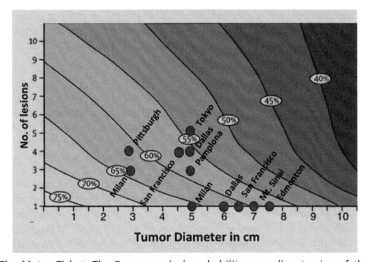

**Fig. 9.** The Metro Ticket: The 5-year survival probability according to size of the largest tumor and number of lesions. The longer the distance, the higher the price. (*Modified from* Mazzaferro V, Llovet JM, Miceli R, et al, for Metroticket Investigator Study Group. Predicting survival after liver transplantation in patients with hepatocellular carcinoma beyond the Milan criteria: a retrospective, exploratory analysis. Lancet Oncol 2009;10(1):39; with permission.)

| Table 2 | | | | |
|---|---|---|---|---|
| Criteria for liver transplantation for HCC at selected centers | | | | |
| | Original | April 2003 | January 2004 | January 2005 |
| Stage I: 1 tumor <2 cm | 15% Risk = MELD 24 | 8% Risk = MELD 20 | 0% Risk = MELD calculated | 0% Risk = MELD calculated |
| Stage II: 1 tumor ≥2 cm but <5 cm or 2–3 tumors <3 cm | 30% Risk = MELD 29 | 15% risk = MELD 24 | 15% Risk = MELD 24 | 15% Risk = MELD 22 |

The major constraint of the Milan criteria as the basis for allocation has been the radiologic staging errors. The National Conference on Liver Allocation in Patients with Hepatocellular Carcinoma in the United States was convened in 2009 to address these and other important allocation issues.[44] A work group of experts in radiology proposed minimum imaging equipment specifications, a standardized imaging protocol, and structured reporting that is currently required by the United Network for Organ Sharing (UNOS)/OPTN in order for a patient to be eligible for automatic HCC MELD exception points. A new OPTN classification of liver nodules was proposed that bases the diagnosis of HCC on the presence of specific, well-defined imaging findings on dynamic contrast-enhanced CT and/or MRI.[44]

Another drawback is that tumor histologic characteristics, such as grade and microvascular invasion, are not available at the time of listing. The current liver organ allocation system does not accurately predict the risk of dropout because of the above-mentioned concerns. The UNOS Liver and Intestinal Transplantation committee is actively working on the development of a more dynamic scoring scheme for patients with HCC because the current HCC policy does not adhere to the general principles for liver allocation adopted with the introduction of the MELD score. That is, the current HCC prioritization rules are categorical and based purely on waiting time and not based on any tumor biology variables or the degree of underlying liver disease. Development of a continuous scoring system for HCC candidates that incorporates tumor size, grade, AFP levels, and calculated laboratory MELD that would better predict the risk of dropout is being debated.

### The Role of Pretransplant Ablative Therapy

Several locoregional therapeutic modalities are being increasingly used as a bridging strategy to prevent wait list drop out from progression of HCC beyond the Milan criteria and to improve posttransplant survival by reducing the risk of HCC recurrence.[50–53] Radiofrequency ablation (RFA), whether laparoscopic or percutaneous; transarterial chemoembolization (TACE), transarterial radioembolization; and stereotactic radiation therapy are modalities commonly used.

The role of ablation in tumors measuring less than 3 cm is controversial, especially if the wait for liver transplantation is less than 6 month because the dropout rate for these patients if they are closely watched is very low.[54] Reports of better posttransplant survival in patients who underwent LRT as compared with those who did not have prompted several centers to consider LRT for all HCC candidates.[55,56] Currently there are no data to favor one modality over another; however, for tumors less than 3 cm, RFA has a higher rate of complete necrosis than TACE. For tumors larger than 3 cm, the likelihood of incomplete necrosis with RFA increases.

In practice, the choice of which locoregional modality of treatment is most appropriate in a given patient depends on the size, location, and the experience of the multidisciplinary team. Typically more than one modality is applied to achieve a complete radiologic response. In general, a complete response can be achieved for smaller tumors after initial therapy; but multiple tumors or larger tumors often require 2 or more sessions.

### Downstaging for Hepatocellular Carcinoma

Downstaging refers to decreasing the tumor size in patients presenting with HCC exceeding the listing criteria, by using LRT. Patients with tumors beyond the Milan criteria can potentially undergo liver transplantation after showing a response to LRT with long-term survival comparable with that of patients with tumors initially meeting the Milan criteria.[57–59]

Accuracy of the imaging techniques is important to determine the response to therapeutic interventions. There is no universal agreement regarding the upper limit for the tumor size and number being considered for downstaging. Furthermore, criteria for a response to downstaging vary widely. The best single-center experience to date on tumor downstaging comes from the UCSF group, in which the inclusion criteria for downstaging and criteria for successful downstaging are well defined.[60] Patients within UCSF criteria without evidence of vascular invasion on imaging studies are candidates for downstaging. Successful downstaging is assessed with multiphasic CT scan or MRI showing that the residual tumor size and number fall within the Milan criteria. It is also recommended that a minimum time-out or observation period of 3 months from the date that imaging is documented to meet the Milan criteria exists before being eligible for active priority listing.[44,60] This observation period will help to identify tumors with aggressive biology that will likely progress despite treatment and can be excluded from consideration for transplantation. An additional requirement for priority listing after tumor downstaging pertains to patients initially presenting with AFP levels greater than 1000 ng/mL. Successful downstaging requires a decrease in the AFP level to less than 500 ng/mL before liver transplantation because the results of many studies show that a preoperative AFP exceeding 1000 ng/mL is a strong predictor of recurrence after transplantation.[40,61]

A systematic review of 8 studies that included more than 700 patients was conducted by Gordon-Weeks and colleagues[62] to analyze the outcome of patients outside the Milan criteria who underwent successful downstaging before liver transplantation. The percentage of patients successfully downstaged ranged from 24% to 69%, and the percentage of patients who eventually underwent transplantation varied from 10% to 57%. Patients downstaged to within the Milan criteria achieved a 5-year survival ranging from 54% to 94% after liver transplantation, which is comparable with results of liver transplantation for patients presenting within the Milan criteria.

Despite these encouraging results, there is concern over too much prioritization for HCC candidates over non-HCC candidates. Although some regions in the United States have adopted a downstaging protocol for priority listing, most regions have not. In some regions, patients receive extra priority on a case-by-case basis but with little uniformity in the decision-making process.

### Living Donor Liver Transplant for Hepatocellular Carcinoma

Living donor liver transplantation (LDLT) is an appropriate option for patients in need of liver transplantation, even in countries with access to deceased donors, because of insufficient organ supply. For patients with HCC, LDLT offers the option of timely transplantation and avoids the risk of disease progression while on the waiting list for a suitable deceased donor organ. Reports from around the world have confirmed that the outcome of LDLT is comparable with deceased donor liver transplant (DDLT) for all indications. HCC recurrence has been shown to be higher after LDLT as compared with DDLT, but the overall patient survival is not different.[63,64] In the Adult-to-Adult Living Donor Liver Transplant (A2ALL) cohort study, the unadjusted 5-year HCC recurrence was significantly higher after LDLT (38%) versus DDLT (11%) and was attributed to more advanced HCC at the time of LDLT and less LRT given before LDLT.[64]

The decision to proceed with LDLT in patients with HCC should be made after careful analysis of the recipient's risk-to-benefit ratio. Donor safety should always be paramount when considering LDLT. Donor deaths occur in even the most experienced hands and are estimated to be approximately 0.5% for right lobe donors and 0.1% for left lobe donors. Moreover, morbidity after living donor partial hepatectomy has been shown to directly correlate with the extent of liver parenchyma removed from the donor and is estimated to be approximately 35% to 40% in right lobe donors and 10% to 20% in left lobe donors.[65–67]

HCC within the Milan criteria is an excellent indication for LDLT in countries where the access to deceased donors is limited. Even in countries where deceased donors are readily available, LDLT is indicated if the risk of progression of disease is high and the wait time exceeds 6 month. The decision to offer LDLT must be individualized and weighed against the disease stage and regional differences, such as waiting time and the risk of dropout. For example, a patient with a 2-cm lesion who can receive ablative therapy in the form of RFA or TACE has a reasonable chance of receiving a DDLT even in regions of the United States with longer waiting times. Conversely, a patient with a 4.9-cm lesion in a region where the waiting time exceeds 6 month has a higher risk of dropping out, and LDLT may provide a timely life-saving transplant. It can be argued that acceptable risks for donors and recipients vary with the availability of deceased donor organs within a given region or country.

LDLT is also a possible option for patients exceeding the accepted listing criteria, as the organ allocation policy that allows for increased priority for liver transplant candidates with HCC does not apply to LDLT. Expansion beyond the accepted criteria, however, comes with a potentially high price of increased recurrence and poor outcome. The concept of double equipoise (ie, equilibrium of risk) describes the balance between the recipient's survival with or without an LDLT and the probability of mortality for the donor.[68] In LDLT, the risk-benefit analysis is not confined to the donor and the recipient but also includes balancing the donor risk and the recipient benefit. The degree of benefit to the recipient should be acceptable to justify the risk to the donor. Currently there is no consensus about an acceptable HCC recurrence risk or acceptable donor risk. More importantly, there is no sense of what risk to the living donor might be considered acceptable for a given risk of recurrence. Liver transplantation for HCC exceeding the Milan criteria but within the UCSF criteria yields a 5-year survival of more than 50%, which some think is an acceptable cutoff for considering LDLT. Further expansion has been shown to be associated with high recurrence and poor outcome and may not justify the risk to the donor.

## HOW THE AUTHORS DO IT

Patients with HCC are evaluated by a group of surgeons, hepatologists, oncologists, radiologists, and radiation oncologists in the authors' multidisciplinary clinic. Radiologic images are reviewed at a dedicated weekly conference; the case is discussed in the presence of all the disciplines; an individualized plan of care is formulated for the patients. Noncirrhotic patients are evaluated for hepatic resection; if they are not suitable candidates for surgery, then they are evaluated for LRT. The authors' algorithm for patients presenting with cirrhosis and HCC is depicted in **Fig. 10**. Patients within the

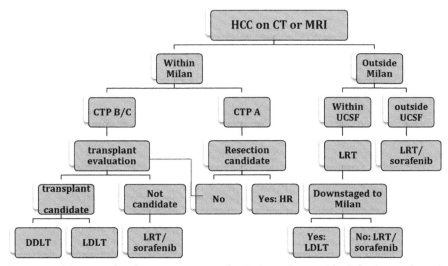

**Fig. 10.** Decision tree for the management of HCC in patients with cirrhosis. HR, hepatic resection.

Milan criteria are evaluated for liver transplantation with the exception of CTP A resection candidates. All of the authors' HCC transplant candidates irrespective of tumor size or number undergo LRT before being activated on the waiting list for a deceased donor liver graft with an aim toward complete radiologic response before transplantation. If residual disease is identified on follow-up imaging, the candidate will undergo additional treatment with LRT. An exception is made for patients with significant hepatic decompensation who are not likely to tolerate treatment. Because the waiting time in the authors' region exceeds 6 months and is often more than1 year, they offer candidates with HCC who are at risk of dropping out the option of LDLT if they identify a suitable living donor. Candidates pursuing LDLT are treated with LRT before transplantation in an attempt to reduce the recurrence of HCC after transplant and to allow patients with aggressive tumor biology to declare themselves. Candidates whose cancer is outside the Milan criteria but within the UCSF criteria are evaluated for downstaging. Patients exceeding the Milan criteria do not receive any priority in the authors' region, and these patients are offered the option of LDLT if they are successfully downstaged to within the Milan criteria and have a suitable living donor. A time-out observation period of 3 months is instituted in these patients from the date that imaging is documented to meet the Milan criteria demonstrating successful downstaging. Patients who meet these criteria proceed to LDLT.

The authors use the same immunosuppression protocol in both HCC and non-HCC recipients. The use of mammalian target of rapamycin inhibitors in HCC recipients has been advocated because of the presumptive benefit of the antiproliferative effects. Currently there are no data to support this practice.

Patients are monitored with measurement of AFP and imaging with either a multiphasic CT scan or MRI at 3 months after transplantation and then annually for 5 years.

## REFERENCES

1. Hu RH, Lee PH, Yu SC, et al. Surgical resection for recurrent hepatocellular carcinoma: prognosis and analysis of risk factors. Surgery 1996;120(1):23–9.

2. Bosch FX, Ribes J, Borras J. Epidemiology of primary liver cancer. Semin Liver Dis 1999;19:271–85.
3. Bismuth H, Chiche L, Castaing D. Surgical treatment of hepatocellular carcinomas in noncirrhotic liver: experience with 68 liver resections. World J Surg 1995;19(1):35–41.
4. Fong Y, Sun RL, Jarnagin W, et al. An analysis of 412 cases of hepatocellular carcinoma at a Western center. Ann Surg 1999;229(6):790.
5. Llovet JM, Fuster J, Bruix J. Intention-to-treat analysis of surgical treatment for early hepatocellular carcinoma: resection versus transplantation. Hepatology 1999;30(6):1434–40.
6. Bruix J, Castells A, Bosch J, et al. Surgical resection of hepatocellular carcinoma in cirrhotic patients: prognostic value of preoperative portal pressure. Gastroenterology 1996;111(4):1018–22.
7. Teh SH, Christein J, Donohue J, et al. Hepatic resection of hepatocellular carcinoma in patients with cirrhosis: Model of End-Stage Liver Disease (MELD) score predicts perioperative mortality. J Gastrointest Surg 2005;9(9):1207–15.
8. Bismuth H, Chiche L, Adam R, et al. Liver resection versus transplantation for hepatocellular carcinoma in cirrhotic patients. Ann Surg 1993;218(2):145–51.
9. Fuster J, Garcia-Valdecasas JC, Grande L, et al. Hepatocellular carcinoma and cirrhosis—results of surgical treatment in a European series. Ann Surg 1996; 223(3):297–302.
10. Iwatsuki S, Starzl TE, Sheahan DG, et al. Hepatic resection versus transplantation for hepatocellular carcinoma. Ann Surg 1991;214(3):221–9.
11. Roayaie S, Haim MB, Emre S, et al. Comparison of surgical outcomes for hepatocellular carcinoma in patients with hepatitis B versus hepatitis C: a Western experience. Ann Surg Oncol 2000;7(10):764–70.
12. Suenaga M, Nakao A, Harada A, et al. Hepatic resection for hepatocellular carcinoma. World J Surg 1992;16(1):97–105.
13. Sasaki Y, Imaoka S, Masutani S, et al. Influence of coexisting cirrhosis on long-term prognosis after surgery in patients with hepatocellular carcinoma. Surgery 1992;112(3):515–21.
14. Lai EC, Fan ST, Lo CM, et al. Hepatic resection for hepatocellular carcinoma. An audit of 343 patients. Ann Surg 1995;221(3):291–8.
15. Schwartz ME, Sung M, Mor E, et al. A multidisciplinary approach to hepatocellular carcinoma in patients with cirrhosis. J Am Coll Surg 1995;180(5):596–603.
16. Nagasue N, Ono T, Yamanoi A, et al. Prognostic factors and survival after hepatic resection for hepatocellular carcinoma without cirrhosis. Br J Surg 2001;88(4): 515–22.
17. Poon RT, Fan ST, Lo CM, et al. Long-term survival and pattern of recurrence after resection of small hepatocellular carcinoma in patients with preserved liver function: implications for a strategy of salvage transplantation. Ann Surg 2002;235(3): 373–82.
18. Belghiti J, Regimbeau JM, Durand F, et al. Resection of hepatocellular carcinoma: a European experience on 328 cases. Hepatogastroenterology 2002;49(43): 41–6.
19. Chen MF, Tsai HP, Jeng LB, et al. Prognostic factors after resection for hepatocellular carcinoma in noncirrhotic livers: univariate and multivariate analysis. World J Surg 2003;27(4):443–7.
20. Laurent C, Blanc JF, Nobili S, et al. Prognostic factors and longterm survival after hepatic resection for hepatocellular carcinoma originating from noncirrhotic liver. J Am Coll Surg 2005;201(5):656–62.

21. Bège T, Le Treut YP, Hardwigsen J, et al. Prognostic factors after resection for hepatocellular carcinoma in nonfibrotic or moderately fibrotic liver. A 116-case European series. J Gastrointest Surg 2007;11(5):619–25.
22. Taura K, Ikai I, Hatano E, et al. Influence of coexisting cirrhosis on outcomes after partial hepatic resection for hepatocellular carcinoma fulfilling the Milan criteria: an analysis of 293 patients. Surgery 2007;142(5):685–94.
23. Cherqui D, Laurent A, Mocellin N, et al. Liver resection for transplantable hepatocellular carcinoma: long-term survival and role of secondary liver transplantation. Ann Surg 2009;250(5):738–46.
24. Lee KK, Kim DG, Moon IS, et al. Liver transplantation versus liver resection for the treatment of hepatocellular carcinoma. J Surg Oncol 2010;101(1):47–53.
25. Mazzaferro V, Regalia E, Doci R, et al. Liver transplantation for the treatment of small hepatocellular carcinomas in patients with cirrhosis. N Engl J Med 1996; 334(11):693–9.
26. Huang YH, Wu JC, Chen CH, et al. Comparison of recurrence after hepatic resection in patients with hepatitis B vs. hepatitis C-related small hepatocellular carcinoma in hepatitis B virus endemic area. Liver Int 2005;25(2):236–41.
27. Kao WY, Su CW, Chau GY, et al. A comparison of prognosis between patients with hepatitis B and C virus-related hepatocellular carcinoma undergoing resection surgery. World J Surg 2011;35(4):858–67.
28. Jaeck D, Bachellier P, Oussoultzoglou E, et al. Surgical resection of hepatocellular carcinoma. Post-operative outcome and long-term results in Europe: an overview. Liver Transpl 2004;10(2 Suppl 1):S58–63.
29. Finkelstein SD, Marsh W, Demetris AJ, et al. Microdissection-based allelotyping discriminates de novo tumor from intrahepatic spread in hepatocellular carcinoma. Hepatology 2003;37(4):871–9.
30. Margarit C, Escartín A, Castells L, et al. Resection for hepatocellular carcinoma is a good option in Child-Turcotte-Pugh class A patients with cirrhosis who are eligible for liver transplantation. Liver Transpl 2005;11(10):1242–51.
31. Belghiti J, Cortes A, Abdalla EK, et al. Resection prior to liver transplantation for hepatocellular carcinoma. Ann Surg 2003;238(6):885–92.
32. Facciuto ME, Koneru B, Rocca JP, et al. Surgical treatment of hepatocellular carcinoma beyond Milan criteria. Results of liver resection, salvage transplantation, and primary liver transplantation. Ann Surg Oncol 2008;15(5):1383–91.
33. Adam R, Azoulay D, Castaing D, et al. Liver resection as a bridge to transplantation for hepatocellular carcinoma on cirrhosis: a reasonable strategy? Ann Surg 2003;238(4):508–18.
34. Belli G, Limongelli P, Fantini C, et al. Laparoscopic and open treatment of hepatocellular carcinoma in patients with cirrhosis. Br J Surg 2009;96(9):1041–8.
35. Tranchart H, Di Giuro G, Lainas P, et al. Laparoscopic resection for hepatocellular carcinoma: a matched-pair comparative study. Surg Endosc 2010;24(5): 1170–6.
36. Cheung TT, Poon RT, Yuen WK, et al. Long-term survival analysis of pure laparoscopic versus open hepatectomy for hepatocellular carcinoma in patients with cirrhosis: a single-center experience. Ann Surg 2013;257(3):506–11.
37. Mazzaferro V, Bhoori S, Sposito C, et al. Milan criteria in liver transplantation for hepatocellular carcinoma: an evidence-based analysis of 15 years of experience. Liver Transpl 2011;17(Suppl 2):S44–57.
38. Freeman RB, Weisner RH, Harper A, et al. The new liver allocation system: moving towards evidence-based transplantation policy. Liver Transpl 2002;8(9): 851–8.

39. Yao FY, Ferrell L, Bass NM, et al. Liver transplantation for hepatocellular carcinoma: expansion of the tumor size limits does not adversely impact survival. Hepatology 2001;33(6):1394–403.

40. Yao FY, Xiao L, Bass NM, et al. Liver transplantation for hepatocellular carcinoma: validation of the UCSF-expanded criteria based on preoperative imaging. Am J Transplant 2007;7(11):2587–96.

41. Duffy JP, Vardanian A, Benjamin E, et al. Liver transplantation criteria for hepatocellular carcinoma should be expanded: a 22-year experience with 467 patients at UCLA. Ann Surg 2007;246(3):502–9.

42. Decaens T, Roudot-Thoraval F, Hadni-Bresson S, et al. Impact of UCSF criteria according to pre- and post-OLT tumor features: analysis of 479 patients listed for HCC with a short waiting time. Liver Transpl 2006;12(12):1761–9.

43. Volk ML, Vijan S, Marrero JA. A novel model measuring the harm of transplanting hepatocellular carcinoma exceeding Milan criteria. Am J Transplant 2008;8(4):839–46.

44. Pomfret EA, Washburn K, Wald C, et al. Report of a national conference on liver allocation in patients with hepatocellular carcinoma in the United States. Liver Transpl 2010;16(3):262–78.

45. Lee SG, Hwang S, Moon DB, et al. Expanded indication criteria of living donor liver transplantation for hepatocellular carcinoma at one large-volume center. Liver Transpl 2008;14(7):935–45.

46. DuBay D, Sandroussi C, Sandhu L, et al. Liver transplantation for advanced hepatocellular carcinoma using poor tumor differentiation on biopsy as an exclusion criterion. Ann Surg 2011;253(1):166–72.

47. Sugawara Y, Tamura S, Makuuchi M. Living donor liver transplantation for hepatocellular carcinoma: Tokyo University series. Dig Dis 2007;25(4):310–2.

48. Zheng SS, Xu X, Wu J, et al. Liver transplantation for hepatocellular carcinoma: Hangzhou experiences. Transplantation 2008;85(12):1726–32.

49. Mazzaferro V, Llovet JM, Miceli R, et al, for Metroticket Investigator Study Group. Predicting survival after liver transplantation in patients with hepatocellular carcinoma beyond the Milan criteria: a retrospective, exploratory analysis. Lancet Oncol 2009;10(1):35–43.

50. Fisher RA, Maluf D, Cotterell AH, et al. Non-resective ablation therapy for hepatocellular carcinoma: effectiveness measured by intention-to-treat and dropout from liver transplant waiting list. Clin Transplant 2004;18(5):502–12.

51. Maddala YK, Stadheim L, Andrews JC, et al. Drop-out rates of patients with hepatocellular cancer listed for liver transplantation: outcome with chemoembolization. Liver Transpl 2004;10(3):449–55.

52. Millonig G, Graziadei IW, Freund MC, et al. Response to preoperative chemoembolization correlates with outcome after liver transplantation in patients with hepatocellular carcinoma. Liver Transpl 2007;13(2):272–9.

53. Pompili M, Mirante VG, Rondinara G, et al. Percutaneous ablation procedures in cirrhotic patients with hepatocellular carcinoma submitted to liver transplantation: assessment of efficacy at explant analysis and of safety for tumor recurrence. Liver Transpl 2005;11(9):1117–26.

54. Freeman RB, Edwards EB, Harper AM. Waiting list removal rates among patients with chronic and malignant liver diseases. Am J Transplant 2006;6(6):1416–21.

55. Lu DS, Yu NC, Raman SS, et al. Percutaneous radiofrequency ablation of hepatocellular carcinoma as a bridge to liver transplantation. Hepatology 2005;41(5):1130–7.

56. Freeman RB Jr, Steffick DE, Guidinger MK, et al. Liver and intestine transplantation in the United States, 1997–2006. Am J Transplant 2008;8(4 Pt 2):958–76.
57. Yao FY, Hirose R, LaBerge JM, et al. A prospective study on downstaging of hepatocellular carcinoma prior to liver transplantation. Liver Transpl 2005;11(12): 1505–14.
58. Chapman WC, Majella Doyle MB, Stuart JE, et al. Outcomes of neoadjuvant transarterial chemoembolization to downstage hepatocellular carcinoma before liver transplantation. Ann Surg 2008;248(4):617–25.
59. Yao FY. Liver transplantation for hepatocellular carcinoma: beyond the Milan criteria. Am J Transplant 2008;8(10):1982–9.
60. Yao FY, Kerlan RK Jr, Hirose R, et al. Excellent outcome following down-staging of hepatocellular carcinoma prior to liver transplantation: an intention-to-treat analysis. Hepatology 2008;48(3):819–27.
61. Figueras J, Ibañez L, Ramos E, et al. Selection criteria for liver transplantation in early-stage hepatocellular carcinoma with cirrhosis: results of a multicenter study. Liver Transpl 2001;7(10):877–83.
62. Gordon-Weeks AN, Snaith A, Petrinic T, et al. Systematic review of outcome of downstaging hepatocellular cancer before liver transplantation in patients outside the Milan criteria. Br J Surg 2011;98(9):1201–8.
63. Vakili K, Pomposelli JJ, Cheah YL, et al. Living donor liver transplantation for hepatocellular carcinoma: increased recurrence but improved survival. Liver Transpl 2009;15(12):1861–6.
64. Kulik LM, Fisher RA, Rodrigo DR, et al. Outcomes of living and deceased donor liver transplant recipients with hepatocellular carcinoma: results of the A2ALL cohort. Am J Transplant 2012;12(11):2997–3007.
65. Barr M, Belghiti J, Villamil F, et al. A report of the Vancouver Forum on the care of the live organ donor: lung, liver, pancreas, and intestine data and medical guidelines. Transplantation 2008;10(81):1373–85.
66. Ghobrial RM, Freise CE, Trotter JF, et al. Donor morbidity after living donation for liver transplantation. Gastroenterology 2008;135(2):468–76.
67. Abecassis MM, Fisher RA, Olthoff KM, et al, the A2ALL Study Group. Complications of living donor hepatic lobectomy - a comprehensive report. Am J Transplant 2012;12(5):1208–17.
68. Miller CM. Ethical dimensions of living donation: experience with living liver donation. Transplant Rev (Orlando) 2008;22(3):206–9.

# Locoregional Therapy of Hepatocellular Carcinoma

Ali Habib, BA[a], Kush Desai, MD[a], Ryan Hickey, MD[a], Bartley Thornburg, MD[a], Robert Lewandowski, MD[a], Riad Salem, MD, MBA[b],*

## KEYWORDS

- Hepatocellular carcinoma • Interventional oncology • Transplantation
- Locoregional therapies • Radioembolization • Transarterial chemoembolization
- Radiofrequency ablation • Percutaneous ethanol injection

## KEY POINTS

- Most hepatocellular carcinomas are not amenable to standard surgical intervention or systemic oncologic therapies.
- Interventional oncology, practiced by a subset of interventional radiologists, offers minimally invasive, locoregional therapies for the treatment of hepatic malignancies.
- Some of these locoregional therapies can be combined, or used in sequence.
- In the setting of transplantation, locoregional therapies offer promise in "bridging" patients to transplantation.
- Large-scale studies in a randomized setting will help better elucidate the appropriate application of locoregional therapies for personalized care of a patient's hepatocellular carcinoma.

## INTRODUCTION

Locoregional therapy has become increasingly important for patients with hepatocellular carcinoma (HCC) because of advances of techniques, survival benefit, and a favorable safety profile. Although curative measures, such as liver transplantation and surgical resection, continue to be the gold standard, approximately 70% to 80% of patients are poor candidates for such invasive procedures.[1] Underlying liver dysfunction, stage of disease at presentation, and comorbidities limit patients from curative intervention. These patients often have extrahepatic spread of disease, cancer-related symptoms, and portal vein invasion, warranting alternative approaches

The authors have nothing to disclose.
[a] Section of Interventional Radiology, Division of Interventional Oncology, Department of Radiology, Northwestern University, Chicago, IL, USA; [b] Vascular and Interventional Radiology, Image-Guided Therapy, Section of Interventional Radiology, Division of Interventional Oncology, Department of Radiology, Northwestern University, 676 North St. Clair, Suite 800, Chicago, IL 60611, USA
* Corresponding author.
*E-mail address:* r-salem@northwestern.edu

that can help decrease rates of disease progression and recurrence. Patients with advanced-stage HCC according to Barcelona Clinic Liver Cancer (BCLC) specifications, could potentially receive sorafenib, a first-line therapy that has improved overall survival (OS) in both the Asia-Pacific and Sorafenib HCC Assessment Randomized Protocol (SHARP) trials.[2,3] However, sorafenib warrants future quality-of-life (QoL) studies to better understand its tolerability. Systemic chemotherapy has not shown survival benefit in patients with advanced HCC. External beam radiation therapy has been used in a similar clinical setting; however, radiation-induced liver disease (RILD) (ie, elevation of liver enzymes, hepatomegaly, and/or ascites) has proven to complicate its use.[4,5] For patients who may not be candidates for therapies due to comorbidities or disease stage, interventional radiology (IR) has allowed for treatment of these patients via locoregional techniques, image-guided therapies that allow for minimally invasive delivery of oncologic and necrotizing agents. The therapies can be divided into catheter-based embolotherapies, such as radioembolization (RE, with Yttrium-90 [$^Y$90]) or transarterial chemoembolization (TACE), and thermal ablative therapies, such as radiofrequency ablation (RFA), microwave ablation (MWA), irreversible electroporation (IRE), cryoablation, and chemical ablation, such as percutaneous ethanol injection (PEI). Potential risks and benefits of these treatments, appropriate patient selection, and determining response to therapy is discussed at length (summarized in **Tables 1–4**), helping elucidate the application of locoregional therapy in the setting of HCC.

**Table 1**
**Candidacy for surgical resection, liver transplantation, or ablative therapies according to Barcelona Clinic Liver Cancer stage**

| | Patient Type | | | | |
|---|---|---|---|---|---|
| **Stage** | **Performance Status** | **Nodules** | **Metastases** | **Associated Disease** | **Treatment** |
| A (Early) | 0 | 3 nodules <3 cm | None | Yes | Ablative |
| B (Intermediate) | 0 | Multinodular | None | X | Chemoembolization |
| C (advanced) | 1–2 | N1 | M1 | Portal invasion | Sorafenib |

| | Patient Type | | | | |
|---|---|---|---|---|---|
| **Surgical Resection Candidate** | **CTP Class** | **Transplant Candidate** | **Extrahepatic Disease** | **Nodules** | **Treatment** |
| Yes | A/B | No | No | Solitary | On operative evaluation if inoperable->ethanol injection, RFA, cryoablation |
| No | C | No | No | If single <5 cm, or up to 4 lesions, each <4 cm | RFA, PEI/ cryoablation, TACE, RE, radiotherapy |
| No | C | Yes | No | X | Bridge to transplant (RFA, TACE, RE) |

*Abbreviations:* CTP, Child-Turcotte-Pugh; M1, distant metastasis; N1, regional lymph node metastasis; PEI, percutaneous ethanol injection; RE, radioembolization; RFA, radiofrequency frequency ablation; TACE, transarterial chemoembolization; X, not included for guidelines.

## DIAGNOSTIC APPROACH TO LOCOREGIONAL THERAPY

To properly identify patients who may benefit from locoregional therapy, a clinical picture should be pieced together by the 4 pillars of oncology: medical oncology, surgical oncology, radiation oncology, and interventional oncology, a subset of IR practice. Open dialogue regarding a patient's candidacy for a particular intervention in the treatment pathway will help tailor care to each patient's unique disease process. To diagnose HCC, a patient should have the "classic" appearance of vascular enhancement and portal venous washout on dynamic imaging, and if there is a discrepancy, an image-guided biopsy is necessary for definitive tumor diagnosis. It is exceptional to core biopsy tumors larger than 2 cm, or where there are elevated serum alpha-fetoprotein (AFP) levels greater than 200 ng/mL, unless the tumor exhibits increased rate of growth. There are many different staging methods available, however the most commonly used is the BCLC, along with the Cancer of the Liver Italian Program, and the Chinese University Prognostic Index.[6,7] The purpose of these staging systems is to appropriately weight clinical factors that have predictive value in HCC prognosis. The challenge of crafting a universal staging system lies in dynamic nature of certain prognostic indicators during the disease process, some which cannot be defined, and others are not often evaluated. Certain factors, such as liver function, performance status, and stage of HCC, all help evaluate a patient's potential for benefit from locoregional therapy. Liver status can be assessed via laboratory, radiological, and pathology studies, in an effort to determine if a patient is cirrhotic, and exhibits hemodynamic and metabolic derangements that alter the clinical approach to HCC. Liver performance is quantitatively measured by the Model for End-stage Liver Disease (MELD) score, as well as the Child-Turcotte-Pugh (CTP) score and class. Besides the liver performance per se, a patient's overall functional ability is captured by the Eastern Cooperative Oncology Group (ECOG) performance status. Early-stage disease is considered curable if a patient has a single tumor of 5 cm or smaller, or up to 3 tumors, none larger than 3 cm,[8,9] while retaining performance status and liver function. Patients may undergo surgical resection, or may be deemed to be transplant candidates based on the Milan criteria.[8] A patient is determined to be end stage if their liver function deteriorates to CTP class C (score 10–15), or if their ECOG performance status is greater than 2,[6] as summarized in **Table 1**. The goals of treatment for patients who are end stage are to maintain QoL, while managing symptoms related to disease progression. It is of note that although there are appropriate treatment recommendations for patients throughout the BCLC spectrum, nearly half are poor candidates because of exclusion criteria.[10] A combined picture of the cancer and underlying liver function helps determine if a patient would be a viable candidate for locoregional therapy; this clinical mosaic drives HCC prognosis.[11]

## ENDOVASCULAR EMBOLOTHERAPIES

For patients who present with BCLC intermediate-stage HCC, in the absence of extrahepatic spread, portal vein invasion, cancer-related symptoms, and with underlying liver function defined as CTP-A (score 5–6) or CTP-B (score 7–9), catheter-based approaches are recommended by the American Association for the Study of Liver Diseases and the European Association for the Study of the Liver (EASL).[11,12] Furthermore, the unique perfusion environment of the liver makes it the ideal organ for endovascular embolotherapies. The hepatic artery and portal vein provide a dual blood supply to the liver; whereas, HCCs are perfused solely by the hepatic artery, thereby allowing for a more selective, catheter-based approach to treatment while sparing surrounding parenchyma. Although different forms of TACE and RE have

**Table 2**
Absolute and relative contraindications to locoregional therapies according patient and tumor characteristics

| TACE (cTACE and DEB-TACE) | RE | RFA | MWA | IRE | Cryoablation | PEI |
|---|---|---|---|---|---|---|
| **Absolute contraindications** | | | | | | |
| Technical contraindications | Technical contraindications | Technical contraindications | Technical contraindications | Technical contraindications | Technical contraindications | Technical contraindications |
| Decompensated cirrhosis | Decompensated cirrhosis | Decompensated cirrhosis | Decompensated cirrhosis | Cardiac arrhythmia/pacemaker | Extrahepatic disease | CTP Class C |
| Hemodynamic derangement in portal venous system | Renal Failure (GFR<30 mL/min, serum creatinine >2 mg/dL) | Active infection | Organ inflammation | Large lesion | Portal venous disease | Extrahepatic disease |
| Large tumor encompassing both lobes | | | Tumor volume >70% of liver | Extrahepatic disease | Tumor size | Portal venous disease |
| Renal failure (GFR<30 mL/min, serum creatinine >2 mg/dL) | | | Platelets: <3 × $10^9/mm^3$ Prothrombin time: >30 s | Portal vein involvement | | Tumor >10% of liver volume |
| | | | Organ failure | Biliary tract occlusion or anomaly | | |
| | | | | Multifocal hepatic disease | | |

**Relative contraindications**

| Occlusion in biliary tract | Occlusion in biliary tract | Tumor >5 cm | Proximity to key structures |
|---|---|---|---|
| Varices | Large tumor encompassing both lobes | | |
| Segmental PVT | Hepatopulmonary shunts | | |
| Tumor >10 cm | | | |

*Abbreviations:* cTACE, conventional TACE; CTP, Child-Turcotte-Pugh; DEB-TACE, drug-eluting beads-TACE; GFR, glomerular filtration rate; IRE, irreversible electroporation; MWA, microwave ablation; PEI, percutaneous ethanol injection; PVT, portal vein thrombus; RE, radioembolization; RFA, radiofrequency ablation; TACE, transarterial chemoembolization.

**Table 3**
Long-term outcomes of patients with hepatocellular carcinoma receiving different locoregional therapies stratified according to Barcelona Clinic Liver Cancer stage: series from 2008 through 2013

| Reference | Therapy | No. of Patients | Median Survival, mo |
|---|---|---|---|
| **Stage A (early, 1–3 nodules <3 cm, performance status 0)** | | | |
| Moreno-Luna, 2013 | cTACE | 23 | 18.6 |
| Hsu, 2011 | cTACE | 73 | 37.9 |
| Lewandowski et al,[41] 2010 | cTACE | 62 | 40 |
| Ho, 2009 | cTACE | 80 | 29.9 |
| Chen, 2009 | cTACE | nr | 16.8 |
| Wang, 2008 | cTACE | 453 | 35.4 |
| Burrel, 2012 | DEB-TACE | 41 | 40.6 |
| Moreno-Luna, 2013 | RE | 12 | 23.9 |
| Salem et al,[73] 2011 | RE | 47 | 45.4 |
| Sangro et al,[76] 2011 | RE | 52 | 24.4 |
| Salem et al,[74] 2010 | RE | 48 | 26.9 |
| Lencioni 2005 | RFA | 206 | 57 |
| Salmi et al,[87] 2008 | RFA | 25 | 92%, 72%, 64% (1, 3, 5 y) |
| Lin et al,[93] 2005 | PEI | 62 | 88%, 66%, 51% (1, 2, 3 y) |
| **Stage B (intermediate, multinodular, performance status 0)** | | | |
| Moreno-Luna, 2013 | RE | 34 | 16.8 |
| Mazzaferro, 2013 | RE | 17 | 18 |
| Sangro et al,[76] 2011 | RE | 87 | 16.9 |
| Hilgard et al,[75] 2010 | RE | 51 | 16.4 |
| Salem et al,[74] 2010 | RE | 83 | 17.2 |

*Summary*

1. LR-2 has features suggestive of but not diagnostic of a benign entity.
2. LR-2 does not need to be reported as an LI-RADS observation.
3. Continued surveillance is generally recommended.

## LIVER IMAGING REPORTING AND DATA SYSTEM 3

LI-RADS 3 includes lesions with features that are not diagnostic for benign entities or LR-4 or LR-5 categories and do not have features suggestive of non-HCC malignancy (**Fig. 8**). Such lesions are compatible with a moderate probability for HCC related to the indeterminate status. This category acts as a placement holder for observations that do not meet criteria for other LI-RADS categories. There may not be a definitive mass, but LR-3 can include nodulelike hepatic arterial phase hyperenhancement (NAPH), or a mass with hepatic arterial phase hypoenhancement or isoenhancement. An isoenhancing or hypoenhancing mass less than 2 cm may have one other major feature, whereas a mass greater than 2 cm may not have any of these features. LR-3 also includes an arterially enhancing mass less than 2 cm in size with none of the other major features. The reporting of observations categorized as LR-3 depends on the presence of LR4, LR5, or OM elsewhere in the liver. These observations are reported if there are no LR4/5 observations present. Management of these lesions is variable depending on size, stability, and clinical considerations.

*Summary*

1. LR-3 category includes lesions that do not unequivocally belong to LR 1/2, LR 4/5, or OM categories.
2. LR-3 lesions include NAPH less than 2 cm without associated features or less than 2 cm arterially hypoenhancing lesions with only one associated major feature or greater than 2 cm lesions with no other major features.
3. These lesions may require customized follow-up, depending on observation size, stability, and clinical considerations.

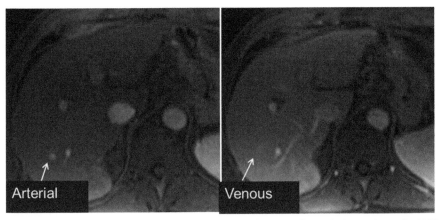

**Fig. 8.** A 6mm arterially enhancing lesion (*arrows*) without washout: indeterminate for HCC: LI-RADS 3.

## LIVER IMAGING REPORTING AND DATA SYSTEM 4

This observation indicates a high probability that a lesion is HCC but there is not 100% certainty (**Fig. 9**). The findings are suggestive but not diagnostic of HCC. There are 2 subtypes based on the size of lesion and enhancement characteristics. LR-4A refers to a mass less than 2 cm in size with arterial phase hypoenhancement or isoenhancement with 2 or more of the following: washout, capsule, threshold growth, or arterial phase hyperenhancement in a mass less than 1 cm with 1 or more of the major features or a 10- to 19-mm mass with only 1 of the other major features.

LR-4B are lesions 2 cm or greater in mass that demonstrate arterial phase hypoenhancement or isoenhancement, 1 or more other major features, or larger than 2 cm in diameter with arterial phase hyperenhancement and no other major feature. LR-4 lesions must be reported. Management may require biopsy, close follow-up, or additional imaging.

### Summary

1. LR-4 indicates a high probability, although not 100% certainty for HCC.
2. LR-4 A lesions are less than 1 cm arterially enhancing lesion with one other major feature, or 10- to 20-mm arterially enhancing lesion with only one other major feature, or less than 2 cm isoenhancing or hypoenhancing lesions with 2 other major features.
3. LR-4B lesions are greater than 2 cm; if arterially hypoenhancing, then associated with 1 or more other major feature, or if arterially hyperenhancing, then associated with no other major feature.

## LIVER IMAGING REPORTING AND DATA SYSTEM 5

There is 100% certainty that a lesion is HCC. LR-5 is essentially equivalent to OPTN 5 (**Figs. 10** and **11**). These lesions demonstrate imaging features diagnostic of HCC or are proven to be HCC at biopsy. The category LR-5 is further subclassified into LR-5A and LR-5B. LR-5A are 10- to 19-mm masses with arterial phase hyperenhancement with 2 or more of following: washout, capsule, and threshold growth.

LR-5B are 2 cm or larger with arterial phase hyperenhancement with 1 or more of the following: washout, capsule, and threshold growth. According to OPTN policy, LR-5

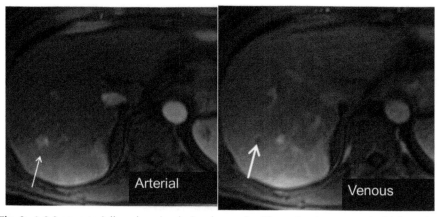

**Fig. 9.** A 0.9-cm arterially enhancing lesion (*arrows*) with washout, no capsule: high probability of HCC: LI-RADS 4 (no transplant exception).

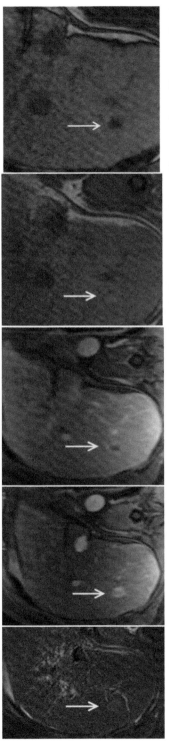

**Fig. 10.** A 1.1-cm T2 hyperintense mass in the right lobe of the liver (*arrows*) with arterial enhancement, washout with a capsule, and intracytoplasmic fat compatible with HCC: definitely HCC: LI-RADS 5 A (eligible for liver transplant).

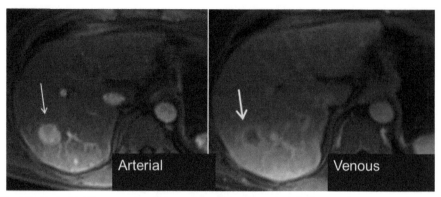

**Fig. 11.** Typical HCC measuring 2.3 cm demonstrating arterial phase enhancement (*arrow*) followed by washout and a capsule (*arrow*) compatible with LI-RADS 5 B (eligible for liver transplant).

lesions must have a diameter of 1 cm or greater, as smaller mass lesions are difficult to characterize at CT and MRI and also difficult to localize for biopsy to obtain histopathology. Because less than 1-cm masses cannot be diagnosed at CT or MRI with 100% certainty as HCC, close follow-up is usually needed for these lesions that are easily characterized as LR-5 A once diameter exceeds 1 cm. These lesions must be reported. LR-5 lesions are treated without biopsy and, if greater than 2 cm, receive HCC exception points for determining priority on the LT list.

### Summary

1. LR-5 lesions are definitely HCC.
2. LR-5A are 1- to 2-cm masses with arterial hyperenhancement and associated with 2 other major features.
3. LR-5B masses are greater than 2-cm masses with one or more other major features.
4. LR-5 is congruent with OPTN 5 nodules, but OPTN classification does not allow less than 1-cm masses to be classified OPTN 5.

### LIVER IMAGING REPORTING AND DATA SYSTEM 5 TREATED

These lesions are LR-5A/B or biopsy-proven HCC that have undergone locoregional treatment (ie, ablation or embolization) that gives them the T designation. These lesions must be reported. LR-5T observations require close follow-up to assess treatment response and to document areas of persistent/recurrent tumor that may require re-treatment. LR-5T observations qualify for continued MELD priority points based on their pretreatment imaging features.

To maintain congruency between LI-RADS and OPTN, LR-5T does not apply to LR4 or lesser observations that have undergone locoregional treatment, or to HCC that has been treated with systemic therapy or resection. HCC undergoing systemic therapy should be assigned their pretreatment LI-RADS category regardless of treatment effect; the pretreatment LI-RADS category is not downgraded.

### Summary

1. LR-5T are locoregionally treated HCCs.
2. LR-5T observations qualify for continued priority points based on their pretreatment imaging features.

3. HCCs undergoing systemic therapy are assigned pretreatment LI-RADS category regardless of treatment effect; the pretreatment LI-RADS category is not downgraded.

## LIVER IMAGING REPORTING AND DATA SYSTEM 5V

This category refers to definite HCCs in which there is extension into or invasion of a portal or hepatic vein. It denotes with 100% certainty that the lesion is HCC invading a vein. These lesions must be reported and are treated without biopsy. They present a contraindication to LT. The term LR-5V is applied even if a parenchymal mass is not identified at imaging. Features that aid the diagnosis include an occluded vein with any of the following:

- Moderately to markedly expanded vascular lumen
- Ill-defined walls to the vein
- Restricted diffusion of water molecules within the tumor
- Contiguity with HCC
- Heterogeneous enhancement of the vein not attributable to mixing artifact
- Nontumoral bland thrombus not enhancing and not expanding the vein lumen to same degree as the tumor does.

### Summary

1. LR-5V is definitely HCC with venous invasion.
2. LR-5V indicates a contraindication to LT.

## NONHEPATOCELLULAR CARCINOMA MALIGNANCY

HCC is the most common malignancy in patients with cirrhosis or other risk factors, such as chronic hepatitis B infection. However, in some cases, other malignancies do occur. Lesions thought to represent a non-HCC malignancy should be categorized OM. Examples of non-HCC malignancy include the following.

### Cholangiocarcinoma

Risk factors for cholangiocarcinoma (CCC) overlap with those for HCC such as cirrhosis, and primary sclerosing cholangitis. CCC may be associated with elevated tumor markers such as cancer antigen 19-9 and carcinoembryonic antigen. Imaging features include arterial phase target enhancement, portal venous and delayed phase central enhancement, with or without markedly restricted diffusion. Liver surface retraction is usually seen commonly with these tumors in addition to biliary obstruction.

### Metastasis

Metastases are extremely rare in cirrhosis and are usually encountered in patients with a history of primary extrahepatic malignancy. There may be elevation of tumor biomarkers depending on the identity of the primary cancer. Imaging features include arterial phase ring or target enhancement, with portal venous and delayed phase central enhancement. Restricted diffusion may or may not be seen. These metastases are generally many and may show central necrosis or ischemia.

### Lymphoma

There is usually a history of extrahepatic lymphoma with secondary involvement of liver. Risk factors include AIDS, immune suppression, and rarely, hepatitis C infection.

**Table 3**
**Comparison of American Association for the Study of Liver Diseases, US Organ Procurement and Transplant Network, and Liver Imaging Reporting and Data System classifications**

|  | AASLD 2011 | OPTN 2014 | LI-RADS 2014 |
|---|---|---|---|
| Overview | Comprehensive management system for HCC. Includes algorithm for US-based surveillance and CT/MRI-based diagnosis of HCC | OPTN policy for liver transplant candidates with HCC (in United States) Includes CT and MRI criteria for HCC to determine eligibility and priority for LT | Comprehensive imaging diagnosis system for HCC |
| Target population | Patients at risk for HCC in a surveillance program | Patients with HCC considered for LT | All patients at risk for HCC |
| Categorization of observations | • HCC<br>• Indeterminate<br>• Benign | Untreated definite HCC<br>• Class 5A: 10–19 mm<br>• Class 5B: 20–50 mm<br>• Class 5X: >50 mm or tumor in vein<br>Treated definite HCC<br>• Class 5T (treated)<br>Nondiagnostic examination<br>• Class 0 | Untreated observations<br>• LR-1: definitely benign<br>• LR-2: probably benign<br>• LR-3: intermediate probability<br>• LR-4: probably HCC<br>• LR-5: definitely HCC<br>• LR-5V: tumor in vein<br>• LR-M: probably malignant, not specific for HCC<br>Treated observations: LR-treated |
| Imaging methods addressed | US for surveillance; CT and MRI with extracellular agents for diagnosis | CT and MRI with extracellular agents | CT, MRI with extracellular agents. Provides guidance for use of MRI with hepatobiliary agents, although these have not been validated prospectively for primary diagnosis of HCC |
| Imaging features addressed | • Arterial phase hyperenhancement<br>• Washout appearance<br>• Diameter<br>These features apply only to ≥10 mm observations detected at surveillance ultrasound | • Arterial phase hyperenhancement<br>• Washout appearance<br>• Capsule appearance<br>• Diameter<br>• Diameter increase over time | • Arterial phase hyperenhancement<br>• Washout appearance<br>• Capsule appearance<br>• Diameter<br>• Diameter increase over time<br>• Visibility at surveillance ultrasound<br>• Multiple ancillary features |
| Intended users | Radiologists with expertise in liver imaging | Radiologists at LT centers | All radiologists |

Adapted from Mitchell DG, Bruix J, Sherman M, et al. LI-RADS (liver imaging reporting and data system): summary, discussion, and consensus of the LI-RADS management working group and future directions. Hepatology 2015;61:1056–65; with permission.

## Posttransplant Lymphoproliferative Disorder

In posttransplant lymphoproliferative disorder (PTLD), there is a history of prior solid organ transplantation, often but not exclusively with an increase in Epstein-Barr virus (EBV)-negative recipients and EBV-positive donors, especially in those with prolonged or repeated high-dose immunosuppression. PTLD usually occurs 2 to 60 months after transplant and extrahepatic involvement is generally common.[25]

Differentiation between HCC and non-HCC malignancies is important because the management and prognosis differ.

## SUMMARY

Major diagnostic criteria for HCC include arterial phase hyperenhancement, portal venous or delayed phase contrast appearance, and capsule appearance, in addition to interval threshold growth. Ancillary features, such as intralesional fat, blood products from intralesional bleeding, and mosaic architecture, also favor a diagnosis of HCC. Tumor entry into a vein is a definitive finding for an HCC even if a parenchymal mass is not clearly visualized. LI-RADS is a form of structured reporting that has been devised to standardize the reporting of CT and MRI imaging findings for HCC in cirrhotic patients. LI-RADS should be applied only for individuals at increased risk for HCC and not for the general population. There are 5 categories of liver observations that are referred to, LR-1, definitely benign; LR 2, probably benign; LR-3, neither definitely benign nor malignant; LR-4, probably HCC; LR-5, definitely HCC.

Other categories include OM, LR-5, a definite HCC that has received locoregional treatment for downgrading, and LR-5V, which refers to advanced HCC with extension into the hepatic or portal veins. Because LI-RADS is adopted for the management of HCC patients, the differences in classification between LI-RADS and the guidelines of the AASLD and OPTN (**Table 3**) must be resolved.

## REFERENCES

1. Lovet JM, Burroughs A, Bruix J. Hepatocellular carcinoma. Lancet 2003;362: 1907–17.
2. Bruix J, Sherman M. Management of hepatocellular carcinoma: an update. Hepatology 2011;53:1020–2.
3. Bruix J, Sherman M, Practice Guidelines Committee, American Association for the Study of Liver Diseases. Management of hepatocellular carcinoma. Hepatology 2005;42:1208–36. Available at: http://www.aasld.org/practiceguidelines/Documents/Bookmarked%20Practice%20Guidelines/HCCUpdate2010.pdf.
4. Willatt MJ, Hussain KH, Adusumilli S, et al. MR imaging of hepatocellular carcinoma in the cirrhotic liver: challenges and controversies. Radiology 2008;247:311–30.
5. Grazioli L, Morana G, Caudana R, et al. Hepatocellular carcinoma: correlation between gadobenate dimeglumine-enhanced MRI and pathologic findings. Invest Radiol 2000;35:25–34.
6. Ebara M, Fukuda H, Kojima Y, et al. Small hepatocellular carcinoma: relationship of signal intensity to histopathologic findings and metal content of the tumor and surrounding hepatic parenchyma. Radiology 1999;210:81–8.
7. Serste T, Barrau V, Ozenne V, et al. Accuracy and disagreement of computed tomography and magnetic resonance imaging for the diagnosis of small hepatocellular carcinoma and dysplastic nodules: role of biopsy. Hepatology 2012;55: 800–6.

8. Forner A, Vilana R, Ayuso C, et al. Diagnosis of hepatic nodules 20 mm or smaller in cirrhosis: prospective validation of the noninvasive diagnostic criteria for hepatocellular carcinoma. Hepatology 2008;47:97–104.

9. Jang HJ, Kim TK, Khalili K, et al. Characterization of 1-to 2-cm liver nodules detected on HCC surveillance ultrasound according to the criteria of the American Association for the Study of Liver Disease: is quadriphasic CT necessary? Am J Roentgenol 2013;201:314–21.

10. Kim TK, Lee KH, Jang HJ, et al. Analysis of gadobenate dimeglumine-enhanced MR findings for characterizing small (1-2-cm) hepatic nodules in patients at high risk for hepatocellular carcinoma. Radiology 2011;259:730–8.

11. Khan AS, Hussain HK, Johnson TD, et al. Value of delayed hypointensity and delayed enhancing rim in magnetic resonance imaging diagnosis of small hepatocellular carcinoma in the cirrhotic liver. J Magn Reson Imaging 2010;32:360–6.

12. Yu JS, Lee JH, Chung JJ, et al. Small hypervascular hepatocellular carcinoma: limited value of portal and delayed phases on dynamic magnetic resonance imaging. Acta Radiol 2008;49:735–43.

13. Martin P, DiMartini A, Feng S, et al. Evaluation for liver transplantation in adults: 2013 practice guideline by the American Association for the Study of Liver Diseases and the American Society of Transplantation. Hepatology 2014;59:1144.

14. Marrero JA, Hussain HK, Nghiem HV, et al. Improving the prediction of hepatocellular carcinoma in cirrhotic patients with an arterially-enhancing liver mass. Liver Transpl 2005;11:281–9.

15. United Network for Organ Sharing. Policy 3.6, organ distribution: allocation of livers. Organ procurement and transplantation network web site. Available at: http://optn.transplant.hrsa.gov/. Accessed November 20, 2014.

16. Mazzaferro V, Regalia E, Doci R, et al. Liver transplantation for the treatment of small hepatocellular carcinomas in patients with cirrhosis. N Engl J Med 1996; 334(11):693–9.

17. Duffy JP, Vardanian A, Benjamin E, et al. Liver transplantation criteria for hepatocellular carcinoma should be expanded: a 22-year experience with 467 patients at UCLA. Ann Surg 2007;246:502–9.

18. Cruite I, Tang A, Sirlin CB. Imaging-based diagnostic systems for hepatocellular carcinoma. AJR Am J Roentgenol 2013;201:41–55.

19. Petruzzi N, Mitchell D, Guglielmo F, et al. Hepatocellular carcinoma likelihood on MRI exams: evaluation of a standardized categorization system. Acad Radiol 2013;20:694–8.

20. Anis M, Irshad A. Imaging of hepatocellular carcinoma: practical guide to differential diagnosis [review]. Clin Liver Dis 2011;15(2):335–52, vii–x.

21. Choi BI, Lee JM. Advancement in HCC imaging: diagnosis, staging and treatment efficacy assessments. J Hepatobiliary Pancreat Sci 2010;17:369–73.

22. Hussain HK, Barr DC, Wald C. Imaging techniques for the diagnosis of hepatocellular carcinoma and the evaluation of response to treatment. Semin Liver Dis 2014;34:398–414.

23. Available at: http://www.acr.org/~/media/ACR/Documents/PDF/QualitySafety/Resources/LIRADS/lirads%20v20131%20w%20note.pdf. Accessed November 20, 2014.

24. Mitchell DG, Bruix J, Sherman M, et al. LI-RADS (liver imaging reporting and data system): summary, discussion, and consensus of the LI-RADS management working group and future directions. Hepatology 2014. http://dx.doi.org/10.1002/hep27304.

25. Koch DG, Christiansen L, Lazarchick J, et al. Posttransplantation lymphoproliferative disorder – the great mimic in liver transplantation: appraisal of the clinicopathologic spectrum and the role of Epstein-Barr virus. Liver Transpl 2007;13:904–12.

# Oncogenic Viruses and Hepatocellular Carcinoma

Ziv Ben Ari, MD[a,b,c,*], Ella Weitzman, MD[a,c], Michal Safran, PhD[a,b]

## KEYWORDS

- Hepatocellular carcinoma • Oncogenic viruses • Hepatitis B • Hepatitis C

## KEY POINTS

- Cirrhosis in patients with chronic hepatitis B virus (HBV) and hepatitis C virus (HCV) infection is not a prerequisite step for hepatic tumorigenesis.
- The role of HCV and HBV in promoting hepatocellular carcinoma (HCC) development by either direct or indirect effects is still speculative, yet there is compelling evidence that both mechanisms exist.
- Vaccination plays a central role in the prevention of HBV-related HCC.
- Current antiviral therapies for HBV and HCV, if successful, can reduce but not completely eliminate the risk of HCC.
- The introduction of the new HCV direct-acting antiviral agents has not been in practice long enough to permit an estimate of their likelihood of reducing HCC incidence.

## INTRODUCTION

Worldwide, approximately 80% of hepatocellular carcinoma (HCC) is caused by hepatitis B virus (HBV) and/or hepatitis C virus (HCV) infection, especially in the setting of established cirrhosis or advanced fibrosis. There are more than half a million new cases of HCC globally and almost the same number of deaths caused by this disease annually[1] because of the very high case-fatality rate.

The risk of developing HCC among carriers of HBV infection ranges from 10- to 100-fold greater compared with the rates in uninfected people, depending on the markers and populations that are evaluated.[2] In HCV infection, the relative risk for developing HCC in patients with serologically confirmed HCV infection is estimated to be 17-fold.[3] The age-adjusted incidence of HCC is increasing in many countries,

The authors have nothing to disclose.
[a] Liver Disease Center, Sheba Medical Center, Derech Sheba No 1, Ramat Gan 52621, Israel;
[b] Liver Research Laboratory, Sheba Medical Center, Ramat Gan, Israel; [c] Sackler School of Medicine, Tel Aviv University, Tel Aviv 69978, Israel
* Corresponding author. Liver Disease Center, Sheba Medical Center, Ramat Gan 52621, Israel.
E-mail address: Ziv.Ben-Ari@sheba.health.gov.il

including the United States, and has been widely attributed to the spread of HCV infection in industrialized countries.[4] The geographic distribution of HCC coincides with the distribution of HBV and HCV infections in those areas. In the United States, Europe, Egypt, and Japan, more than 60% of HCC is associated with HCV and about 20% is related to HBV, whereas nonalcoholic fatty liver disease and other causes contribute to the remainder. In Africa and Asia, where HBV is endemic, 60% of HCC is associated with HBV, 20% is related to HCV, and the remainder is distributed among other risk factors (for example aflatoxin).[1,5] Men are more susceptible to HCC than women; older age, family history of HCC, and advanced disease are also associated with its development. Other risk factors for HCC, apart from viral hepatitis B and C, include alcohol consumption and nonalcoholic fatty liver disease. Although recent clinical observations and translational research have enhanced our understanding of the molecular mechanisms driving the initiation and progression of HCC, much remains unknown. The role of HCV and HBV in promoting HCC development either directly or indirectly is still speculative.[6,7] The indirect pathways include the development of HCC on a background of chronic inflammation and the associated regenerative wound-healing response that is linked to the development of fibrosis and cirrhosis. The more direct pathways refer to alteration in cellular homeostasis caused by integration of the virus (notably HBV DNA) into the host's genome or modifications in cell signaling by specific HBV or HCV viral-encoded proteins.[6,7] The evidence, as described later, is compelling that molecular derangements that are hepatocarcinogenic exist in viral infection; but the cause-and-effect relationships have yet to be confirmed.

In Taiwan, HBV vaccination has decreased the incidence of new infections and HCC; however, there is no vaccine for HCV. Suppression of HBV replication and a sustained viral response (SVR) in the treatment of HCV are associated with a reduction in HCC incidence among treated populations. There is an ongoing controversy regarding the role of antiviral therapy in reducing HCC incidence in cirrhotic patients with HBV.[8–12] Also a small subset of patients with HCV with advanced fibrosis or cirrhosis who achieve SVR remain at a heightened risk for HCC development.[13–18] None of the new HCV direct-acting antiviral agents have been in use long enough to evaluate their effect in reducing HCC incidence.

## PATHOGENESIS

Current data indicate that HCC tumors are highly complex and heterogeneous resulting from the aberrant function of multiple molecular pathways. The role of HCV or HBV in promoting HCC development by either direct or indirect activity and their relative importance to the pathogenesis of HCC have not been clearly defined.[6,7]

### Hepatitis B Virus

Although HBV integration into the host's genome is not essential for viral replication, there is substantial evidence showing that such HBV DNA genomic integration occurs.[19–22] Since the development of new whole-genome sequencing methods, several studies have been done to evaluate the relative extent and the functional impact of such integrations on the development of HCC. Whole-genome sequencing analysis of HCC in patients with HBV revealed that, although HBV sequences were present in both the tumor and their adjacent nontumorous liver tissue, HBV signals were more frequent in the tumor than in the nontumorous tissue.[23,24] Furthermore, although HBV integration in the nontumorous tissue occurs in many sites, in the tumor, most of the insertions are at major integration sites.[23] These findings suggest that, although in the nontumorous tissue hepatocytes are heterogeneous, HCC tumors are more likely to result from a clonal expansion. Furthermore, most breaking points of HBV integration in the HCC samples were near coding genes.

### Hepatitis B Virus DNA Viral Integration into the Host's Genome

There are 3 main consequences of HBV DNA viral integration into the host's genome:

### Alterations in the transcriptional levels of adjacent genes

Results of recent studies have provided a long, growing list of HBV integration events and have uncovered 3 cancer-associated genes that were found at frequent integration sites in HBV-positive tumors: TERT,[20,23–26] MLL4,[21,23] and CCNE1.[24] Regardless of whether HBV integration was at the promoter, intron, or exon sites, all 3 genes showed upregulated expression in the tumor relative to nontumorous tissue.

### Genome instability

To evaluate genome instability in HBV-infected HCC tissue, Sung and colleagues[24] measured the somatic copy number variations (CNVs) adjacent to HBV integration sites. They found that CNVs were significantly increased at HBV break point locations where chromosomal instability was likely induced, suggesting that HBV integration might alter chromosomal stability and cause changes in the CNVs.[24] One of the consequences of HBV integration that leads to genome instability and alteration in molecular signaling is a heterozygous deletion of a cluster of caspase and caspase-recruiting domain family genes. These genes, which are important for the execution of apoptosis caused by viral integration, colocalized precisely within the junction of a large DNA copy number loss. Jiang and colleagues,[23] following RNA-sequencing (RNA-seq) analysis, revealed downregulation in the expression levels of these genes.

### Viral-human fusion transcripts

This phenomenon is common in HBV-associated HCC tumors. According to RNA-seq analysis, the viral arm of such chimeric transcripts is mapped preferentially to a region between 1500 and 2000 base pairs on the viral genome located toward the end of the HBx gene.[23] Lau and colleagues[27] performed transcriptome sequencing of 6 HBV-positive HCC cell lines. They identified a viral-human chimeric fusion transcript that functions like a long noncoding RNA to promote HCC. Multiple instances of chimeric transcripts resulting from HBV integration were detected, many of which were from the human intergenic regions that contained a portion of a repetitive element, such as a LINE or SINE. The most intriguing and abundant fusion was the HBx-LINE1 chimera, detected is 23% of the HBV-associated HCC tissues examined. The HBx-LINE1 chimera functioned as a hybrid RNA. In addition, they also demonstrated that HBx-LINE1 can promote tumor growth likely through the activation of Wnt/b-catenin signaling.[27]

### HBx

HBx is a 17-kD protein encoded by the X open reading frame of HBV. HBx can complex with cellular proteins and transcriptionally transactivates virus gene expression and replication.[28] Furthermore, HBx protects virus-infected cells from immune-mediated destruction during repeated bouts of hepatitis.[29] HBx is thought to play a pivotal role in the hepatocarcinogenesis abilities of HBV by interfering with several cellular functions.

### Epigenetic effects

HBx was shown in several studies to induce promoter hypermethylation and, as a consequence, to downregulate the expression of tumor suppressor genes. DNA methylation is an epigenetic tool that allows cells to repress the transactivation of certain genes. Methylation of CpG sites within the promoters of genes can lead to their silencing. The DNMT family of genes executes DNA methylation.[30] HBx can upregulate CpG methylation by transactivation of DNMT1 and DNMT3A expression.[31,32] Among others, P16INK4A,[31,33,34] E-cadherin,[32,35,36] and IGFBP3[30] were repressed in HBV-infected hepatocytes by the hypermethylation mechanism induced by upregulation of the DNMT genes. Both SFRP1 and SFRP5, antagonists of the Wnt signaling pathway, were epigenetically silenced by HBx in hepatoma cell lines. Downregulation of SFRP1 and SFRP5 correlated positively with DNMT1 overexpression.[37] HBx can alter the methylation status of specific genes by the recruitment of DNMT1 and DNMT3A to specific methylation sites.[38,39] However, other studies demonstrated an opposite effect of HBx, namely, the downregulation of levels of methylation on specific promoters and, as a consequence, upregulated expression of those genes.[40,41] Recently, the effect of HBx on a novel epigenetic regulatory element, the highly methylated CpG islands (mCGIs), was demonstrated.[42] Severe hypomethylation of intragenic mCGIs was observed in HBx liver before the full development of HCC. Furthermore, hypomethylation of mCGIs was caused by the downregulation of Dnmt3L and Dnmt3a expression levels because of the binding of HBx to their promoters, along with histone deacetylase 1 (HDAC1). These events led to the downregulation of many developmental regulators that could facilitate tumorigenesis.[42]

The cell regulates gene expression by acetylation of histones in the nucleosome. These reactions are typically catalyzed by enzymes with histone acetyltransferase (HAT) or HDAC activity. p300/CBP is a transcriptional coactivator complex of proteins that harbors intrinsic HAT activity.[43,44] HBx can bind directly to the CREB-binding domain of CREB-responsive promoters of endogenous cellular genes, such as interleukin (IL) 8 and PCNA; increase the recruitment of p300 to these promoters; and, as a result, upregulate those gene expressions.[45] Conversely, HBx was shown to inhibit the expression of other genes (CDH1 and IGFBP3) by recruitment of HDAC complexes to their promoters.[46,47]

### MicroRNA

MicroRNAs (miRNAs) can be important mediators of HBV infection leading to HCC development and progression. HBx regulates miRNAs activity and is associated with both the downregulation and upregulation of different miRNAs expression. Wang and colleagues[48] reported that HBx upregulated the expression of 7 miRNAs and downregulated 11 miRNAs. Eight out of the 9 members of the let-7 family were downregulated in the HBx-transfected cells. The most highly expressed let-7 family member, let-7a, negatively regulated cellular proliferation partly through targeting STAT3.[48] HBx was shown to upregulate the oncoprotein astrocyte elevated gene-1 via downregulation of miR-375 and miR-136 in HBx-transfected cells.[49] Additionally, Zhang and colleagues[50] have shown that HBx directly targeted miR-205. HBx inhibits miR-205 expression probably by hypermethylation of its promoter. The forced miR-205 expression remarkably inhibited HBx-enhanced proliferation of hepatoma cells in vitro and in vivo, suggesting that miR-205 is a potential tumor-suppressive gene in HCC.[50] Conversely, Liu and colleagues[51] have shown that HBxΔ127 (a naturally occurring HBx mutant) was able to significantly increase miR-215 expression relative to wild-type HBx in hepatoma HepG2 and H7402 cells. Upregulation of miR-215 targeted the protein tyrosine phosphatase receptor type T, a tumor suppressor gene, indicating that HBxΔ127 strongly enhances proliferation of hepatoma cells.[51]

Yip and colleagues[52] infected nontumorigenic human hepatocytes with lentivirus-expressing full-length and carboxyl-terminal truncated HBx (Ct-HBx) for cell growth assay and miRNA profiling. Ct-HBx decreased, whereas full-length HBx increased the expression of a set of miRNAs with growth-suppressive functions. Ct-HBx inhibited the transcriptional activity of some of these miRNA promoters.[52]

### Apoptosis

HBx protein contributes to the development of HCC by its effects on apoptosis. HBx has both proapoptotic and antiapoptotic effects. The p53 gene and other tumor suppressor genes mediate both effects, at least partially.[53] These contradictory effects might be explained by the evidence that high levels of HBx protein promote apoptosis, whereas low levels inhibit apoptosis.[54] Knoll and colleagues[55] showed that, in HCC tumor cell lines differing in their p53 status, HBx was proapoptotic but exhibited opposite effects in nontumor cells. In normal cells, p53 and p73 were retained in the cytoplasm, whereas, in hepatoma cells, HBx led to nuclear translocation of p53 and p73, followed by enhanced transactivation of p53-dependent promoters, supporting the dual function of HBx.[55]

### DNA repair pathways and genetic instability

Gene array analysis comparing mRNA expression in fetal hepatic cell lines transfected with the HBx gene found increased expression of a large group of genes that are involved in cellular DNA damage repair and checkpoint signaling, such as DDB1, UGT1A9, UNG, XRCC1, XRCC3, XRCC4, and RAD17.[56] HBx required binding to UV-damaged DNA binding protein 1 (DDB1)–ubiquitin ligase, a protein involved in DNA repair and cell cycle regulation, in order to stimulate transcription from the viral episomal DNA genome.[57,58] HBx also induced lagging chromosomes during mitosis, leading to formation of aberrant mitotic spindles and multinucleated cells. These effects required the binding of HBx to DDB1 and were unexpectedly attributable to HBx interfering with S-phase progression and not directly with mitotic events. The binding of HBx to DDB1 may induce genetic instability in regenerating hepatocytes and, thereby, contribute to HCC development.[59]

### Hepatitis C Virus

HCV, a positive-strand RNA virus, replicates in the cytoplasm and does not integrate into the host genome. Thus, HCV has a far lower direct oncogenic potential than HBV. It is currently thought that the main mechanism leading to HCC development in HCV infection is the indirect effect of chronic inflammation resulting from immune responses against infected hepatocytes, associated with apoptosis and enhanced hepatocellular proliferation, which leads to fibrosis with eventual progression to cirrhosis and the subsequent development of HCC.[4] Data from several studies have implicated the direct role of HCV-specific mechanisms by both HCV structural and nonstructural proteins that are also involved in hepatocellular carcinogenesis.[4] Transgenic mice expressing the HCV polyprotein develop liver cancer in the absence of inflammation or immune recognition of the transgene, thus, supporting a direct role for HCV proteins in carcinogenesis.[60] Other evidence suggests that HCV protein expression may have broader cocarcinogenic effects. No single viral protein has been shown to consistently cause liver cancer when expressed at a low abundance comparable with that present in most patients with HCV-related liver disease.

### Core protein

In 1998, Moriya and colleagues[60] published the results of experiments with 2 independent transgenic mouse lines, each with a complementary DNA fragment containing the complete core gene of HCV genotype 1b. The expression of HCV core protein in both lines resulted in progressive morphologic and biochemical changes that ultimately resulted in the development of HCC. Chronic hepatitis, with continuous cell death and regeneration, was not an absolute prerequisite for the development of HCC, indicating that the HCV core protein probably has a direct role in the development of HCC.[60] HCV core protein induced spontaneous, persistent, age-dependent, and heterogeneous activation of PPARα in transgenic mice, which may contribute to multicentric hepatocarcinogenesis.[61] Furthermore, in order to demonstrate the molecular mechanism of HCV core protein induction of hepatocyte growth regulation, microarray analysis of RNA purified from primary human hepatocytes and HCV core gene transfected hepatocytes suggested that the expression of HCV core protein resulted in an increase in expression of IL-6, gp130, leptin receptor, and STAT3. Upregulation of these genes in turn may regulate c-Myc and cyclin D1, downstream the STAT3 signaling pathway.[62] Core protein also activates the Wnt/β-catenin cascade, which is known to play a role in the development of HCC. In HCCs samples, 40% to 70% were shown to harbor nuclear accumulation of the β-catenin protein, the hallmark of the Wnt/β-catenin pathway activation.[63] One of the genes that was overexpressed in cells transfected with the core protein is the Wnt1 gene.[64] Recently, Huang and colleagues[65] have shown that cell lines transfected with HCV core protein significantly suppressed miR-152 expression. Reduction in miR-152 expression upregulated Wnt1 transcript expression leading to proliferation of liver cancer cells.[65] The core protein also activates the Wnt signaling pathway by silencing SFRP1, a regulator of this pathway.[66] HCV core protein markedly increased the expression level and binding of DNMT1 and HDAC1 to the SFRP1 promoter region, resulting in epigenetic silencing of SFRP1 expression. Silencing of SFRP1 may lead to the activation of the Wnt signaling pathway and, thus, contribute to HCC aggressiveness.[66] HCV core protein can also activate the transforming growth factor-β (TGF-β) singling pathway.[67] Stellate cells growing in coculture with hepatoma cells expressing HCV core were activated by TGF-β, indicating a dual impact of HCV core on liver fibrosis and liver carcinogenesis, acting both in an autocrine manner by modulating the TGF-β responses in hepatocytes and by affecting stellate cell activation in a paracrine mechanism via TGF-β activation.[67] Additionally, HCV core protein can upregulate and stabilize the levels of hypoxia-inducible factor 1α in Huh7.5.1 cells and transactivate the expression of vascular endothelial growth factor, one of the important angiogenic factors associated with the maintenance of liver carcinogenesis.[68]

### NS3

Results of experiments, both with tissue culture and nude mice models, have shown that NS3 has a direct role in the induction of cellular transformation.[69,70] Furthermore, results indicated that the serine protease activity of NS3 is crucial for this transformation.[70] The importance of the serine protease domain was emphasized by the authors' findings that significant amino acid changes were defined at the catalytic domain of the NS3 serine protease gene isolated from HCC tissue.[71] These changes were not detected in nontumorous tissues or in serum. In addition, NS3 protein can specifically repress the promoter activity of p21 in a dose-dependent manner probably via a protein–protein interaction with p53.[72] Furthermore, the NS3 N-terminal peptide significantly upregulated the phosphorylation of p44/42[MAPK] but did not affect the expression of the total MAPK protein resulting in proliferation and transformation of hepatocytes.[73] The same group later demonstrated that the NS3 protein can promote cell growth and contribute to hepatocarcinogenesis by the activation of ERK/AP-1 and NF-κB/cyclin D1 cascades.[74] Cheng and colleagues,[75] showed that NS3 interacts with Smad3 and represses TGF-β/Smad3-mediated transactivation and growth inhibition and, thus, antagonizes the host defenses during hepatocarcinogenesis.[75] However, recently it was shown that NS3 in the presence of NS4A interacted with

SMURF2, a negative regulator of TGF-β signaling.[76] As a result, cells expressing the combination of NS3 and NS4A stimulate TGF-β induction and increase the expression of SMAD-dependent genes compared with control cells, pointing to the tumor suppressor function of SMURF2 as an interesting target to prevent HCC progression.[76] NS3 protease mimics TGF-β2 and directly exerts its activity via binding to and activating TβRI, thereby, enhancing liver fibrosis.[77]

### NS5A

NS5A is an HCV nonstructural protein that was shown to have transformation abilities in tissue culture and nude mice.[78] NS5A binds directly to p53 and inhibits its transcriptional activity and, thereby, downregulates endogenous p21/waf1 expression.[79,80] As a result, p53-induced apoptosis was abrogated by NS5A, thereby, contributing to the hepatocarcinogenesis of HCV.[80] Moreover, NS5A downregulates the expression of GADD45α in a P53-dependent manner and subsequently triggers cellular proliferation.[81] GADD45 proteins serve as tumor suppressors. Defects in the GADD45 signaling pathway can be related to the initiation and progression of malignancies.[82] NS5A can also affect the Wnt/β-catenin cascade by stabilization of β-catenin and stimulation of β-catenin–dependent transcription by activation of PI3K.[83,84] NS5A also binds directly to β-catenin and stimulates its activity.[85] NS5A stabilization of β-catenin stimulated the expression of c-Myc that led to increased production of reactive oxygen species, mitochondrial perturbation, enhanced DNA damage, and aberrant cell-cycle arrest—all suggesting that HCV has a direct effect in liver tumorigenesis.[86]

### NS5B

NS5B the viral RNA-dependent RNA polymerase nonstructural protein forms a cytoplasmic complex with the retinoblastoma tumor suppressor protein (Rb) and, thereby, strongly negatively regulated HCV infection in cultured cells.[87] NS5B recruits E6-associated protein to the process.[88] The recruitment leads to polyubiquitination of Rb and Rb degradation through the proteasome. The end result is activation of E2F-responsive promoters, which would be expected to stimulate entry into the S phase of the cell cycle. The disruption of Rb/E2F regulatory pathways in cells infected with HCV is likely to promote hepatocellular proliferation and chromosomal instability, factors important for the development of liver cancer.[88] These findings, which are unique among RNA viruses and may share attributes in common with many DNA tumor viruses, suggest a novel theoretic framework for the origins of liver cancer.[87]

### MicroRNAs and hepatitis C virus–associated cancer

HCV replication critically depends on miR-122.[89] There is some evidence that miR-122 may have tumor suppressor properties. Expression of miR-122 has been shown to be low or undetectable in the human hepatoma cell lines, Hep3B and HepG2, in which its overexpression inhibited tumor formation in nude mice.[90,91] Although several studies have profiled miRNA expression in HCC, it remains unclear whether miR-122 abundance is altered in HCV-associated HCC and what the exact role is of miRNAs in the development of HCC.

## RISK OF HEPATOCELLULAR CARCINOMA IN A NONCIRRHOTIC LIVER
### Hepatitis B Virus

Cirrhosis in patients with chronic HBV infection is only present in about 70% to 80% of HBV-related HCC cases[92,93] and, thus, is not a prerequisite for tumorigenesis, especially in Asian and African patients. Patients with HBV can develop HCC with minimal liver damage. The REVEAL-HBV study demonstrated that 1932 inactive noncirrhotic HBV carriers, followed for a mean period of 13.1 years, were at a substantial risk of developing HCC.[94] The multivariate adjusted hazard ratio for carriers of inactive HBV, compared with controls, was 4.6 (95% confidence interval 2.5–8.3) for HCC. The REVEAL-HBV study also evaluated the risk of HCC across a biological gradient of serum HBV DNA levels.[95] The incidence of HCC was significantly associated with serum HBV DNA levels in a dose-response manner from less than 300 (undetectable) to greater than 1,000,000 copies per milliliter. The serum level of HBV DNA was a prominent predictor of HCC risk, independent of the presence of cirrhosis ($P<.001$). Liu and colleagues[96] reported that the accumulation of mutations in the basal core promoter and a high viral load ($10^{4-5}$ copies per milliliter) were independent predictors of HCC development in the absence of cirrhosis.

### Occult Hepatitis B Virus

In occult HBV infection, HBV virus can continue to replicate at low levels causing persistent inflammation and injury, which may contribute to the development of HCC,[97] implying that the occult viral strains maintained the transcriptional activity and the pro-oncogenic property of the overt (termed *clear* by the investigators) HBV infection (ie, showing HBsAg positivity).[98] However, knowledge of the role of occult HBV in the development of HCC is still very limited and often confounded by current therapy and testing methodology.[99]

HBV infection can trigger hepatic carcinogenesis independent of the development of cirrhosis. Different molecular mechanisms may be involved underlying the development of HCC with and without cirrhosis. For instance, as previously mentioned, the HBV viral genome can directly integrate into the host human genome and act as an oncogenic factor, a process that is independent of the chronic inflammation that commonly characterizes cirrhosis.[100] By using comparative genomic hybridization,[101] it has been observed that copy number gains in 8q and 20q and the loss of 4q were more frequent in HBV-associated HCCs with no underlying cirrhosis then in cirrhotic HCCs. Telomere length has emerged as a promising risk predictor of various cancers, including HCC. Longer relative telomere length in circulating cell-free serum DNA was significantly associated with an increased risk of noncirrhotic HBV-related HCC.[102] HBx protein increased both the expression of telomere reverse transcriptase and telomerase activity, the enzyme responsible for the maintenance of telomere length, thus, prolonging the lifespan of hepatocytes and contributing to malignant transformation.[103]

### Hepatitis C Virus

To date there are very few data on HCC arising in HCV infected but noncirrhotic livers.[104–110] Of HCV-related HCC, 6% to 17% were reported in noncirrhotic livers.[104–107] In the prospective HALT-C trial of 1005 chronically infected patients in the United States, 17% of HCCs were found in the absence of advanced fibrosis.[107] The mechanism of HCV-associated HCC arising in noncirrhotic livers is not clear. There is general agreement that ongoing necroinflammation resulting from HCV infection seems to contribute significantly to the risk of developing HCC, independent of hepatic fibrosis. Elevated levels of transaminases, a marker for liver inflammation, correlate with HCC risk among patients with HCV independently of fibrosis stage.[111] As stated earlier, several HCV gene products (core, NS3, NS4B, and NS5A) possess a transformation potential to alter several potentially oncogenic pathways suggesting that HCV also has a direct hepatocarcinogenic potential. The development of HCC in persons with noncirrhotic fibrosis raises the question of whether such patients should undergo HCC surveillance, as is recommended for persons with established cirrhosis. Currently, screening in noncirrhotic fibrosis is optional.

## PREVENTION OF HEPATOCELLULAR CARCINOMA IN PATIENTS WITH CHRONIC VIRAL HEPATITIS B AND C
### Hepatitis B Virus Vaccine

It is now well established that vaccination against hepatitis B is very effective in preventing HBV infection. Control and significant reduction in incidence of new HBV infections as well as a reduced incidence of HCC have been repeatedly reported in countries in East Asia and Africa. Data from Taiwan have shown convincingly that rates of childhood HCC have decreased significantly since the implementation of universal infant vaccination in Taiwan in 1984.[112] The prevention of HCC by HBV vaccination extends from childhood to early adulthood; failure to prevent HCC resulted mostly from incomplete HBV vaccination or unsuccessful control of HBV infection in highly infectious mothers.[113] In a recently published follow-up study, the 30-year outcomes of the HBV Taiwanese immunization program were evaluated and HCC incidence decreased by more than 80% for individuals aged 5 to 29 years.[114] Likewise, a reduction in HCC has been demonstrated among Thai and native Alaskan children who received hepatitis B vaccination at birth.[115,116] Hepatitis B vaccination is now a part of the National Infant Immunization Schedule in 162 countries and constitutes the first example of cancer prevented by vaccination, although confirming the mortality reductions from HBV-associated HCC may require several decades.

### Hepatitis B Virus Antiviral Therapy: Interferon and Nucleoside/Nucleotide Analogues

It has been difficult to prove that HBV treatment reduces the incidence of HCC. Prevention of HCC in patients with HBV with a maintained virological response to therapy is not, as yet, convincingly demonstrated because it takes many years for long-term outcomes, such as HCC development, to present. The exclusion of patients from treatment while continuing to observe them clinically is obviously unethical and untenable.[10] All therapeutic trials designed to assess antiviral efficacy of anti-HBV regimens adopted surrogate end points and, therefore, were underpowered to capture hard end points of hepatitis B infection, including HCC. The two accepted treatment modalities are interferon-$\alpha$ (IFN-$\alpha$) given subcutaneously for a limited time period and nucleoside/nucleotide analogues given orally on a long-term basis. These treatments are effective in suppressing viral activity and improving disease markers in short-term studies. There are no studies directly comparing IFN-$\alpha$ and nucleoside/nucleotide analogues.

#### Interferon-$\alpha$ therapy

Results of long-term follow-up studies of IFN-$\alpha$ therapy were inconsistent regarding the reduction of HCC development, probably related to IFN-$\alpha$'s moderate suppressive ability on HBV replication.[117,118] Although in some studies there was prevention of HCC by IFN,[119–122] in others no benefits of IFN therapy were demonstrated.[123–125] Patients with less severe disease were included in these IFN studies in order to improve patient compliance, which resulted in a selection bias.[118] There were also differences in the duration of follow-up between patients who responded to INF-$\alpha$ versus nonresponders. Moreover, in most of the studies, hepatitis B e antigen (HBeAg) seroconversion was used as the end point of treatment, although most patients continued to have detectable HBV DNA after HBeAg seroconversion.[117] Currently it can be surmised that the beneficial effect of IFN-$\alpha$ in reducing the development of HCC is limited to patients with cirrhosis who are sustained responders, although they compose a relatively small proportion of patients studied.[117,118]

### Nucleoside/Nucleotide analogues

In the long-term studies of treatment with lamivudine (and adefovir), there was a consistent reduction in the development of liver cancer in patients who achieved a virological response irrespective of the presence of cirrhosis; but in some cases, nonetheless, HCC still developed. This beneficial effect is blunted by the development of HBV resistance. In a systematic review of studies of NUC treatment of patients with HBV,[8] it was clearly determined that HCC was prevented in patients with chronic hepatitis but not in those with cirrhosis and, in general, in patients who could not achieve complete virological suppression. This finding was also confirmed by a cohort study from Greece in which cirrhotic patients on long-term lamivudine were shown to remain at risk of developing liver cancer.[126] Recently the effect of the more potent anti-HBV drugs, such as entecavir and tenofovir, was evaluated in terms of HCC prevention in responders with cirrhosis.[9,12,127–129] In a large US-based longitudinal observational cohort study in 2671 patients with HBV,[9] HBV antiviral therapy (94% received NUCs: lamivudine, entecavir, tenofovir, telbivudine, or adefovir) was associated with a significantly decreased risk of HCC (follow-up 9 years) than those who did not receive antiviral therapy (adjusted hazard ratio, 0.39; 95% confidence interval, 0.27–0.56; $P<.001$). The beneficial effects were not associated with the fibrosis stage (using various surrogates to estimate the severity of underlying liver disease).[9] Treated patients with viral loads greater than 20,000 IU/mL had a significantly lower risk of HCC than untreated patients with comparable viral loads. In a recent Japanese study,[12] entecavir significantly reduced the incidence of HCC among chronic HBV-infected patients and did so to a greater extent than lamivudine did. Patients at higher risk for HCC (ie, those with cirrhosis) derived greater benefit from treatment compared with lower-risk subjects. However, this was not the case in a large nationwide Greek study[127] that included 321 patients treated with entecavir for a median of 40 months; the HCC risk remained increased in entecavir-treated HBeAg-negative patients with HBV with cirrhosis. In another multicenter study from Italy,[128] patients with compensated cirrhosis and undetectable serum HBV DNA during 5 years of entecavir monotherapy showed an annual rate of HCC of approximately 2.5%, which is similar to the HCC rates in untreated HBeAg-negative patients in Europe. A prediction model (REACH-B risk calculator) was used to compare the incidence of HCC in 641 patients treated for 6 years with tenofovir in the tenofovir long-term registration trial.[129] In non-cirrhotic patients, the effect of tenofovir became noticeable at approximately 2 years of therapy and became significant (55% reduction) at 6 years. But the benefit was less pronounced in cirrhotic patients.[129]

Persistence of HCC risk in cirrhotic patients responding to NUCs therapy may be the consequence of the extended survival provided by NUCs, or it can be assumed that HBV-related liver carcinogenesis is promoted by cellular events that are established early during chronic infection with HBV and are independent of the onset of cirrhosis.[118]

### Hepatitis C Virus Antiviral Therapy

In chronic HCV infection, HCC is usually associated with advanced fibrosis or cirrhosis. There is limited evidence for the role of IFN-based therapy in the prophylaxis of HCC in patients with chronic HCV, as most studies were primarily designed to assess the antiviral effect of treatment and not the long-term impact on the natural history of the disease. HCV eradication decreases the risk of HCC in antiviral responders compared with that observed in patients failing therapy.[130–134] Significantly lower incidences of HCC and mortality were observed in sustained virological responders (both for IFN monotherapy and IFN/ribavirin in combination), but not in nonresponders, when compared with untreated patients.[130] Preexisting cirrhosis, nonresponse, HCV genotype-1, and age were associated with HCC,[130] as well as steatosis, male sex, diabetes, and alcohol consumption.[131] SVR had a strong independent positive influence on the incidence of HCC in 127 HCV patients with bridging fibrosis and 180 with cirrhosis, treated with pegylated IFN (pegIFN) and ribavirin.[132] In a recent Japanese multicenter study of 1013 patients with HCV (noncirrhosis n = 863 and cirrhosis n = 150),[133] SVR and complete viral suppression during treatment in relapsers were associated with a lower risk of HCC development in cirrhotic patients when compared with nonresponders. In a meta-analysis that combined data from 30 studies,[134] the incidence of HCC was 1.05% per person-year in those with SVRs compared with 3.3% in those without an SVR. In patients with advanced fibrosis (Ishak fibrosis score 4–6), the cumulative occurrence of HCC after 10 years was 21.8% without an SVR and 5.1% with an SVR.[17] Results of several studies suggested that low-dose IFN may delay the development of HCC[135,136] even in patients with cirrhosis. However, this latter finding remains controversial; there are also inconclusive and negative studies.[107,137,138] In the HALT-C cohort, HCV-positive patients with bridging fibrosis or cirrhosis who did not respond to PegIFN and ribavirin, maintenance PegIFN for 3.5 years did not reduce the incidence of HCC.[107] A lower incidence of HCC in patients randomized to long-term low-dose PegIFN only emerged after 5 to 7 years of follow-up.[137] Maintenance therapy with PegIFN α-2b in the Evaluation of PegIntron in Control of Hepatitis C Cirrhosis (EPIC) 3 program was deemed unwarranted in cirrhotic patients with chronic HCV,[138] as there was no decrease in the development of HCC with therapy. Altogether, long-term suppressive therapy with IFN to prevent HCC is not currently a realistic strategy especially with the emergence of the new HCV direct-acting antiviral agents, even though none of them have been in use long enough to evaluate their effect in reducing HCC incidence.

### Risk for Hepatocellular Carcinoma Development in Patients Without Cirrhosis After Successful Antiviral Therapy

Whether there is an increased risk for HCC development among noncirrhotic patients after successful antiviral therapy remain unclear.[14] In a recently published study a total of 642 patients with an SVR after PegIFN/RBV therapy were studied in Taiwan for a median follow-up period of 53.0 months (range: 6–133 months).[139] Of the 556 noncirrhotic patients, only 17 (3.1%) versus 16 (18.6%) of the 86 cirrhotic patients developed HCC (P<.001). Older noncirrhotic patients with high-baseline γ-glutamyl transferase levels had as great a risk for HCC development as cirrhotic patients.[139]

### Advanced fibrosis/patients with cirrhosis achieving sustained viral response and risk for hepatocellular carcinoma

There is clear evidence that patients with advanced fibrosis or cirrhosis who achieve SVR remain at heightened risk for HCC.[13,15,16,140,141] In a Japanese study,[13] 1193 patients with HCV-related chronic liver disease and IFN monotherapy or IFN plus ribavirin-induced SVR were followed up for a mean period of 8.3 years. The crude rates of hepatocarcinogenesis at 5, 10, and 15 years were 1.5%, 2.4%, and 4.1%, respectively. Moreover, HCC was diagnosed in 26% of 562 consecutive SVR patients, more than 10 years after completion of IFN therapy. F2 fibrosis (ie, the presence of periportal or portal septa) was detected in 42% of these patients.[15] Patients with the risk factors of advanced age at HCV eradication and heavy alcohol intake were at heightened risk for the development of HCC within 5 years after HCV eradication.[141] Van der Meer and colleagues[17] reported the results of an international, multicenter, long-term follow-up study from 5 large tertiary care hospitals in Europe and Canada of 530 patients with chronic HCV infection who started an IFN-based treatment regime between 1990 and 2003, following histologic proof of advanced hepatic fibrosis or cirrhosis. Patients who achieved SVR had a lower incidence of HCC (0.55 vs 1.01 per 100 person-years), liver failure (0.31 vs 3.62 per 100 person-years), liver-related mortality (0.23 vs 3.20 per 100 person-years), and, most importantly, all-cause mortality (1.01 vs 2.93 per 100 person-years) than patients who did not achieve SVR. A recent Swedish study[142] prospectively evaluated the long-term effect of antiviral therapy on the risk of developing HCC in a cohort of 351 patients with HCV with Child-Turcotte-Pugh class A cirrhosis. The incidence of HCC was significantly reduced in patients who achieved SVR (1.0 per 100 person-years) compared with those who failed treatment (2.3 per 100 person-years) or those who were never treated (4.0 per 100 person-years). The incidence of HCC was similar in the first 3 years and the subsequent 3 years after viral clearance. In both studies,[17,142] better outcomes were detected in patients who achieved SVR; however, they have also documented that some patients were still at risk of developing HCC, with an incidence of approximately 0.5% to 1.0% per year. Investigators of the HALT-C study[107] showed that patients with bridging fibrosis had a 0.82% risk per year of developing HCC. These findings suggest that long-term screening for HCC should be done in patients with cirrhosis even after achieving SVR. However, the guidelines from the American Association for the Study of Liver Disease do not recommend screening such patients because the incidence is less than the cost-effectiveness analysis threshold of 1.5% per year.[143]

## REFERENCES

1. El-Serag HB, Rudolph KL. Hepatocellular carcinoma: epidemiology and molecular carcinogenesis. Gastroenterology 2007;132:2557–76.
2. Nguyen VT, Law MG, Dore GJ. Hepatitis B-related hepatocellular carcinoma: epidemiological characteristics and disease burden. J Viral Hepat 2006;16: 453–63.
3. de Martel C, Ferlay J, Franceschi S, et al. Global burden of cancers attributable to infections in 2008: a review and synthetic analysis. Lancet Oncol 2012;13(6): 607–15.
4. Lemon SM, McGivern DR. Is hepatitis C virus carcinogenic? Gastroenterology 2012;142:1274–8.
5. Venook AP, Papandreou C, Furuse J, et al. The incidence and epidemiology of hepatocellular carcinoma: a global and regional perspective. Oncologist 2010; 15:S5–13.
6. Shlomai A, de Jong YP, Rice CM. Virus associated malignancies: the role of viral hepatitis in hepatocellular carcinoma. Semin Cancer Biol 2014;26:78–88.
7. Arzumanyan A, Reis HM, Feitelson MA. Pathogenic mechanisms in HBV- and HCV-associated hepatocellular carcinoma. Nat Rev Cancer 2013;13(2): 123–35.
8. Papatheodoridis GV, Lampertico P, Manolakopoulos S, et al. Incidence of hepatocellular carcinoma in chronic hepatitis B patients receiving nucleos(t)ide therapy: a systematic review. J Hepatol 2010;53(2):348–56.
9. Gordon SC, Lamerato LE, Rupp LB, et al. Antiviral therapy for chronic hepatitis B virus infection and development of hepatocellular carcinoma in a US population. Clin Gastroenterol Hepatol 2014;12(5):885–93.
10. Sherman M. Does hepatitis B treatment reduce the incidence of hepatocellular carcinoma? Hepatology 2013;58(1):18–20.

11. Thiele M, Gluud LL, Krage A. Antiviral therapy in hepatitis B has no effect on mortality and decreases incidence of HCC only in patients with cirrhosis. A meta-analysis of 27 trials and 7,034 patients. Hepatology 2012;56(S1):642A.

12. Hosaka T, Suzuki F, Kobayashi M, et al. Long-term entecavir treatment reduces hepatocellular carcinoma incidence in patients with hepatitis B virus infection. Hepatology 2013;58:98–107.

13. Hirakawa M, Ikeda K, Arase Y, et al. Hepatocarcinogenesis following HCV RNA eradication by interferon in chronic hepatitis patients. Intern Med 2008;47: 1637–43.

14. Yoshida H, Shiratori Y, Moriyama M, et al. Interferon therapy reduces the risk for hepatocellular carcinoma: national surveillance program of cirrhotic and noncirrhotic patients with chronic hepatitis C in Japan. IHIT study group. Inhibition of Hepatocarcinogenesis by Interferon Therapy. Ann Intern Med 1999;131:174–81.

15. Yamashita N, Ohho A, Yamasaki A, et al. Hepatocarcinogenesis in chronic hepatitis C patients achieving a sustained virological response to interferon: significance of lifelong periodic cancer screening for improving outcomes. J Gastroenterol 2014;49:1504–13.

16. Maylin S, Martinot-Peignoux M, Moucari R, et al. Eradication of hepatitis C virus in patients successfully treated for chronic hepatitis C. Gastroenterology 2008; 135:821–9.

17. van der Meer AJ, Veldt BJ, Feld JJ, et al. Association between sustained virological response and all-cause mortality among patients with chronic hepatitis C and advanced hepatic fibrosis. JAMA 2012;308:2584–93.

18. Dienstag JL, Ghany MG, Morgan TR, et al. A prospective study of the rate of progression in compensated, histologically advanced chronic hepatitis C. Hepatology 2011;54(2):396–405.

19. Gozuacik D, Murakami Y, Saigo K, et al. Identification of human cancer-related genes by naturally occurring hepatitis B virus DNA tagging. Oncogene 2001; 20(43):6233–40.

20. Murakami Y, Saigo K, Takashima H, et al. Large scaled analysis of hepatitis B virus (HBV) DNA integration in HBV related hepatocellular carcinomas. Gut 2005;54(8):1162–8.

21. Saigo K, Yoshida K, Ikeda R. Integration of hepatitis B virus DNA into the myeloid/lymphoid or mixed-lineage leukemia (MLL4) gene and rearrangements of MLL4 in human hepatocellular carcinoma. Hum Mutat 2008;29(5):703–8.

22. Mason WS, Liu C, Aldrich CE, et al. Clonal expansion of normal-appearing human hepatocytes during chronic hepatitis B virus infection. J Virol 2010;84(16): 8308–15.

23. Jiang Z, Jhunjhunwala S, Liu J, et al. The effects of hepatitis B virus integration into the genomes of hepatocellular carcinoma patients. Genome Res 2012; 22(4):593–601.

24. Sung WK, Zheng H, Li S, et al. Genome-wide survey of recurrent HBV integration in hepatocellular carcinoma. Nat Genet 2012;44(7):765–9.

25. Paterlini-Bréchot P, Saigo K, Murakami Y, et al. Hepatitis B virus-related insertional mutagenesis occurs frequently in human liver cancers and recurrently targets human telomerase gene. Oncogene 2003;22(25):3911–6.

26. Fujimoto A, Totoki Y, Abe T, et al. Whole-genome sequencing of liver cancers identifies etiological influences on mutation patterns and recurrent mutations in chromatin regulators. Nat Genet 2012;44(7):760–4.

27. Lau CC, Sun T, Ching AK, et al. Viral-human chimeric transcript predisposes risk to liver cancer development and progression. Cancer Cell 2014;25(3):335–49.

28. Keasler VV, Hodgson AJ, Madden CR, et al. Enhancement of hepatitis B virus replication by the regulatory X protein in vitro and in vivo. J Virol 2007;81(6): 2656–62.

29. Feitelson MA, Reis HM, Tufan NL, et al. Putative roles of hepatitis B x antigen in the pathogenesis of chronic liver disease. Cancer Lett 2009;286(1):69–79.

30. Park IY, Sohn BH, Yu E, et al. Aberrant epigenetic modifications in hepatocarcinogenesis induced by hepatitis B virus X protein. Gastroenterology 2007;132(4): 1476–94.

31. Zhu YZ, Zhu R, Fan J, et al. Hepatitis B virus X protein induces hypermethylation of p16(INK4A) promoter via DNA methyltransferases in the early stage of HBV-associated hepatocarcinogenesis. J Viral Hepat 2010;17(2):98–107.

32. Lee JO, Kwun HJ, Jung JK, et al. Hepatitis B virus X protein represses E-cadherin expression via activation of DNA methyltransferase 1. Oncogene 2005; 24(44):6617–25.

33. Jung JK, Arora P, Pagano JS, et al. Expression of DNA methyltransferase 1 is activated by hepatitis B virus X protein via a regulatory circuit involving the p16INK4a-cyclin D1-CDK 4/6-pRb-E2F1 pathway. Cancer Res 2007;67(12): 5771–8.

34. Park SH, Jung JK, Lim JS, et al. Hepatitis B virus X protein overcomes all-trans retinoic acid-induced cellular senescence by downregulating levels of p16 and p21 via DNA methylation. J Gen Virol 2011;92(Pt 6):1309–17.

35. Liu J, Lian Z, Han S, et al. Downregulation of E-cadherin by hepatitis B virus X antigen in hepatocellular carcinoma. Oncogene 2006;25(7):1008–17.

36. Osada T, Sakamoto M, Ino Y, et al. E-cadherin is involved in the intrahepatic metastasis of hepatocellular carcinoma. Hepatology 1996;24(6):1460–7.

37. Xie Q, Chen L, Shan X, et al. Epigenetic silencing of SFRP1 and SFRP5 by hepatitis B virus X protein enhances hepatoma cell tumorigenicity through Wnt signaling pathway. Int J Cancer 2014;135(3):635–46.

38. Zhao J, Wu G, Bu F, et al. Epigenetic silence of ankyrin-repeat-containing, SH3-domain-containing, and proline-rich-region- containing protein 1 (ASPP1) and ASPP2 genes promotes tumor growth in hepatitis B virus-positive hepatocellular carcinoma. Hepatology 2010;51(1):142–53.

39. Zheng DL, Zhang L, Cheng N, et al. Epigenetic modification induced by hepatitis B virus X protein via interaction with de novo DNA methyltransferase DNMT3A. J Hepatol 2009;50(2):377–87.

40. Tong A, Gou L, Lau QC, et al. Proteomic profiling identifies aberrant epigenetic modifications induced by hepatitis B virus X protein. J Proteome Res 2009;8(2): 1037–46.

41. Tang SH, Hu W, Hu JJ, et al. Hepatitis B virus X protein promotes P3 transcript expression of the insulin-like growth factor 2 (IGF2) gene via inducing hypomethylation of P3 promoter in hepatocellular carcinoma. Liver Int 2015;35:608–19.

42. Lee SM, Lee YG, Bae JB, et al. HBx induces hypomethylation of distal intragenic CpG islands required for active expression of developmental regulators. Proc Natl Acad Sci U S A 2014;111(26):9555–60.

43. Bannister AJ, Kouzarides T. The CBP co-activator is a histone acetyltransferase. Nature 1996;384(6610):641–3.

44. Ogryzko VV, Schiltz RL, Russanova V, et al. The transcriptional coactivators p300 and CBP are histone acetyltransferases. Cell 1996;87(5):953–9.

45. Cougot D, Wu Y, Cairo S, et al. The hepatitis B virus X protein functionally interacts with CREB-binding protein/p300 in the regulation of CREB-mediated transcription. J Biol Chem 2007;282(7):4277–87.

46. Shon JK, Shon BH, Park IY, et al. Hepatitis B virus-X protein recruits histone deacetylase 1 to repress insulin-like growth factor binding protein 3 transcription. Virus Res 2009;139(1):14–21.
47. Arzumanyan A, Friedman T, Kotei E, et al. Epigenetic repression of E-cadherin expression by hepatitis B virus x antigen in liver cancer. Oncogene 2012;31(5): 563–72.
48. Wang Y, Lu Y, Toh ST, et al. Lethal-7 is down-regulated by the hepatitis B virus x protein and targets signal transducer and activator of transcription 3. J Hepatol 2010;53(1):57–66.
49. Zhao J, Wang W, Huang Y, et al. HBx Elevates oncoprotein AEG-1 expression to promote cell migration by downregulating miR-375 and miR-136 in malignant hepatocytes. DNA Cell Biol 2014;33:715–22.
50. Zhang T, Zhang J, Cui M, et al. Hepatitis B virus X protein inhibits tumor suppressor miR-205 through inducing hypermethylation of miR-205 promoter to enhance carcinogenesis. Neoplasia 2013;15(11):1282–91.
51. Liu F, You X, Chi X, et al. Hepatitis B virus X protein mutant HBxΔ127 promotes proliferation of hepatoma cells through up-regulating miR-215 targeting PTPRT. Biochem Biophys Res Commun 2014;444(2):128–34.
52. Yip WK, Cheng AS, Zhu R, et al. Carboxyl-terminal truncated HBx regulates a distinct microRNA transcription program in hepatocellular carcinoma development. PLoS One 2011;6(8):e22888.
53. Kew MC. Hepatitis B virus x protein in the pathogenesis of hepatitis B virus-induced hepatocellular carcinoma. J Gastroenterol Hepatol 2011;26(Suppl 1): 144–52.
54. Ye L, Dong N, Wang Q, et al. Progressive changes in hepatoma cells stably transfected with hepatitis B virus X gene. Intervirology 2008;51(1):50–8.
55. Knoll S, Fürst K, Thomas S, et al. Dissection of cell context-dependent interactions between HBx and p53 family members in regulation of apoptosis: a role for HBV-induced HCC. Cell Cycle 2011;10(20):3554–65.
56. Chen HY, Tang NH, Lin N, et al. Hepatitis B virus X protein induces apoptosis and cell cycle deregulation through interfering with DNA repair and checkpoint responses. Hepatol Res 2008;38(2):174–82.
57. van Breugel PC, Robert EI, Mueller H, et al. Hepatitis B virus X protein stimulates gene expression selectively from extrachromosomal DNA templates. Hepatology 2012;56(6):2116–24.
58. Guo L, Wang X, Ren L, et al. HBx affects CUL4-DDB1 function in both positive and negative manners. Biochem Biophys Res Commun 2014;450(4): 1492–7.
59. Martin-Lluesma S, Schaeffer C, Robert EI, et al. Hepatitis B virus X protein affects S phase progression leading to chromosome segregation defects by binding to damaged DNA binding protein 1. Hepatology 2008;48(5): 1467–76.
60. Moriya K, Fujie H, Shintani Y, et al. The core protein of hepatitis C virus induces hepatocellular carcinoma in transgenic mice. Nat Med 1998;4(9):1065–7.
61. Tanaka N, Moriya K, Kiyosawa K, et al. Hepatitis C virus core protein induces spontaneous and persistent activation of peroxisome proliferator-activated receptor alpha in transgenic mice: implications for HCV-associated hepatocarcinogenesis. Int J Cancer 2008;122(1):124–31.
62. Basu A, Meyer K, Lai KK, et al. Microarray analyses and molecular profiling of Stat3 signaling pathway induced by hepatitis C virus core protein in human hepatocytes. Virology 2006;349(2):347–58.

63. Pez F, Lopez A, Kim M, et al. Wnt signaling and hepatocarcinogenesis: molecular targets for the development of innovative anticancer drugs. J Hepatol 2013; 59(5):1107–17.

64. Fukutomi T, Zhou Y, Kawai S, et al. Hepatitis C virus core protein stimulates hepatocyte growth: correlation with upregulation of wnt-1 expression. Hepatology 2005;41(5):1096–105.

65. Huang S, Xie Y, Yang P, et al. HCV core protein-induced down-regulation of microRNA-152 promoted aberrant proliferation by regulating Wnt1 in HepG2 cells. PLoS One 2014;9(1):e81730.

66. Quan H, Zhou F, Nie D, et al. Hepatitis C virus core protein epigenetically silences SFRP1 and enhances HCC aggressiveness by inducing epithelial-mesenchymal transition. Oncogene 2014;33(22):2826–35.

67. Benzoubir N, Lejamtel C, Battaglia S, et al. HCV core-mediated activation of latent TGF-β via thrombospondin drives the crosstalk between hepatocytes and stromal environment. J Hepatol 2013;59(6):1160–8.

68. Zhu C, Liu X, Wang S, et al. Hepatitis C virus core protein induces hypoxia-inducible factor 1α-mediated vascular endothelial growth factor expression in Huh7.5.1 cells. Mol Med Rep 2014;9(5):2010–4.

69. Sakamuro D, Furukawa T, Takegami T. Hepatitis C virus nonstructural protein NS3 transforms NIH 3T3 cells. J Virol 1995;69(6):3893–6.

70. Zemel R, Gerechet S, Greif H, et al. Cell transformation induced by hepatitis C virus NS3 serine protease. J Viral Hepat 2001;8(2):96–102.

71. Zemel R, Kazatsker A, Greif F, et al. Mutations at vicinity of catalytic sites of hepatitis C virus NS3 serine protease gene isolated from hepatocellular carcinoma tissue. Dig Dis Sci 2000;45(11):2199–202.

72. Kwun HJ, Jung EY, Ahn JY, et al. p53-dependent transcriptional repression of p21(waf1) by hepatitis C virus NS3. J Gen Virol 2001;82(Pt 9):2235–41.

73. Feng DY, Sun Y, Cheng RX, et al. Effect of hepatitis C virus nonstructural protein NS3 on proliferation and MAPK phosphorylation of normal hepatocyte line. World J Gastroenterol 2005;11(14):2157–61.

74. Li B, Li X, Li Y, et al. The effects of hepatitis C virus non-structural protein 3 on cell growth mediated by extracellular signal-related kinase cascades in human hepatocytes in vitro. Int J Mol Med 2010;26(2):273–9.

75. Cheng PL, Chang MH, Chao CH, et al. Hepatitis C viral proteins interact with Smad3 and differentially regulate TGF-beta/Smad3-mediated transcriptional activation. Oncogene 2004;23(47):7821–38.

76. Verga-Gérard A, Porcherot M, Meyniel-Schicklin L, et al. Hepatitis C virus/human interactome identifies SMURF2 and the viral protease as critical elements for the control of TGF-β signaling. FASEB J 2013;27(10):4027–40.

77. Sakata K, Hara M, Terada T, et al. HCV NS3 protease enhances liver fibrosis via binding to and activating TGF-β type I receptor. Sci Rep 2013;3:3243.

78. Ghosh AK, Steele R, Meyer K, et al. Hepatitis C virus NS5A protein modulates cell cycle regulatory genes and promotes cell growth. J Gen Virol 1999;80(Pt 5):1179–83.

79. Majumder M, Ghosh AK, Steele R, et al. Hepatitis C virus NS5A physically associates with p53 and regulates p21/waf1 gene expression in a p53-dependent manner. J Virol 2001;75(3):1401–7.

80. Lan KH, Sheu ML, Hwang SJ, et al. HCV NS5A interacts with p53 and inhibits p53-mediated apoptosis. Oncogene 2002;21(31):4801–11.

81. Cheng D, Zhao L, Zhang L, et al. p53 controls hepatitis C virus non-structural protein 5A-mediated downregulation of GADD45α expression via the NF-κB and PI3K-Akt pathways. J Gen Virol 2013;94(Pt 2):326–35.

82. Tamura RE, de Vasconcellos JF, Sarkar D, et al. GADD45 proteins: central players in tumorigenesis. Curr Mol Med 2012;12(5):634–51.
83. He Y, Nakao H, Tan SL, et al. Subversion of cell signaling pathways by hepatitis C virus nonstructural 5A protein via interaction with Grb2 and P85 phosphatidylinositol 3-kinase. J Virol 2002;76(18):9207–17.
84. Street A, Macdonald A, McCormick C, et al. Hepatitis C virus NS5A-mediated activation of phosphoinositide 3-kinase results in stabilization of cellular beta-catenin and stimulation of beta-catenin-responsive transcription. J Virol 2005; 79(8):5006–16.
85. Milward A, Mankouri J, Harris M. Hepatitis C virus NS5A protein interacts with beta-catenin and stimulates its transcriptional activity in a phosphoinositide-3 kinase-dependent fashion. J Gen Virol 2010;91(Pt 2):3.
86. Higgs MR, Lerat H, Pawlotsky JM. Hepatitis C virus-induced activation of β-catenin promotes c-Myc expression and a cascade of pro-carcinogenetic events. Oncogene 2013;32(39):4683–93.
87. McGivern DR, Lemon SM. Virus-specific mechanisms of carcinogenesis in hepatitis C virus associated liver cancer. Oncogene 2011;30(17):1969–83.
88. Munakata T, Liang Y, Kim S, et al. Hepatitis C virus induces E6AP-dependent degradation of the retinoblastoma protein. PLoS Pathog 2007;3(9):1335–47.
89. Jopling CL, Yi M, Lancaster AM, et al. Modulation of hepatitis C virus RNA abundance by a liver-specific MicroRNA. Science 2005;309(5740):1577–81.
90. Bai S, Nasser MW, Wang B, et al. MicroRNA-122 inhibits tumorigenic properties of hepatocellular carcinoma cells and sensitizes these cells to sorafenib. J Biol Chem 2009;284(46):32015–27.
91. Llovet JM, Burroughs A, Bruix J. Hepatocellular carcinoma. Lancet 2003;362: 1907–17.
92. Fattovich G, Stroffolini T, Zagni I, et al. Hepatocellular carcinoma in cirrhosis: incidence and risk factors. Gastroenterology 2004;127:S35–50.
93. Simonetti RG, Camma C, Fiorello F, et al. Hepatocellular carcinoma. A worldwide problem and the major risk factors. Dig Dis Sci 1991;36:962–72.
94. Chen JD, Yang HI, Iloeje UH, et al. Carriers of inactive hepatitis B virus are still at risk for hepatocellular carcinoma and liver-related death. Gastroenterology 2010;138(5):1747–54.
95. Chen CJ, Yang HI, Su J, et al. Risk of hepatocellular carcinoma across a biological gradient of serum hepatitis B virus DNA level. JAMA 2006;295(1): 65–73.
96. Liu CJ, Chen BF, Chen PJ, et al. Role of hepatitis B virus precore/core promoter mutations and serum viral load on noncirrhotic hepatocellular carcinoma: a case–control study. J Infect Dis 2006;194:594–9.
97. Chemin I, Trépo C. Clinical impact of occult HBV infections. J Clin Virol 2005; 34(Suppl 1):S15–21.
98. De Mitri MS, Cassini R, Bernardi M. Hepatitis B virus-related hepatocarcinogenesis: molecular oncogenic potential of clear or occult infections. Eur J Cancer 2010;46(12):2178–86.
99. Huang X, Hollinger FB. Occult hepatitis B virus infection and hepatocellular carcinoma: a systematic review. J Viral Hepat 2014;21(3):153–62.
100. Buendia MA. Hepatitis B viruses and hepatocellular carcinoma. Adv Cancer Res 1992;59:167–226.
101. Wong N, Lai P, Lee SW, et al. Assessment of genetic changes in hepatocellular carcinoma by comparative genomic hybridization analysis: relationship to disease stage, tumor size, and cirrhosis. Am J Pathol 1999;154:37–43.

102. Fu X, Wan S, Hann HW, et al. Relative telomere length: a novel non-invasive biomarker for the risk of non-cirrhotic hepatocellular carcinoma in patients with chronic hepatitis B infection. Eur J Cancer 2012;48(7):1014–22.

103. Zhang X, Dong N, Zhang H, et al. Effects of hepatitis B virus X protein on human telomerase reverse transcriptase expression and activity in hepatoma cells. J Lab Clin Med 2005;145:98–104.

104. el-Refaie A, Savage K, Bhattacharya S, et al. HCV-associated hepatocellular carcinoma without cirrhosis. J Hepatol 1996;24(3):277–85.

105. Yeh MM, Daniel HD, Torbenson M. Hepatitis C-associated hepatocellular carcinomas in non-cirrhotic livers. Mod Pathol 2010;23(2):276–83.

106. De Mitri MS, Poussin K, Baccarini P. HCV-associated liver cancer without cirrhosis. Lancet 1995;345(8947):413–5.

107. Lok AS, Seeff LB, Morgan TR, et al. Incidence of hepatocellular carcinoma and associated risk factors in hepatitis C-related advanced liver disease. Gastroenterology 2009;136:138–48.

108. Herr W, Gerken G, Poralla T, et al. Hepatitis C virus associated primary hepatocellular carcinoma in a noncirrhotic liver. Clin Investig 1993;71:49–53.

109. Nash KL, Woodall T, Brown AS, et al. Hepatocellular carcinoma in patients with chronic hepatitis C virus infection without cirrhosis. World J Gastroenterol 2010; 16:4061–5.

110. Albeldawi M, Soliman M, Lopez R, et al. Hepatitis C virus-associated primary hepatocellular carcinoma in non-cirrhotic patients. Dig Dis Sci 2012;57(12): 3265–70.

111. Lee MH, Yang HI, Lu SN, et al. Hepatitis C virus seromarkers and subsequent risk of hepatocellular carcinoma: long-term predictors from a community-based cohort study. J Clin Oncol 2010;28(30):4587–93.

112. Lavanchy D. Viral hepatitis: global goals for vaccination. J Clin Virol 2012;55: 296–302.

113. Chang MH, You SL, Chen CJ, et al. Decreased incidence of hepatocellular carcinoma in hepatitis B vaccinees: a 20-year follow-up study. J Natl Cancer Inst 2009;101:1348–55.

114. Chiang CJ, Yang YW, You SL, et al. Thirty-year outcomes of the national hepatitis B immunization program in Taiwan. JAMA 2013;310(9):974–6.

115. Wichajarn K, Kosalaraksa P, Wiangnon S. Incidence of hepatocellular carcinoma in children in Khon Kaen before and after national hepatitis B vaccine program. Asian Pac J Cancer Prev 2008;9:507–9.

116. Lanier AP, Holck P, Ehrsam Day G, et al. Childhood cancer among Alaska natives. Pediatrics 2003;112:e396.

117. Lai CL, Yuen MF. Prevention of hepatitis B virus-related hepatocellular carcinoma with antiviral therapy. Hepatology 2013;57(1):399–408.

118. Iavarone M, Colombo M. HBV infection and hepatocellular carcinoma. Clin Liver Dis 2013;17(3):375–97.

119. Miyake Y, Kobashi H, Yamamoto K. Meta-analysis: the effect of interferon on development of hepatocellular carcinoma in patients with chronic hepatitis B virus infection. J Gastroenterol 2009;44(5):470–5.

120. Yang YF, Zhao W, Zhong YD, et al. Interferon therapy in chronic hepatitis B reduces progression to cirrhosis and hepatocellular carcinoma: a meta-analysis. J Viral Hepat 2009;16(4):265–71.

121. Sung JJ, Tsoi KK, Wong VW, et al. Meta-analysis: treatment of hepatitis B infection reduces risk of hepatocellular carcinoma. Aliment Pharmacol Ther 2008; 28(9):1067–77.

122. Shen YC, Hsu C, Cheng CC, et al. A critical evaluation of the preventive effect of antiviral therapy on the development of hepatocellular carcinoma in patients with chronic hepatitis C or B: a novel approach by using meta-regression. Oncology 2012;82(5):275–89.

123. Cammà C, Giunta M, Andreone P, et al. Interferon and prevention of hepatocellular carcinoma in viral cirrhosis: an evidence-based approach. J Hepatol 2001; 34(4):593–602.

124. Zhang CH, Xu GL, Jia WD, et al. Effects of interferon treatment on development and progression of hepatocellular carcinoma in patients with chronic virus infection: a meta-analysis of randomized controlled trials. Int J Cancer 2011;129(5): 1254–64.

125. Jin H, Pan N, Mou Y, et al. Long-term effect of interferon treatment on the progression of chronic hepatitis B: Bayesian meta-analysis and meta-regression. Hepatol Res 2011;41(6):512–23.

126. Papatheodoridis GV, Manolakopoulos S, Touloumi G, et al. Virological suppression does not prevent the development of hepatocellular carcinoma in HBeAg-negative chronic hepatitis B patients with cirrhosis receiving oral antiviral(s) starting with lamivudine monotherapy: results of the nationwide HEPNET Greece cohort study. Gut 2011;60:1109–16.

127. Papatheodoridis GV, Manolakopoulos S, Touloumi G, et al. Hepatocellular carcinoma risk in HBeAg-negative chronic hepatitis B patients with or without cirrhosis treated with entecavir: HepNet. Greece cohort. J Viral Hepat 2015; 22:118–25.

128. Lampertico P, Soffredini R, Vigano M, et al. Entecavir treatment for NUC naïve, field practice patients with chronic hepatitis B: excellent viral suppression and safety profile over 5 years of treatment. Hepatology 2012;56(S1): 370A.

129. Kim WR, Berg T, Loomba R, et al. Long term tenofovir disoproxil fumarate (TDF) therapy and the risk of hepatocellular carcinoma. J Hepatol 2013;58:S19.

130. Yu ML, Lin SM, Chuang WL, et al. A sustained virological response to interferon or interferon/ribavirin reduces hepatocellular carcinoma and improves survival in chronic hepatitis C: a nationwide, multicenter study in Taiwan. Antivir Ther 2006;11:985–94.

131. Tanaka A, Uegaki S, Kurihara H, et al. Hepatic steatosis as a possible risk factor for the development of hepatocellular carcinoma after eradication of hepatitis C virus with antiviral therapy in patients with chronic hepatitis C. World J Gastroenterol 2007;13(39):5180–7.

132. Cardoso AC, Moucari R, Figueiredo-Mendes C, et al. Impact of peginterferon and ribavirin therapy on hepatocellular carcinoma: incidence and survival in hepatitis C patients with advanced fibrosis. J Hepatol 2010;52(5):652–7.

133. Ogawa E, Furusyo N, Kajiwara E, et al. Efficacy of pegylated interferon alpha-2b and ribavirin treatment on the risk of hepatocellular carcinoma in patients with chronic hepatitis C: a prospective, multicenter study. J Hepatol 2013;58(3): 495–501.

134. Morgan RL, Baack B, Smith BD, et al. Eradication of hepatitis C virus infection and the development of hepatocellular carcinoma: a meta-analysis of observational studies. Ann Intern Med 2013;158(5 Pt 1):329–37.

135. Toyoda H, Kumada T, Nakano S, et al. Effect of the dose and duration of interferon-therapy on the incidence of hepatocellular carcinoma in noncirrhotic patients with a nonsustained response to interferon for chronic hepatitis C. Oncology 2001;61:134–42.

136. Ikeda K, Saitoh S, Kobayashi M, et al. Long-term interferon therapy for 1 year or longer reduces the hepatocellular carcinogenesis rate in patients with liver cirrhosis caused by hepatitis C virus: a pilot study. J Gastroenterol Hepatol 2001;16:406–15.

137. Lok AS, Everhart JE, Wright EC, et al. Maintenance peginterferon therapy and other factors associated with hepatocellular carcinoma in patients with advanced hepatitis C. Gastroenterology 2011;140:840–9.

138. Bruix J, Poynard T, Colombo M, et al. Maintenance therapy with peginterferon alfa-2b does not prevent hepatocellular carcinoma in cirrhotic patients with chronic hepatitis C. Gastroenterology 2011;140(7):1990–9.

139. Huang CF, Yeh ML, Tsai PC, et al. Baseline gamma-glutamyl transferase levels strongly correlate with hepatocellular carcinoma development in non-cirrhotic patients with successful hepatitis C virus eradication. J Hepatol 2014;61(1): 67–74.

140. Scherzer TM, Reddy KR, Wrba F, et al. Hepatocellular carcinoma in long-term sustained virological responders following antiviral combination therapy for chronic hepatitis C. J Viral Hepat 2008;15(9):659–65.

141. Nagaoki Y, Aikata H, Miyaki D, et al. Clinical features and prognosis in patients with hepatocellular carcinoma that developed after hepatitis C virus eradication with interferon therapy. J Gastroenterol 2011;46(6):799–808.

142. Aleman S, Rahbin N, Weiland O, et al. A risk for hepatocellular carcinoma persists long-term after sustained virologic response in patients with hepatitis C-associated liver cirrhosis. Clin Infect Dis 2013;57(2):230–6.

143. Bruix J, Sherman M. Management of hepatocellular carcinoma: an update. Hepatology 2011;53:1020–2.

# Nonalcoholic Fatty Liver Disease, Diabetes, Obesity, and Hepatocellular Carcinoma

Mazen Noureddin, MD[a], Mary E. Rinella, MD[b],*

## KEYWORDS

- Nonalcoholic steatohepatitis • Cirrhosis • Noncirrhotic • Insulin resistance
- Hepatocellular carcinoma • Obesity • Diabetes • Chemoprevention

## KEY POINTS

- Obesity, type 2 diabetes mellitus (T2DM), and insulin resistance are strongly associated with nonalcoholic fatty liver disease (NAFLD) and increased incidence of hepatocellular carcinoma (HCC).
- HCC incidence is increasing as NAFLD becomes the most common cause of liver disease.
- HCC can develop in NAFLD patients without cirrhosis so cancers may be missed given the high prevalence of NAFLD and the limitations of current screening strategies.
- Activation of pathways that promote inflammation, insulin resistance, angiogenesis, and cellular proliferation seen in these diseases promote the development of HCC.
- Clinical studies to prevent the development of HCC in patients with obesity, T2DM or NAFLD are critically needed.

## INTRODUCTION

Nonalcoholic fatty liver disease (NAFLD) is now the most common liver disease in the United States, with more than 80 million Americans affected. It represents a spectrum of diseases ranging from isolated hepatic steatosis (IHS) to steatosis in association with inflammation and cellular injury—the progressive subtype of NAFLD referred to as nonalcoholic steatohepatitis (NASH). NASH is often but not always associated with varying degrees of fibrosis that can develop into cirrhosis and all of its associated complications.[1,2] The prevalence of the disease parallels the epidemic of the metabolic syndrome, namely obesity, type 2 diabetes mellitus (T2DM) and its other

Financial Support: USC Research Center of Liver Diseases, P30 DK48522. Dr M.E. Rinella has provided consulting services for Abbvie, Fibrogen, Takeda, and NGM pharmaceuticals. Dr M. Noureddin has nothing to disclose.
[a] Division of Gastrointestinal and Liver Diseases, USC Keck School of Medicine, 2011 Zonal Avenue, HMR 101, Los Angeles, CA 90033, USA; [b] Division of Gastroenterology and Hepatology, Northwestern University Feinberg School of Medicine, 676 North Saint Clair, Arkes Pavillion 14-005, Chicago, IL 60611, USA
* Corresponding author.
E-mail address: m-rinella@northwestern.edu

manifestations worldwide. It is no surprise that the mechanisms underlying the metabolic syndrome, insulin resistance, and obesity are also important in the development of both IHS and NASH.[3]

Hepatocellular carcinoma (HCC), known to occur most commonly in the setting of cirrhosis, is also increasing in incidence, and is now the second leading cause of cancer deaths worldwide.[4] Historically, the risk factors for HCC in the United States have primarily included alcoholic cirrhosis, hepatitis B virus (HBV) infection, hemochromatosis, and hepatitis C virus (HCV) infection. Because of its link to the HCV epidemic, HCC is considered the fastest growing cause of cancer mortality overall in the United States as well.[5] However, the clinical landscape of HCV is changing rapidly into a future where cure is not only probable, but will be nearly universal for those who have access to therapy. No doubt, this will reduce the development of HCV-related HCC in the future. Results of recent studies demonstrate that HCC is more prevalent in the setting of obesity and insulin resistance, and may occur in NAFLD patients without cirrhosis.[4] Therefore, if the incidence of obesity, diabetes, and NASH continues to increase, and the HCV-related association decreases with effective treatment strategies, NAFLD could become the most common cause of HCC in the United States and other developed countries. Indeed, in a recent retrospective cohort study that evaluated trends in HCC etiology among adult liver transplant recipients from 2002 to 2012, the number of patients undergoing liver transplant for HCC secondary to NASH increased by nearly 4-fold, whereas the number of patients with HCC secondary to HCV increased by only 2-fold.[6] During that same 10-year period, the prevalence of NASH-related HCC increased steadily, becoming the second leading etiology of HCC-related liver transplant in the United States (increasing from 8.3% in 2002 to 10.3% in 2007 and to 13.5% in 2012).

To clarify these relationships, this review discusses the pathophysiologic mechanisms that underpin the close relationship between obesity, insulin resistance, NAFLD, and the progression to HCC, both in the presence and absence of cirrhosis.

## OBESITY, DIABETES, NONALCOHOLIC FATTY LIVER DISEASE, AND NONALCOHOLIC STEATOHEPATITIS AS RISK FACTORS FOR HEPATOCELLULAR CARCINOMA

The results of several studies have elucidated the relative risk of several disease processes that are implicated in the pathogenesis of HCC. In a population-based study, authors analyzed 6991 cases from the Surveillance, Epidemiology, and End Results–Medicare databases that link cancer registry data and Medicare enrollment during the period from1994 to 2007.[7] The authors estimated the population-attributable fractions (PAFs), that is, the proportions of cases that can be attributed to specific risk factors. They found that T2DM and/or obesity had the greatest PAF (36.6%), followed by alcohol-related disorders (23.5%), HCV (22.4%), HBV (6.3%), and rare genetic disorders (3.2%; **Fig. 1**). Although the relative risk of HCV for HCC incidence (39.9) was higher than the relative risk of T2DM and/or obesity (2.47), the high prevalence of T2DM and obesity in the United States accounted for more cases of HCC than HCV. However, the exact PAF of NAFLD remains to be determined, because NAFLD cases per se were not identified in the Surveillance, Epidemiology, and End Results database. Although the study was limited to age groups 68 years or older, it represented about 25% of the general population of the United States.[7]

In other studies, a direct relationship between obesity and HCC has been demonstrated. Available data suggest that obesity increases the risk of HCC 1.5- to 4-fold (**Table 1**).[8–10] In Danish and Korean studies, an association between obesity and an increased relative risk of HCC (1.9 and 1.56, respectively) was seen.[9,11] Data

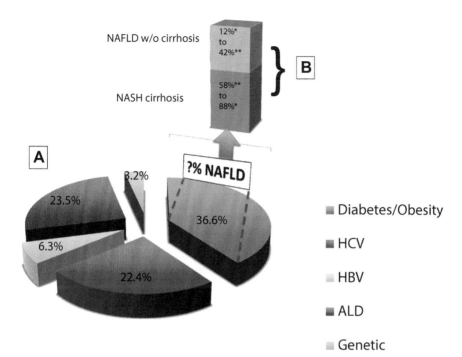

**Fig. 1.** Risk factors for hepatocellular carcinoma (HCC) incidence in the United States. (*A*) Risk factors of HCC in the United States (presented as percentage). In a study by Welzel and colleagues of 6991 cases from the Surveillance, Epidemiology, and End Results (SEER)–Medicare databases from 1994 to 2007 the authors estimated the PAFs, that is, the proportions of cases that can be attributed to specific risk factors. The PAF owing to type 2 diabetes mellitus (T2DM) and/or obesity was the highest (36.6%), followed by alcohol-related disorders (23.5%), HCV (22.4%), HBV (6.3%), and rare genetic disorders (3.2%). Although the contribution of NAFLD is not exactly known, it is thought to contribute to the majority of the obesity and diabetes cases. (*B*) A breakdown of cases of HCC occurring in the setting of NAFLD in the presence or absence of cirrhosis to HCC. ALD, alcoholic liver disease; HBV, hepatitis B virus; HCV, hepatitis C virus; NAFLD, nonalcoholic fatty liver disease; NASH, nonalcoholic steatohepatitis. (*Data from* [*A*] Welzel TM, Graubard BI, Quraishi S, et al. Population-attributable fractions of risk factors for hepatocellular carcinoma in the United States. Am J Gastroenterol 2013;108(8):1314–21; [*B*] *Hashimoto E, Yatsuji S, Tobari M, et al. Hepatocellular carcinoma in patients with nonalcoholic steatohepatitis. J Gastroenterol 2009;44 Suppl 19:89–95; and **Mittal S, Sada YH, El-Serag HB, et al. Temporal trends of non-alcoholic fatty liver disease-related hepatocellular carcinoma in the veteran affairs population. Clin Gastroenterol Hepatol 2014;146(5):S–917.)

from the United States also suggest that with obesity there is a significantly elevated relative risk of death from many cancers including HCC (4.52 for men; see **Table 1**).[8] One large meta-analysis included 7 cohort studies in 5037 overweight subjects (body mass index of 25–30 kg/m$^2$) and 10 studies in 6042 obese subjects (body mass index of $\geq$30 kg/m$^2$). The authors found that, compared with normal weight people, HCC risk increased 17% in those who were overweight and 89% in those who were obese.[12] Furthermore, in a study from Japan that looked at the recurrence of HCC after ablation therapy in NASH patients, the authors found that increased visceral fat was an independent risk factor for recurrence of HCC at 3 years (75.1% vs 43.1% with low visceral fat).[13] The mechanism through which obesity leads to increased HCC is thought to be related

**Table 1**
**Risk of obesity, diabetes, and NAFLD on incidence of HCC**

| Author, Year | Location | Cases | Study Type | Risk Measurement | Reported Risk |
|---|---|---|---|---|---|
| **Obesity** | | | | | |
| Moller et al,[9] 1994 | Denmark | 43,965 | Case control | RR | 1.9 |
| Wolk et al,[10] 2001 | Sweden | 28,129 | Case control | SIR | 2.4 |
| Calle et al,[8] 2003 | USA | 90,000 | Prospective | RR | 1.68 (F), 4.52 (M) |
| Oh et al,[11] 2005 | Korea | 781,283 | Prospective | RR | 1.56 |
| Larsson et al,[12] 2007 | NA | 11,079 | Meta-analysis | RR | 1.89 |
| **Diabetes** | | | | | |
| Adami et al,[15] 1996 | Sweden | 153,852 | Case control | SIR | 4.1 |
| Wideroff et al,[17] 1997 | Denmark | 109,581 | Case control | SIR | 4 (M), 2.1 (F) |
| El-Serag et al,[16] 2004 | USA | 824,263 | Case control | HRR | 2.16 |
| Yang et al,[18] 2011 | NA | NR | Meta-analysis | RR | 1.87 |
| Wang et al,[111] 2012 | NA | NR | Meta-analysis | RR | 2.31 |
| **NAFLD/NASH** | | | | | |
| Adams et al,[26] 2005 | USA | 420 | Prospective | Prevalence | 0.5% |
| Ekstedt et al,[24] 2006 | Sweden | 129 | Prospective | Prevalence | 2.3% |
| Rafiq et al,[25] 2009 | USA | 173 | Retrospective | Prevalence | 0% NAFLD and 2.8% NASH |
| Ascha et al,[28] 2010 | USA | 195 | Retrospective | Prevalence | 12.8% in NASH cirrhosis |

*Abbreviations:* CC, cryptogenic cirrhosis; F, female; HCC, hepatocellular carcinoma; HRR, hazard rate ratios; M, male; NAFLD, non-alcoholic fatty liver disease; NASH, non-alcoholic steatohepatitis; OR, odds ratio; RR, relative risk; SIR, standardized incidence ratio.
*Data from* Refs.[8–12,15–19,24–26,28]

both to a direct effect of obesity on insulin resistance and the perpetuation of a proinflammatory milieu, as well as via its role in the development and progression of liver disease in patients with NAFLD. In a 2008 review of studies of the epidemiology of NAFLD, Lazo and Clark[14] found that, on average, 76% (range, 33%–99%) of obese patients undergoing bariatric surgery are reported to have steatosis and 37% (range, 9.8%–72.5%) NASH.

In a similar trend seen in many studies, T2DM was associated with a substantially increased risk of HCC (see **Table 1**). In a large cohort from Sweden consisting of 153,852 diabetics, the risk of HCC was increased 4-fold. Even after exclusion of other risk factors for HCC, such as cirrhosis and viral hepatitis, T2DM was associated with a 3-fold increased risk of HCC.[15] In a large study from the Veterans Administration (VA) hospitals in the United States similar conclusions were drawn. Of 173,643 diabetic patients and 650,620 nondiabetic controls followed over 10 to 15 years, the incidence of HCC was increased more than 2-fold in diabetic patients, with the risk remaining significant even after the exclusion of patients with other causes of liver disease, including NAFLD.[16] One limitation of these studies is that other causes of liver disease, such as alcohol and viral hepatitis, could have been underestimated because diagnosis identification codes were used to identify patients. In a large Danish study of 109,581 patients hospitalized for T2DM, the standardized incidence ratio for HCC was 4 in men and 2.1 in women.[17] Two large meta-analyses in 2011 confirmed that the relative risks of T2DM for the development of HCC were 1.87 and 2.31, respectively.[18,19] Most recently, a 2014 meta-analysis of 21 studies that included a total of

9767 HCC patients evaluated the association of T2DM with overall and disease-free survival in HCC.[20] In this study the pooled hazard ratios were 1.46 for overall survival and 1.57 for disease-free survival for patients with DM. Although it is possible that the increased HCC risk associated with diabetes seen in these studies may be mediated through the development of NAFLD, the presence of multiple pathogenic mechanisms common to obesity, insulin resistance and NAFLD[21] suggests that this link may not be mediated through NAFLD per se.[12]

Data from several retrospective and prospective studies demonstrate a direct relationship between NASH and HCC. Retrospective results suggest that between 4% and 27% of NASH patients develop HCC at one point[22,23]; however, the true prevalence of HCC across the whole spectrum of NAFLD remains unknown. In prospective studies, the reported prevalence of HCC was 0% to 0.5% in patients with IHS, and as high as 12.8% in those with NASH.[24–26] In a cross-sectional study of 4406 HCC patients, 59% had NAFLD/NASH, 36% T2DM, and 22% HCV infection.[27] In this context, it is noteworthy that patients with HCV cirrhosis develop HCC at a higher rate than those with NAFLD/NASH. Ascha and colleagues[28] followed 195 patients with NASH cirrhosis and 315 patients with HCV cirrhosis for 3.2 years and identified HCC in 12.8% and 20.3% of patients in the NASH and HCV groups, respectively. Here, the yearly cumulative incidence of HCC was 2.6% in patients with NASH-associated cirrhosis, whereas it was 4.0% in those with HCV-associated cirrhosis. Bhala and colleagues[29] studied patients with advanced fibrosis and cirrhosis, including 247 owing to NASH and 264 owing to HCV, who were followed for a mean of 85.6 months. They found that NAFLD patients had a lower incidence of HCC compared with those with HCV (2.4% vs 6.8%; $P<.03$). In comparison to Ascha and associates' study,[28] Bhala and colleagues attributed the lower incidence of HCC in both their NASH and HCV populations to potential differences in population risk factors and the fact that only those with biopsy-proven NASH were included in the Ascha and colleagues study.

NASH is increasing in importance as an indication for liver transplantation (LT) and may exceed HCV as an indication numerically over the next decade. Interestingly, although HCC may occur more commonly in patients with HCV cirrhosis, the rate at which patients are transplanted for HCC in the setting of NASH is increasing rapidly. Indeed, in a recent retrospective cohort study that evaluated trends in HCC as an etiology among adult LT recipients from 2002 to 2012, the authors found that the number of patients undergoing LT for HCC secondary to NASH increased by nearly 4-fold, whereas the number of LT patients with HCC secondary to HCV increased by only 2.5-fold in the Model of End-stage Liver Disease era of LT listing.[6] As noted, during that 10-year period, NASH-related HCC increased steadily, becoming the second leading etiology of HCC-related LT in the United States.

## HEPATOCELLULAR CARCINOMA IN NONALCOHOLIC FATTY LIVER DISEASE WITHOUT CIRRHOSIS

The fact that fibrosis and cirrhosis are not necessary for the development of HCC in NASH patients indicates that obesity, insulin resistance, and the proinflammatory milieu of NASH may mediate carcinogenesis directly. Evidence of the development of HCC in noncirrhotic patients continues to accumulate in case reports or case series (**Table 2**).[29–52] In a recent study analyzing 1419 HCC cases that were related to NASH (120 cases), HCV (1013), and alcohol (286) in the VA system, cirrhosis was present in only 58.3% of NASH-related HCC cases.[51] The researchers also found less robust adherence to HCC surveillance in NASH patients than in patients with HCV or alcoholic liver disease, and attributed the high rate of incidence of HCC in NASH without

**Table 2**
Reports of HCC incidence in NAFLD/NASH without cirrhosis

| Study, Year | No. of Cases | Average Age (y) | Gender | Fibrosis | Comorbidities | Tumor |
|---|---|---|---|---|---|---|
| Zen et al,[30] 2001 | 1 | 62 | F | Pericellular | DM | Multifocal |
| Orikasa et al,[31] 2001 | 1 | 67 | F | Bridging | DM | Solitary |
| Bencheqroun et al,[32] 2004 | 1 | 68 | M | F2 | DM | Solitary |
| Bullock et al,[33] 2004 | 2 | 64/74 | M | None (F0) | DM, HTN, obesity | Solitary |
| Gonzalez et al,[34] 2004 | 1 | 73 | M | F1 | DM, HTN, obesity | Solitary |
| Cuadrado et al,[35] 2005 | 1 | 71 | M | Portal | DM, obesity | Solitary |
| Sato et al,[36] 2005 | 1 | 64 | M | Bridging | Obesity, dyslipidemia | Solitary |
| Hai et al,[37] 2006 | 1 | 72 | M | F2 | DM | Solitary |
| Ichikawa et al,[38] 2006 | 2 | 60/66 | M/F | F2–F3 | DM, obesity | Solitary |
| Hashizume et al,[39] 2007 | 3 | 54/72/82 | M | F1–F3 | DM, HTN, obesity | Solitary (2), Multifocal (1) |
| Guzman et al,[40] 2008 | 3 | 45/57/70 | M (1), F (2) | F0 | DM, HTN, obesity, dyslipidemia | Multifocal |
| Chagas et al,[41] 2009 | 1 | 65 | M | F1 | Obesity, dyslipidemia | Multifocal |
| Paradis et al,[42] 2009 | 16 | NR | M (16) | F0–F3 | DM, HTN, obesity, dyslipidemia | NR |
| Kawada et al,[43] 2009 | 6 | 59–81 | M (3), F (3) | F2–F3 | DM, HTN, obesity, dyslipidemia | Solitary |
| Hashimoto et al,[44] 2009 | 4/34 (12%) | NR | M, F | F1–F2 | NR | NR |
| Takuma et al,[45] 2010 | 7 | 67–75 | M (3), F (3) | F1–F3 | DM, HTN, obesity, dyslipidemia | Solitary (5), multifocal (2) |
| Tokushige et al,[46] 2010 | 10 | NR | NR | F1 (1), F2 (3), F3 (10) | NR | NR |
| Yasui et al,[47] 2011 | 43 | NR | M (77%) | F1 (10), F2 (15), F3 (18) | DM, HTN, obesity, dyslipidemia | Solitary (72%) |
| Ikura et al,[49] 2011 | 1 | 72 | M | F1 | HTN | Solitary |
| Ertle et al,[52] 2011 | 10 | 69 | M (89%) | F0–F3 | DM, HTN, obesity, dyslipidemia | NR |
| Mittal et al,[51] 2014 | ≈50 | NR | NR | NR | DM, HTN, obesity, dyslipidemia | NR |

*Abbreviations:* DM, diabetes; F, female; HTN, hypertension; M, male; NR, not reported.
*Data from* Refs.[30–47,49,51,52]

cirrhosis (41.7%) to the lower rate of surveillance, because there is currently no recommendation for surveillance in this population. There is also the incorrect perception that NASH patients without cirrhosis are unlikely to develop HCC. Interestingly, despite the lack of surveillance and resulting early detection, the 1-year survival rate did not differ among the different etiologies of HCC.[53]

Interesting insights into possible areas of further research can be derived from NASH–HCC studies in which potential differences between NASH- and HCV-associated HCC are suggested. In the Mittal and colleagues'[51] analysis of the VA population previously discussed, the authors noted that patients with NASH more often had fewer alpha-fetoprotein–secreting tumors. The authors speculated that less aggressive tumor biology in NASH-related HCC could be partially explained by this finding, but it could also be related to the short period of survival rate estimation of only 1 year. A Japanese group also reported lower alpha-fetoprotein synthesis in NASH-associated HCC (35.3%) compared with 69.6% of tumors in patients with HCV.[48] Furthermore, they found that 52.9% of patients with NASH-related HCC had elevated des-gamma-carboxy prothrombin, a biomarker of HCC, compared with 41.3% of patients with HCV-related HCC.[46] This result suggests that the tumor markers and cancer biology in NASH-related HCC may differ from HCV-related HCC, and should be investigated further.

Results of several studies support the possibility that NASH-related HCC may behave differently in certain subpopulations. Limited available data suggest that risk factors for the development of NASH without cirrhosis include older age, male gender, and the metabolic syndrome (see **Table 2**). Indeed, HCC was even reported to develop in patients with the metabolic syndrome and features of IHS without steatohepatitis or fibrosis.[40] In a study of 87 Japanese NASH patients with HCC, Yasui and colleagues[47] found that 56% of patients were noncirrhotic. The authors stratified the data by gender and noted that men developed HCC at a less advanced stage of liver fibrosis than women. Hashimoto and colleagues[44] examined 34 cases of NASH-related HCC and found that there was a prevalence of advanced age, male gender, obesity, and T2DM; 12% of the patients had stage 1 or 2 fibrosis and 88% had advanced fibrosis (stage 3–4). These HCC patients tended to be older, male, and to have the metabolic syndrome. Although there are currently no recommendations to initiate HCC screening in noncirrhotic NASH, mounting data suggest that it should be a concern, particularly for older men with the metabolic syndrome. Inexpensive and reliable methods of HCC detection are needed to capture reliably patients at risk for HCC before the development of cirrhosis. Revisiting the surveillance guidelines may be warranted.

## PATHOGENESIS OF HEPATOCELLULAR CARCINOMA IN OBESITY, DIABETES, AND NONALCOHOLIC FATTY LIVER DISEASE

Although the precise pathogenesis by which obesity and insulin resistance foster the development of HCC is not defined clearly, several mechanisms could operate in the setting of NAFLD. The inflammatory milieu associated with obesity and insulin resistance is characterized by abundant oxidative stress, activation of the unfolded protein response (UPR), and other inflammatory processes, including activation of the innate immune system. Many of these pathways could play a major role in the tumorigenicity and development of DNA damage, which provide a favorable setting for the development of HCC.[53] Insulin resistance and obesity promote an aberrant adipocytokine profile, including increased interleukin-6, leptin, and tumor necrosis factor (TNF)-α and decreased adiponectin, which seems to contribute to increased cellular proliferation, angiogenesis, inhibition of apoptosis, and worsening insulin resistance.[54,55]

## Insulin Resistance

In a prospective study of 6237 French men, hyperinsulinemia was associated with an approximately 3-fold increased risk for HCC.[56] In addition to its role in glucose and lipid metabolism, insulin has pleotropic effects that regulate inflammatory and other pathways. Insulin-like growth factor-1 (IGF-1) and insulin receptor substrate-1 (IRS-1), an important substrate of IGF-1, are downstream targets of insulin that are crucial to cellular proliferation (**Fig. 2**).[57,58] Human HCC cells overexpress both IGF-1[59] and IRS-1.[60] IRS-1–mediated signals may act as survival factors and protect against transforming growth factor β1–induced apoptosis in HCC, which may contribute to hepatic oncogenesis.[61] In addition, IRS-1 can promote hepatocyte proliferation via mitogen-activated protein kinase and phosphatidylinositol–3 kinase (PI3K), important pathways in HCC development.[61] Interestingly, cirrhotic patients with HCC and impaired glucose metabolism that causes postprandial hyperinsulinemia have accelerated HCC growth.[62] The PI3K/phosphatase and tensin homolog (PTEN)/Akt axis is a key regulator of critical cellular functions such as insulin and other growth factor signaling, glucose and lipid homeostasis, and apoptosis.[63]

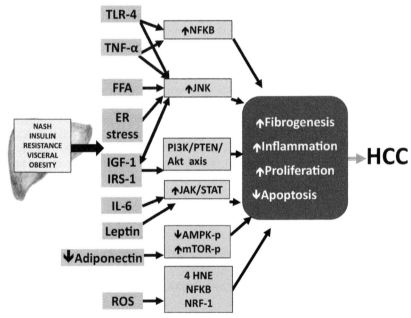

**Fig. 2.** Potential pathways linking NASH to HCC. The inflammatory milieu associated with obesity, insulin resistance and NASH leads to the activation of multiple pathways that impair insulin signaling, induce oxidative stress, ER stress and other inflammatory processes. These in turn lead to the activation of oncogenic signaling pathways such as PI3K/PTEN/Akt, JAK/STAT, NF-κB, mTOR, 4HNE and NRF-1. In concert, these pathways promote cellular proliferation, increased angiogenesis, decreased apoptosis that can then foster the development of HCC. 4 HNE, trans-4-hydroxy-2-nonenal; AMPK-p, activated protein kinase; ER, endoplasmic reticulum; FFA, free fatty acids; IGF-1, insulin-like growth factor-1; IL-6, interleukin-6; IRS-1, insulin receptor substrate-1; mTOR-p, mammalian target of rapamycin complex 1; NF-κB, nuclear factor kappa B; NRF-1, nuclear factor erythroid 2-related factor; PI3k, phosphatidylinositol-3 kinase; PTEN, PI3K/phosphatase and tensin homolog; TLR, Toll-like receptors; TNF-α, tumor necrosis factor-α.

PTEN acts as a phosphoinositide phosphatase which terminates PI3K-propagated signaling.[63] Thus, PTEN is a tumor suppressor that is dysregulated in obesity, insulin resistance, and T2DM, thus offering another mechanism through which NAFLD, T2DM, and insulin resistance could promote tumor growth in the setting of HCC.[63]

### c-Jun amino-terminal kinases

The c-Jun amino-terminal kinases (JNKs) are associated with development of NASH and hepatic carcinogenesis.[64-67] Free fatty acids, reactive oxygen species and TNF-α are increased in the setting of hyperinsulinemia and are activators of JNK1, which in turn phosphorylates IRS-1 (see **Fig. 1**). JNK1 activation and the subsequent phosphorylation of IRS-1 are very important factors in obesity-induced insulin resistance and increased hepatic inflammation and apoptosis; JNK2 has been shown not to play a role.[64,65,68] Puri and colleagues[64] have shown that the extent of JNK activation is associated with the level of histologic activity in NASH patients. Several studies have described an important role of JNK1 in the development of HCC.[66,67,69] Chang and colleagues[66] demonstrated enhanced JNK1 activation in 55% of human HCC samples compared with non-HCC liver tissue. JNK1 plays an important role in the development of HCC, partially through activation of the mammalian target of rapamycin mTOR complex 1, which is involved in several human cancers.[70,71]

### Endoplasmic Reticulum Stress

Emerging data suggest that endoplasmic reticulum (ER) stress plays an important role in NASH and HCC.[72-74] The ER regulates protein synthesis and folding for a variety of cellular processes. Various stressors, such as nutrient or glucose deprivation, viral infections, disrupted calcium homeostasis, protein glycosylation, and excess fatty acids, can promote the accumulation of unfolded or misfolded proteins in the ER lumen and activation of an adaptive response called the UPR, which can result in salvage or further injury and apoptosis, depending on the trigger and milieu.[75-77] JNK is a downstream target of the inositol-requiring enzyme-1, a branch of the UPR that has been shown to perpetuate inflammatory processes and insulin resistance.[76] Both ER stress and the subsequent activation of the UPR have been found to play a role in HCC.[78] Although the exact mechanism is not understood completely, it is thought to be owing to the effect of the activation of extracellular signal-regulated protein kinase (ERK) which is highly expressed in HCC via PIK13 activation. ER stress also activates the nuclear factor erythroid 2-related factor 2 and transcription factor-6, both of which regulate the small heterodimer partner nuclear receptor, leading to its suppression. This in turn activates cyclin D1 and hence increases tumorigenicity and hepatocyte proliferation.[79,80]

Insulin resistance is also associated with increased oxidative stress. The generation of reactive oxygen species leads to upregulation of proinflammatory cytokines such as TNF-α. This upregulation then can promote tumor growth via both anti-apoptotic action and further upregulation of proinflammatory cytokines through activation of nuclear factor-kappa B (NF-κB).[81] Oxidative stress may favor tumorigenesis via inflammation and dysregulated cell proliferation; however, it may also directly induce cancer-promoting gene mutations. Trans-4-hydroxy-2-nonenal (4HNE), a product of lipid peroxidation, is important in cancers that are caused by mutations of the p53 gene (see **Fig. 2**).[82] The p53 pathway targets include wild-type p53 activated fragment (p21WAF), a cyclin-dependent kinase inhibitor and the growth arrest DNA damage gene, GADD45, a p53-regulated and DNA damage-inducible protein, and the 14-3-3 protein, which plays a role in G2/M arrest.[83] Nuclear respiratory factor-1 (Nrf-1) is an essential transcription factor in the prevention of oxidative injury. Nrf-1 knockout mice develop NASH and progress to HCC owing to increased oxidative stress.[84] In a human study, Maki and colleagues[85] showed a higher incidence and recurrence of HCC in patients with high levels of 8-Oxo-2'-deoxyguanosine (8-OHdG) and 4HNE in liver tissue, suggesting that oxidative stress may influence HCC carcinogenesis or tumor biological behavior.

### Leptin

Leptin, a product of the obese (*ob*) gene, is a regulator of food intake and energy expenditure via hypothalamic-mediated mechanisms.[86] The importance of leptin in angiogenesis, hematopoiesis, and lipid and carbohydrate metabolism as well as in immune systems, has been demonstrated recently.[86,87] Furthermore, leptin has a direct effect on hepatic stellate cells and is likely to play an important role in the progression of liver fibrosis in NASH.[87] The leptin receptor has 6 isoforms, of which obRB is the most important. Leptin levels are increased in obese individuals, suggesting a state of leptin resistance.[86] Suppressors of cytokine signaling and insulin resistance are associated with leptin resistance, with higher levels of leptin found in NASH patients and in patients with HCC.[88,89] In a human study, the expression of leptin and its receptor in both adjacent nontumor liver tissue and HCC tissue was explored using immunohistochemical staining. It was found that adjacent nontumorous liver tissue expressed higher levels of leptin and its receptor than the HCC tissue.[89] The authors suggested that leptin might act as an endocrine growth factor that stimulates hepatocytes toward the initiation and progression of HCC.

Available evidence suggests that leptin mediates its effect through the Jak2/Stat 3 pathway, which in turn augments cyclin D1 protein expression, leading to cellular proliferation and thereby the development of HCC.[90] In addition, leptin inhibits apoptosis by inhibiting transforming growth factor-$\beta$1. Therefore, leptin may mediate HCC oncogenesis via stimulation of proliferation and inhibition of proapoptotic pathways. Interestingly, these pathways also lead to increased methionine adenosyl transferase (MAT) 2A and MAT2b gene expression, which are known to play a role in hepatocyte proliferation.[91] Finally, leptin promotes fibrogenesis by stimulating hepatic stellate cells. Stellate cells are critical mediators of fibrogenesis and angiogenesis via multiple pathways including ERK/Akt, nuclear factor kappa D (NF-$\kappa$D), and hypoxia-inducible factor 1, each of which has been associated with the development of HCC.[87,92]

### S-Adenosylmethionine

Recently, a role for abnormal levels of S-adenosylmethionine (SAMe) in the development of NASH and HCC has been proposed.[93] SAMe is the principal biological methyl donor made in all mammalian cells. The liver plays a central role in the homeostasis of SAMe.[93,94] SAMe is endogenously produced from methionine and adenosine triphosphate by MAT.[93] MAT has 2 subunits, $\alpha$1 and $\alpha$2, encoded by MAT1A and MAT2A. MAT1A is expressed mostly in differentiated liver and encodes the $\alpha$1 subunit, whereas MAT2A encodes for the catalytic subunit $\alpha$2, which is distributed widely. Mice deficient in MAT1A develop NASH and HCC. Deletion of MAT1A may impair very-low-density lipoprotein (VLDL) assembly, leading to the synthesis of small, lipid-poor VLDL particles and decreased secretion of triglycerides. Additionally, low SAMe levels promote proinflammatory cytokine release and development of NASH.[93] Several abnormal pathways have also been identified in MAT1A-knockout mice that can contribute to HCC formation, including (1) a decrease in apurinic/apyrimidinic endonuclease activity, which leads to DNA instability and malignant transformation, (2) increased liver kinase B1 activity, which induces the activation of 5' adenosine monophosphate-activated protein kinase (AMPK) and enhanced hepatocyte proliferation, (3) leptin signaling, which induces MAT2A and MAT2b genes via activation of these survival pathways and promotes enhanced cell proliferation (the MAT2A-encoded protein induces leptin's mitogenic response by raising intracellular SAMe levels, leading to polyamine biosynthesis and growth), and (4) activation of the ERK pathway, which is highly expressed in HCC.[93]

These pathways suggest that the tumorigenic process is closely related to insulin resistance, oxidative stress and changes in adiponectin and leptin levels which precede the development of fibrosis. Thus, it is plausible that HCC development in NASH patients without cirrhosis is the result of the activation of these pathways.

### Toll-Like Receptors

TLRs are a family of pattern-recognition receptors that recognize pathogen-associated molecular patterns and endogenous components that result from cell death, known as damage-associated molecular patterns, and activate the innate immune system.[95–97] Ten members of the TLR family have been identified. They play a role in ligand recognition after which a signal via myeloid differentiation factor (MyD)88 leads to activation of NF-κB and production of proinflammatory cytokines, including TNF-α and IL-6.[96,98] The MyD88-dependent pathways activate JNK signaling as well. TLR4 may play a specific role in HCC progression by increasing proliferation, preventing apoptosis, and increasing production of cytokines (TNF-α and interleukin-6).[99,100]

### Potential Chemoprevention of Hepatocellular Carcinoma in Obesity and Nonalcoholic Fatty Liver Disease

There is currently no effective chemoprevention to decrease the incidence of HCC, irrespective of disease etiology, with the possible exceptions of the treatment of HBV and HCV infection.[101] With soaring numbers of NAFLD/NASH patients and the incremental increase in HCC, chemopreventive agents are crucially needed. Indeed, with increasing evidence that HCC can develop in NASH without cirrhosis, the lack of clear recommendations for surveillance in this population and the absence of effective treatments for NASH is concerning. Preliminary data point to statins, metformin, and SAMe as potentially effective chemopreventive compounds. Clinical trials are urgently needed to evaluate methods to prevent or hinder the development of HCC in patients with NASH.

### Statins

In previous studies, a beneficial effect of statins in reducing the risk of HCC has been shown.[102–104] Multiple mechanisms have been proposed from animal studies, including (1) statin inhibition of cell proliferation via inhibition of v-myc avian myelocytomatosis viral oncogene homolog (MYC) protein phosphorylation which seems to play a role in liver tumorigenicity (atorvastatin blocked MYC and suppressed tumor initiation in an animal model of MYC-induced HCC and in human cell lines of HCC[105]), (2) induction of apoptosis (simvastatin was found to induce apoptosis selectively in living cancer cells but not in normal cells[106,107]), and (3) inhibition of angiogenesis.[107]

In a randomized trial of 91 patients with HCC who were treated with local therapy followed by randomization to either 40 mg of atorvastatin or placebo, survival was increased in the atorvastatin group (18 vs 9 months; $P = .006$).[104] In a matched case-control study conducted within a VA cohort of patients with T2DM, the incidence of HCC was reported at least 6 months after entry in the cohort.[103] Statin use was recorded by searching filled prescriptions. The study identified 1303 HCC cases and 5212 controls and found a significant reduction in the incidence of HCC (range,

25%–40%) in statin-treated diabetic patients. This beneficial effect was evident in patients with and without cirrhosis. This study was limited by many confounding variables, including in particular that patients with T2D have lipid abnormalities and that NAFLD was not identified per se given the lack of a diagnostic code for NAFLD in the VA system. In a recent nationwide case-control study from Sweden, 3994 HCC patients treated with statins (determined from the national drug registry) were compared with 19,970 controls matched by age and sex.[102] In this study, the odds ratio for HCC among statin users was 0.88, suggesting a modest effect of statins on decreasing the risk of HCC.[102] Although these data are intriguing, they have important limitations and the true effect of statins on chemoprevention in HCC will need to be ascertained through carefully conducted, randomized, controlled trials.

## Metformin

Although metformin may not have significant efficacy in the treatment of NASH itself, it may have a role in decreasing the risk of HCC. In several studies, insulin sensitizers in patients with T2DM may have reduced the risk of HCC.[108–114] Metformin has an antitumor effect in HCC through the suppression of the mTOR pathway which occurs via 2 mechanisms. The first mechanism involves inhibition of mitochondrial oxidative phosphorylation leading to AMPK activation and subsequent mTOR pathway suppression; the second mechanism works via glycemic control leading to inhibition of IGF-R and thus inactivation of the mTOR pathway in insulin-responsive cancers.[115] A large Italian case control study compared 610 HCC patients treated with metformin with 618 untreated cirrhotic patients and 1696 controls.[109] Metformin use was associated with a decreased incidence of HCC in diabetic patients (odds ratio, 0.15). Given the complex relationship between T2DM, HCC, and cirrhosis and the fact that this was a retrospective case control study, a definitive conclusion cannot be drawn from this research. Two recent meta-analyses included 10 studies with 22,650 cases of HCC in 334,307 patients with T2DM. Metformin use was associated with a 50% reduction in the incidence of HCC, whereas sulfonylurea and insulin use increased HCC incidence by 62% and 161%, respectively.[111] Similarly, another metaanalysis of 17 case-controlled studies and 32 cohort studies of HCC reported a combined relative risk estimate of 2.31 for HCC among diabetic patients. In these studies, sulphonylureas and treatment with insulin increased the risk of HCC. The authors attributed this increased risk to the effects of hyperinsulinemia on stimulating oncogenesis. In another study, survival in 135 patients with early stage HCC who underwent radiofrequency ablation was assessed; of the 53 diabetic patients, 21 were treated with metformin and 32 were not. The authors found that the survival rate after ablation was less in diabetic patients compared with nondiabetic patients (1 year, 82.8% vs 93.9%; 3 years, 55.1% vs 80.2%; 5 years, 41.3% vs 64.7%; $P = .004$) and that survival was further decreased in diabetics who were not on metformin (hazard ratio, −0.24; $P = .02$) compared with those who were.[112] Large, randomized trials are needed to better understand the role of metformin or other antidiabetic drugs in HCC chemoprevention.

## S-Adenosylmethionine

Lu and colleagues[116] examined the effect of SAMe for chemoprevention of HCC in animal models. Here, SAMe led to inhibition of HCC progression and showed proapoptotic and antiangiogenic properties. Because of the potential direct effect of SAMe on HCC pathogenesis and its proapoptotic and antiangiogenic properties,[93,117] there is an ongoing phase II clinical trial using SAMe as a chemopreventive agent in HCC patients with hepatitis C in the setting of NAFLD.

## SUMMARY

HCC and NAFLD are growing epidemics that seem to be interrelated and pose an important burden to public health. Obesity, T2DM, and NAFLD clearly augment the risk of HCC via multiple pathways, many of which are common to all 3 conditions. Resultant dysregulation of adipocytokines, oxidative stress, and insulin resistance contribute to a proinflammatory milieu that fosters the development of HCC via many oncogenic pathways. Mounting evidence that cirrhosis is not a requisite for tumor development in NASH should make us take pause and urge for strategies to identify such patients at an early stage. Furthermore, effective chemopreventive strategies are urgently needed to temper the increase of HCC in patients with obesity, T2DM, and NAFLD.

## REFERENCES

1. Williams CD, Stengel J, Asike MI, et al. Prevalence of nonalcoholic fatty liver disease and nonalcoholic steatohepatitis among a largely middle-aged population utilizing ultrasound and liver biopsy: a prospective study. Gastroenterology 2011;140(1):124–31.
2. Rinella ME, Loomba R, Caldwell SH, et al. Controversies in the diagnosis and management of NAFLD and NASH. Gastroenterol Hepatol (N Y) 2014;10(4): 219–27.
3. Harrison SA, Torgerson S, Hayashi PH. The natural history of nonalcoholic fatty liver disease: a clinical histopathological study. Am J Gastroenterol 2003;98(9): 2042–7.
4. El-Serag HB, Rudolph KL. Hepatocellular carcinoma: epidemiology and molecular carcinogenesis. Gastroenterology 2007;132(7):2557–76.
5. Seefe LB. Introduction: the burden of hepatocellular carcinoma. Gastroenterology 2004;127(5 Suppl 1):S1–4.
6. Wong RJ, Cheung R, Ahmed A. Nonalcoholic steatohepatitis is the most rapidly growing indication for liver transplantation in patients with hepatocellular carcinoma in the U.S. Hepatology 2014;59(6):2188–95.
7. Welzel TM, Graubard BI, Quraishi S, et al. Population-attributable fractions of risk factors for hepatocellular carcinoma in the United States. Am J Gastroenterol 2013;108(8):1314–21.
8. Calle EE, Rodriguez C, Walker-Thurmond K, et al. Overweight, obesity, and mortality from cancer in a prospectively studied cohort of U.S. adults. N Engl J Med 2003;348(17):1625–38.
9. Moller H, Mellemgaard A, Lindvig K, et al. Obesity and cancer risk: a Danish record-linkage study. Eur J Cancer 1994;30A(3):344–50.
10. Wolk A, Gridley G, Svensson M, et al. A prospective study of obesity and cancer risk (Sweden). Cancer Causes Control 2001;12(1):13–21.
11. Oh SW, Yoon YS, Shin SA. Effects of excess weight on cancer incidences depending on cancer sites and histologic findings among men: Korea National Health Insurance Corporation Study. J Clin Oncol 2005;23(21):4742–54.
12. Larsson SC, Wolk A. Overweight, obesity and risk of liver cancer: a meta-analysis of cohort studies. Br J Cancer 2007;97(7):1005–8.
13. Ohki T, Tateishi R, Shiina S, et al. Visceral fat accumulation is an independent risk factor for hepatocellular carcinoma recurrence after curative treatment in patients with suspected NASH. Gut 2009;58(6):839–44.
14. Lazo M, Clark JM. The epidemiology of nonalcoholic fatty liver disease: a global perspective. Semin Liver Dis 2008;28(4):339–50.

15. Adami HO, Chow WH, Nyren O, et al. Excess risk of primary liver cancer in patients with diabetes mellitus. J Natl Cancer Inst 1996;88(20):1472–7.

16. El-Serag HB, Tran T, Everhart JE. Diabetes increases the risk of chronic liver disease and hepatocellular carcinoma. Gastroenterology 2004;126(2):460–8.

17. Wideroff L, Gridley G, Mellemkjaer L, et al. Cancer incidence in a population-based cohort of patients hospitalized with diabetes mellitus in Denmark. J Natl Cancer Inst 1997;89(18):1360–5.

18. Yang WS, Va P, Bray F, et al. The role of pre-existing diabetes mellitus on hepatocellular carcinoma occurrence and prognosis: a meta-analysis of prospective cohort studies. PLoS One 2011;6(12):e27326.

19. Wang WM, Xu Y, Yang XR, et al. Prognostic role of diabetes mellitus in hepatocellular carcinoma patients after curative treatments: a meta-analysis. Hepatobiliary Pancreat Dis Int 2011;10(4):346–55.

20. Wang YG, Wang P, Wang B, et al. Diabetes mellitus and poorer prognosis in hepatocellular carcinoma: a systematic review and meta-analysis. PLoS One 2014;9(5):e95485.

21. Neuschwander-Tetri BA, Caldwell SH. Nonalcoholic steatohepatitis: summary of an AASLD Single Topic Conference. Hepatology 2003;37(5):1202–19.

22. Ratziu V, Bonyhay L, Di Martino V, et al. Survival, liver failure, and hepatocellular carcinoma in obesity-related cryptogenic cirrhosis. Hepatology 2002;35(6):1485–93.

23. Siegel AB, Zhu AX. Metabolic syndrome and hepatocellular carcinoma: two growing epidemics with a potential link. Cancer 2009;115(24):5651–61.

24. Ekstedt M, Franzen LE, Mathiesen UL, et al. Long-term follow-up of patients with NAFLD and elevated liver enzymes. Hepatology 2006;44(4):865–73.

25. Rafiq N, Bai C, Fang Y, et al. Long-term follow-up of patients with nonalcoholic fatty liver. Clin Gastroenterol Hepatol 2009;7(2):234–8.

26. Adams LA, Lymp JF, St Sauver J, et al. The natural history of nonalcoholic fatty liver disease: a population-based cohort study. Gastroenterology 2005;129(1):113–21.

27. Sanyal A, Poklepovic A, Moyneur E, et al. Population-based risk factors and resource utilization for HCC: US perspective. Curr Med Res Opin 2010;26(9):2183–91.

28. Ascha MS, Hanouneh IA, Lopez R, et al. The incidence and risk factors of hepatocellular carcinoma in patients with nonalcoholic steatohepatitis. Hepatology 2010;51(6):1972–8.

29. Bhala N, Angulo P, van der Poorten D, et al. The natural history of nonalcoholic fatty liver disease with advanced fibrosis or cirrhosis: an international collaborative study. Hepatology 2011;54(4):1208–16.

30. Zen Y, Katayanagi K, Tsuneyama K, et al. Hepatocellular carcinoma arising in non-alcoholic steatohepatitis. Pathol Int 2001;51(2):127–31.

31. Orikasa H, Ohyama R, Tsuka N, et al. Lipid-rich clear-cell hepatocellular carcinoma arising in non-alcoholic steatohepatitis in a patient with diabetes mellitus. J Submicrosc Cytol Pathol 2001;33(1–2):195–200.

32. Bencheqroun R, Duvoux C, Luciani A, et al. Hepatocellular carcinoma without cirrhosis in a patient with nonalcoholic steatohepatitis. Gastroenterol Clin Biol 2004;28(5):497–9.

33. Bullock RE, Zaitoun AM, Aithal GP, et al. Association of non-alcoholic steatohepatitis without significant fibrosis with hepatocellular carcinoma. J Hepatol 2004;41(4):685–6.

34. Gonzalez L, Blanc JF, Sa Cunha A, et al. Obesity as a risk factor for hepatocellular carcinoma in a noncirrhotic patient. Semin Liver Dis 2004;24(4):415–9.

35. Cuadrado A, Orive A, Garcia-Suarez C, et al. Non-alcoholic steatohepatitis (NASH) and hepatocellular carcinoma. Obes Surg 2005;15(3):442–6.
36. Sato K, Ueda Y, Ueno K, et al. Hepatocellular carcinoma and nonalcoholic steatohepatitis developing during long-term administration of valproic acid. Virchows Arch 2005;447(6):996–9.
37. Hai S, Kubo S, Shuto T, et al. Hepatocellular carcinoma arising from nonalcoholic steatohepatitis: report of two cases. Surg Today 2006;36(4):390–4.
38. Ichikawa T, Yanagi K, Motoyoshi Y, et al. Two cases of non-alcoholic steatohepatitis with development of hepatocellular carcinoma without cirrhosis. J Gastroenterol Hepatol 2006;21(12):1865–6.
39. Hashizume H, Sato K, Takagi H, et al. Primary liver cancers with nonalcoholic steatohepatitis. Eur J Gastroenterol Hepatol 2007;19(10):827–34.
40. Guzman G, Brunt EM, Petrovic LM, et al. Does nonalcoholic fatty liver disease predispose patients to hepatocellular carcinoma in the absence of cirrhosis? Arch Pathol Lab Med 2008;132(11):1761–6.
41. Chagas AL, Kikuchi LO, Oliveira CP, et al. Does hepatocellular carcinoma in non-alcoholic steatohepatitis exist in cirrhotic and non-cirrhotic patients? Braz J Med Biol Res 2009;42(10):958–62.
42. Paradis V, Zalinski S, Chelbi E, et al. Hepatocellular carcinomas in patients with metabolic syndrome often develop without significant liver fibrosis: a pathological analysis. Hepatology 2009;49(3):851–9.
43. Kawada N, Imanaka K, Kawaguchi T, et al. Hepatocellular carcinoma arising from non-cirrhotic nonalcoholic steatohepatitis. J Gastroenterol 2009;44(12): 1190–4.
44. Hashimoto E, Yatsuji S, Tobari M, et al. Hepatocellular carcinoma in patients with nonalcoholic steatohepatitis. J Gastroenterol 2009;44(Suppl 19):89–95.
45. Takuma Y, Nouso K. Nonalcoholic steatohepatitis-associated hepatocellular carcinoma: our case series and literature review. World J Gastroenterol 2010; 16(12):1436–41.
46. Tokushige K, Hashimoto E, Yatsuji S, et al. Prospective study of hepatocellular carcinoma in nonalcoholic steatohepatitis in comparison with hepatocellular carcinoma caused by chronic hepatitis C. J Gastroenterol 2010;45(9):960–7.
47. Yasui K, Hashimoto E, Komorizono Y, et al. Characteristics of patients with nonalcoholic steatohepatitis who develop hepatocellular carcinoma. Clin Gastroenterol Hepatol 2011;9(5):428–33 [quiz: e50].
48. Wakai T, Shirai Y, Sakata J, et al. Surgical outcomes for hepatocellular carcinoma in nonalcoholic fatty liver disease. J Gastrointest Surg 2011;15(8): 1450–8.
49. Ikura Y, Mita E, Nakamori S. Hepatocellular carcinomas can develop in simple fatty livers in the setting of oxidative stress. Pathology 2011;43(2):167–8.
50. Arase Y, Kobayashi M, Suzuki F, et al. Difference in malignancies of chronic liver disease due to non-alcoholic fatty liver disease or hepatitis C in Japanese elderly patients. Hepatol Res 2012;42(3):264–72.
51. Mittal S, Sada YH, El-Serag HB, et al. Temporal trends of non-alcoholic fatty liver disease-related hepatocellular carcinoma in the veteran affairs population. Clin Gastroenterol Hepatol 2015;13(3):594–601.
52. Ertle J, Dechene A, Sowa JP, et al. Non-alcoholic fatty liver disease progresses to hepatocellular carcinoma in the absence of apparent cirrhosis. Int J Cancer 2011;128(10):2436–43.
53. Michelotti GA, Machado MV, Diehl AM. NAFLD, NASH and liver cancer. Nat Rev Gastroenterol Hepatol 2013;10(11):656–65.

54. Grundy SM, Brewer HB Jr, Cleeman JI, et al. Definition of metabolic syndrome: report of the National Heart, Lung, and Blood Institute/American Heart Association conference on scientific issues related to definition. Circulation 2004;109(3): 433–8.
55. Harrison SA. Liver disease in patients with diabetes mellitus. J Clin Gastroenterol 2006;40(1):68–76.
56. Balkau B, Kahn HS, Courbon D, et al. Hyperinsulinemia predicts fatal liver cancer but is inversely associated with fatal cancer at some other sites: the Paris prospective study. Diabetes Care 2001;24(5):843–9.
57. Moore MA, Park CB, Tsuda H. Implications of the hyperinsulinaemia-diabetes-cancer link for preventive efforts. Eur J Cancer Prev 1998;7(2):89–107.
58. Kaburagi Y, Yamauchi T, Yamamoto-Honda R, et al. The mechanism of insulin-induced signal transduction mediated by the insulin receptor substrate family. Endocr J 1999;(46 Suppl):S25–34.
59. Kim SO, Park JG, Lee YI. Increased expression of the insulin-like growth factor I (IGF-I) receptor gene in hepatocellular carcinoma cell lines: implications of IGF-I receptor gene activation by hepatitis B virus X gene product. Cancer Res 1996; 56(16):3831–6.
60. Tanaka S, Mohr L, Schmidt EV, et al. Biological effects of human insulin receptor substrate-1 overexpression in hepatocytes. Hepatology 1997;26(3):598–604.
61. Tanaka S, Wands JR. Insulin receptor substrate 1 overexpression in human hepatocellular carcinoma cells prevents transforming growth factor beta1-induced apoptosis. Cancer Res 1996;56(15):3391–4.
62. Saito K, Inoue S, Saito T, et al. Augmentation effect of postprandial hyperinsuli-naemia on growth of human hepatocellular carcinoma. Gut 2002;51(1):100–4.
63. Peyrou M, Bourgoin L, Foti M. PTEN in liver diseases and cancer. World J Gastroenterol 2010;16(37):4627–33.
64. Puri P, Mirshahi F, Cheung O, et al. Activation and dysregulation of the unfolded protein response in nonalcoholic fatty liver disease. Gastroenterology 2008; 134(2):568–76.
65. Hirosumi J, Tuncman G, Chang L, et al. A central role for JNK in obesity and insulin resistance. Nature 2002;420(6913):333–6.
66. Chang Q, Zhang Y, Beezhold KJ, et al. Sustained JNK1 activation is associated with altered histone H3 methylations in human liver cancer. J Hepatol 2009; 50(2):323–33.
67. Hui L, Zatloukal K, Scheuch H, et al. Proliferation of human HCC cells and chemically induced mouse liver cancers requires JNK1-dependent p21 downregulation. J Clin Invest 2008;118(12):3943–53.
68. Schattenberg JM, Singh R, Wang Y, et al. JNK1 but not JNK2 promotes the development of steatohepatitis in mice. Hepatology 2006;43(1):163–72.
69. Abdelmalek MF, Sanderson SO, Angulo P, et al. Betaine for nonalcoholic fatty liver disease: results of a randomized placebo-controlled trial. Hepatology 2009;50(6):1818–26.
70. Fujishita T, Aoki M, Taketo MM. JNK signaling promotes intestinal tumorigenesis through activation of mTOR complex 1 in Apc(Delta716) mice. Gastroenterology 2011;140(5):1556–63.e6.
71. Zhou L, Huang Y, Li J, et al. The mTOR pathway is associated with the poor prognosis of human hepatocellular carcinoma. Med Oncol 2010;27(2):255–61.
72. Rinella ME, Siddiqui MS, Gardikiotes K, et al. Dysregulation of the unfolded protein response in db/db mice with diet-induced steatohepatitis. Hepatology 2011;54(5):1600–9.

73. Henkel A, Green RM. The unfolded protein response in fatty liver disease. Semin Liver Dis 2013;33(4):321-9.
74. Dai R, Chen R, Li H. Cross-talk between PI3K/Akt and MEK/ERK pathways mediates endoplasmic reticulum stress-induced cell cycle progression and cell death in human hepatocellular carcinoma cells. Int J Oncol 2009;34(6):1749-57.
75. Ozcan U, Cao Q, Yilmaz E, et al. Endoplasmic reticulum stress links obesity, insulin action, and type 2 diabetes. Science 2004;306(5695):457-61.
76. Xu C, Bailly-Maitre B, Reed JC. Endoplasmic reticulum stress: cell life and death decisions. J Clin Invest 2005;115(10):2656-64.
77. Kharroubi I, Ladriere L, Cardozo AK, et al. Free fatty acids and cytokines induce pancreatic beta-cell apoptosis by different mechanisms: role of nuclear factor-kappaB and endoplasmic reticulum stress. Endocrinology 2004;145(11): 5087-96.
78. Vandewynckel YP, Laukens D, Geerts A, et al. The paradox of the unfolded protein response in cancer. Anticancer Res 2013;33(11):4683-94.
79. Shuda M, Kondoh N, Imazeki N, et al. Activation of the ATF6, XBP1 and grp78 genes in human hepatocellular carcinoma: a possible involvement of the ER stress pathway in hepatocarcinogenesis. J Hepatol 2003;38(5):605-14.
80. Zhang Y, Hagedorn CH, Wang L. Role of nuclear receptor SHP in metabolism and cancer. Biochim Biophys Acta 2011;1812(8):893-908.
81. Pikarsky E, Porat RM, Stein I, et al. NF-kappaB functions as a tumour promoter in inflammation-associated cancer. Nature 2004;431(7007):461-6.
82. Hu W, Feng Z, Eveleigh J, et al. The major lipid peroxidation product, trans-4-hydroxy-2-nonenal, preferentially forms DNA adducts at codon 249 of human p53 gene, a unique mutational hotspot in hepatocellular carcinoma. Carcinogenesis 2002;23(11):1781-9.
83. Taylor WR, Stark GR. Regulation of the G2/M transition by p53. Oncogene 2001; 20(15):1803-15.
84. Xu Z, Chen L, Leung L, et al. Liver-specific inactivation of the Nrf1 gene in adult mouse leads to nonalcoholic steatohepatitis and hepatic neoplasia. Proc Natl Acad Sci U S A 2005;102(11):4120-5.
85. Maki A, Kono H, Gupta M, et al. Predictive power of biomarkers of oxidative stress and inflammation in patients with hepatitis C virus-associated hepatocellular carcinoma. Ann Surg Oncol 2007;14(3):1182-90.
86. Kelesidis T, Kelesidis I, Chou S, et al. Narrative review: the role of leptin in human physiology: emerging clinical applications. Ann Intern Med 2010;152(2):93-100.
87. Tilg H, Moschen AR. Evolution of inflammation in nonalcoholic fatty liver disease: the multiple parallel hits hypothesis. Hepatology 2010;52(5):1836-46.
88. Dotsch J, Rascher W, Meissner U. New insights into leptin resistance by modifying cytokine receptor signal transduction. Eur J Endocrinol 2005;152(3):333-4.
89. Wang XJ, Yuan SL, Lu Q, et al. Potential involvement of leptin in carcinogenesis of hepatocellular carcinoma. World J Gastroenterol 2004;10(17):2478-81.
90. Fruhbeck G. Intracellular signalling pathways activated by leptin. Biochem J 2006;393(Pt 1):7-20.
91. Ramani K, Yang H, Xia M, et al. Leptin's mitogenic effect in human liver cancer cells requires induction of both methionine adenosyltransferase 2A and 2beta. Hepatology 2008;47(2):521-31.
92. Friedman SL. Molecular regulation of hepatic fibrosis, an integrated cellular response to tissue injury. J Biol Chem 2000;275(4):2247-50.
93. Lu SC, Mato JM. S-adenosylmethionine in liver health, injury, and cancer. Physiol Rev 2012;92(4):1515-42.

94. Mato JM, Martinez-Chantar ML, Lu SC. S-adenosylmethionine metabolism and liver disease. Ann Hepatol 2013;12(2):183–9.
95. Chen CJ, Kono H, Golenbock D, et al. Identification of a key pathway required for the sterile inflammatory response triggered by dying cells. Nat Med 2007; 13(7):851–6.
96. Takeuchi O, Akira S. Pattern recognition receptors and inflammation. Cell 2010; 140(6):805–20.
97. Zhang Q, Raoof M, Chen Y, et al. Circulating mitochondrial DAMPs cause inflammatory responses to injury. Nature 2010;464(7285):104–7.
98. Seki E, Brenner DA. Toll-like receptors and adaptor molecules in liver disease: update. Hepatology 2008;48(1):322–35.
99. Yu LX, Yan HX, Liu Q, et al. Endotoxin accumulation prevents carcinogen-induced apoptosis and promotes liver tumorigenesis in rodents. Hepatology 2010;52(4):1322–33.
100. Dapito DH, Mencin A, Gwak GY, et al. Promotion of hepatocellular carcinoma by the intestinal microbiota and TLR4. Cancer Cell 2012;21(4):504–16.
101. Hosaka T, Suzuki F, Kobayashi M, et al. Long-term entecavir treatment reduces hepatocellular carcinoma incidence in patients with hepatitis B virus infection. Hepatology 2013;58(1):98–107.
102. Bjorkhem-Bergman L, Backheden M, Soderberg Lofdal K. Statin treatment reduces the risk of hepatocellular carcinoma but not colon cancer-results from a nationwide case-control study in Sweden. Pharmacoepidemiol Drug Saf 2014;23(10):1101–6.
103. El-Serag HB, Johnson ML, Hachem C, et al. Statins are associated with a reduced risk of hepatocellular carcinoma in a large cohort of patients with diabetes. Gastroenterology 2009;136(5):1601–8.
104. Kawata S, Yamasaki E, Nagase T, et al. Effect of pravastatin on survival in patients with advanced hepatocellular carcinoma. A randomized controlled trial. Br J Cancer 2001;84(7):886–91.
105. Cao Z, Fan-Minogue H, Bellovin DI, et al. MYC phosphorylation, activation, and tumorigenic potential in hepatocellular carcinoma are regulated by HMG-CoA reductase. Cancer Res 2011;71(6):2286–97.
106. Spampanato C, De Maria S, Sarnataro M, et al. Simvastatin inhibits cancer cell growth by inducing apoptosis correlated to activation of Bax and down-regulation of BCL-2 gene expression. Int J Oncol 2012;40(4):935–41.
107. Gao J, Jia WD, Li JS, et al. Combined inhibitory effects of celecoxib and fluvas-tatin on the growth of human hepatocellular carcinoma xenografts in nude mice. J Int Med Res 2010;38(4):1413–27.
108. Singh S, Singh PP, Singh AG, et al. Anti-diabetic medications and the risk of hepatocellular cancer: a systematic review and meta-analysis. Am J Gastroenterol 2013;108(6):881–91 [quiz: 892].
109. Donadon V, Balbi M, Mas MD, et al. Metformin and reduced risk of hepatocellular carcinoma in diabetic patients with chronic liver disease. Liver Int 2010;30(5):750–8.
110. Donadon V, Balbi M, Valent F, et al. Glycated hemoglobin and antidiabetic strategies as risk factors for hepatocellular carcinoma. World J Gastroenterol 2010;16(24):3025–32.
111. Wang P, Kang D, Cao W, et al. Diabetes mellitus and risk of hepatocellular carcinoma: a systematic review and meta-analysis. Diabetes Metab Res Rev 2012;28(2):109–22.

112. Chen TM, Lin CC, Huang PT, et al. Metformin associated with lower mortality in diabetic patients with early stage hepatocellular carcinoma after radiofrequency ablation. J Gastroenterol Hepatol 2011;26(5):858–65.
113. Lai SW, Chen PC, Liao KF, et al. Risk of hepatocellular carcinoma in diabetic patients and risk reduction associated with anti-diabetic therapy: a population-based cohort study. Am J Gastroenterol 2012;107(1):46–52.
114. Hassan MM, Curley SA, Li D, et al. Association of diabetes duration and diabetes treatment with the risk of hepatocellular carcinoma. Cancer 2010; 116(8):1938–46.
115. Bhat M, Sonenberg N, Gores GJ. The mTOR pathway in hepatic malignancies. Hepatology 2013;58(2):810–8.
116. Lu SC, Ramani K, Ou X, et al. S-adenosylmethionine in the chemoprevention and treatment of hepatocellular carcinoma in a rat model. Hepatology 2009; 50(2):462–71.
117. Anstee QM, Day CP. S-adenosylmethionine (SAMe) therapy in liver disease: a review of current evidence and clinical utility. J Hepatol 2012;57(5):1097–109.

# Surgical Resection and Liver Transplantation for Hepatocellular Carcinoma

Mohamed E. Akoad, MD, Elizabeth A. Pomfret, MD, PhD*

## KEYWORDS

- Hepatic resection • Liver transplantation • Hepatocellular carcinoma
- Living donor liver transplantation • Locoregional therapy • Downstaging

## KEY POINTS

- Hepatic resection offers the best long-term outcome in patients without chronic liver disease and a diagnosis of hepatocellular carcinoma (HCC).
- Treatment options for patients with HCC and underlying cirrhosis include hepatic resection, liver transplantation, locoregional therapy, and chemotherapy.
- Hepatic resection in patients with cirrhosis is associated with a higher incidence of tumor recurrence.
- Liver transplantation offers the best long-term survival and the lowest incidence of tumor recurrence in patients with cirrhosis and early HCC.

## HEPATIC RESECTION FOR HEPATOCELLULAR CARCINOMA

More than 80% of hepatocellular carcinoma (HCC) arises in the background of cirrhosis with an annual incidence of 1% to 6%. It is estimated, however, that 10% to 15% may arise in patients with normal livers.[1–4] The cause of HCC in patients with a normal liver is undetermined most of the time. In patients infected with hepatitis B virus, most cases of HCC arise in the setting of cirrhosis, yet 20% to 30% of HCC can develop in patients with normal livers. Rarely, HCC develops in patients with chronic hepatitis C without chronic inflammation or fibrosis. The presence of HCC is also associated with prolonged excessive alcohol intake, metabolic disease, and iron overload. Fibrolamellar HCC is an uncommon variant that typically develops in patients without chronic liver disease (**Fig. 1**). It has distinct radiologic and histologic characteristics and is not associated with an elevated alpha-fetoprotein (AFP) level.

The authors have nothing to disclose.

Department of Transplantation and Hepatobiliary Diseases, Lahey Hospital and Medical Center, 41 Mall Road, 4 West, Burlington, MA 01805, USA

* Corresponding author.

*E-mail address:* Elizabeth.A.Pomfret@lahey.org

Clin Liver Dis 19 (2015) 381–399

http://dx.doi.org/10.1016/j.cld.2015.01.007     **liver.theclinics.com**

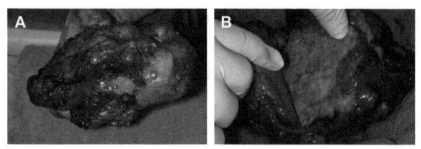

**Fig. 1.** Resected specimen of fibrolamellar HCC (*A, B*).

Fibrolamellar HCC develops in a younger age group (20–40 years) and has a slightly better prognosis.

Surveillance screening with serial imaging studies is not routinely done in patients without chronic liver disease, thus tumors in this population are often large in size (median size 8–10 cm), symptomatic, and require a major hepatic resection (**Fig. 2**). Unlike patients with chronic liver disease, hepatic resection is well tolerated and offers the best option for long-term survival.

HCC arising in the setting of chronic liver disease is often diagnosed at an earlier stage as a result of serial surveillance imaging studies. Treatment options depend on many factors, including size and number of lesions, cause of liver disease, the severity of hepatic dysfunction, and the presence of portal hypertension and cirrhosis.

### Patient Evaluation

Patients with HCC referred for surgery are carefully evaluated to assess resectability based on anatomic considerations, underlying hepatic function, and the patients' overall medical condition. The success of a partial hepatectomy depends on the ability to achieve a complete resection with negative margins while leaving behind an adequate liver remnant.

Unlike most solid tumors whereby the prognosis and subsequent treatment options depend on the staging at the time of presentation, the prognosis and treatment

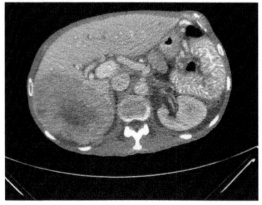

**Fig. 2.** A large HCC measuring 12 × 10 cm occupying most of the right lobe in a patient with no underlying cirrhosis.

| | | | |
|---|---|---|---|
| Moreno-Luna, 2013 | cTACE | 13 | 13 |
| Jung, 2013 | cTACE | | 27 |
| Lewandowski et al,[41] 2010 | cTACE | 73 | 17.4 |
| Chen, 2009 | cTACE | nr | 15.6 |
| Ho, 2009 | cTACE | 163 | 16.8 |
| Wang, 2008 | cTACE | 741 | 18.2 |
| Burrell, 2012 | DEB-TACE | 63 | 42.8 |
| **Stage C (advanced, portal vein invasion, N1, M1, performance status 1–2)** | | | |
| Mazzaferro, 2013 | RE | 35 | 13 |
| Moreno-Luna, 2013 | RE | 14 | 8.4 |
| Sangro et al,[76] 2011 | RE | 183 | 10 |
| Salem et al,[74] 2010 | RE | 107 | 7.3 |
| Inarrairegui, 2010 | RE | 25 | 10 |
| Moreno-Luna, 2013 | cTACE | 19 | 10.1 |
| Jung, 2013 | cTACE | | 9 |
| Chung, 2011 | cTACE | 83 | 5.6 |
| Luo, 2011 | cTACE | 44/40 | 5.3/10.2 |
| Lewandowski et al,[41] 2010 | cTACE | 23 | 6.6 |
| Ho, 2009 | cTACE | 48 | 13.6 |
| Chen, 2009 | cTACE | nr | 12.7 |
| Wang, 2008 | cTACE | 200 | 6.8 |
| Chang et al,[111] 2011 | Cryoablation | 190 | 7.5 |

*Abbreviations:* cTACE, conventional TACE; CTP, Child-Turcotte-Pugh; DEB-TACE, drug-eluting beads-TACE; M1, distant metastasis; N1, regional lymph node metastasis; PEI, percutaneous ethanol injection; RE, radioembolization; RFA, radiofrequency ablation; TACE, transarterial chemoembolization.
*Adapted from* Sangro B, Salem R. Transarterial chemoembolization and radioembolization. Semin Liver Dis 2014;34(04):435–41; with permission.

**Table 4**
Summary of characteristics and long-term outcomes of large mixed-case series of patients with hepatocellular carcinoma receiving intra-arterial therapies, radiofrequency ablation, and cryoablation (2000–2013)

| Reference | Therapy | Patients | Stage (BCLC) | Liver Function (CTP-A/B/C) | Tumor Burden, % | Performance Status ECOG >0, % | Response Rate WHO | Response Rate EASL | Response Duration (TTP, mo) | Survival, mo |
|---|---|---|---|---|---|---|---|---|---|---|
| Mazzaferro 2013 | RE | 52 | 0/33/67/0 | 83/17/0 | 3 | 40 | 40 WHO | 40 EASL | 11 | 15 |
| Sangro et al,[76] 2011 | RE | 325 | 16/27/56/1 | 83/17/0 | 24 | 46 | | | | 12.8 |
| Hilgard et al,[75] 2010 | RE | 108 | 2745/51/0 | 77/22/0 | 27 | 49 | 15 WHO | 40 EASL | 10 | 16.4 |
| Salem et al,[74] 2010 | RE | 291 | 17/28/52/3 | 45/53/3 | 27 | 44 | 42 WHO | 57 EASL | 7.9 | 16.2 |
| Sieghart, 2013 | cTACE | 107 | 11/89/0/0 | 67/33/0 | 26 | 36 | | | | |
| Meyer, 2013 | cTACE | 44 | 27/44/29/0 | 79/21/0 | 34 | | | | 7.5 | 16.3 |
| Lewandowski et al,[41] 2010 | cTACE | 172 | 36/42/20/2 | 56/42/2 | 43 | 48 | 31 WHO | 64 EASL | 7.9 | 8.6 |
| Lammer et al,[49] 2010 | cTACE | 108 | 29/79/0/0 | 82/18/0 | 37 | 53 | | 43 EASL | | |
| Malagari, 2012 | DEB-TACE | 173 | 39/61/0/0 | 59/41/0 | 64 | 11 | | | | 48.7 (mean) |
| Burrel, 2012 | DEB-TACE | 104 | 24/69/0/0 | 95/5/0 | | 0 | | | | 48.6 |
| Lammer et al,[49] 2010 | DEB-TACE | 93 | | 83/17/0 | 31 | 35 | | 51 EASL | | |
| Livraghi et al,[88] 2000 | RFA | 114 | 0/75/51/0 | 100/14/0 | | | | | | |
| Hasegawa et al,[89] 2008 | RFA | | 2189/833/0/0 | 2288/734/0 | | | | | 26.0%, 55.4% (1, 2 y) | 98.3%, 94.5% (1, 2 y) |
| Chen, 2010 | Cryoablation | 40 | 12/24/4/0 | | | | | | 32.4%, 79.2% (1, 3 y) | 81.4%, 63.0% (1, 3 y) |

*Abbreviations:* cTACE, conventional transarterial chemoembolization; CTP, Child-Turcotte-Pugh; DEB-TACE, drug-eluting beads- transarterial chemoembolization; EASL, European Association for the Study of the Liver; ECOG, Eastern Cooperative Oncology Group; RE, radioembolization; RFA, radiofrequency ablation; TTP, time to progression; WHO, World Health Organization.

*Adapted from* Sangro B, Salem R. Transarterial chemoembolization and radioembolization. Semin Liver Dis 2014;34(04):435–41; with permission.

shown varying efficacy and safety profiles in the treatment of HCC, each has its own technique, and different levels of appropriateness for specific patients (see **Table 2**). After treatment, assessment of response is an essential component of determining the next steps in the therapeutic pathway. The unique aspect of evaluating locoregional therapy is that different tumors are exposed to varying amounts of a therapeutic, necessitating a more focused evaluation of response from the tumor treated, with eventual inclusion of untreated tumors when all planned treatment has been completed.[13] Patients are treated every 4 to 6 weeks as needed until therapy is complete. Many factors, such as size and extent of necrosis, allow for better understanding of tumor response. However, tumor size is still the gold standard, which was first determined by the World Health Organization with its bidirectional measurement, then with the Response Evaluation Criteria in Solid Tumors (RECIST), which incorporated unidirectional measurement, and most recently, the modified RECIST (mRECIST), which is proposed to include imaging criteria to accurately assess tumor response.[14–16] RECIST assessment of target or nontarget lesions allows for determination of complete response, partial response, progressive disease, or stable disease, based on disappearance of lesions, appearance of new lesions, or changes in size of the target lesion (which is defined as the largest measured dimension), to determine response to therapy based on imaging and laboratory values. mRECIST takes into account enhancement of lesions on the arterial phase of imaging as a prognostic indicator.

### Transarterial Chemoembolization

TACE is an endovascular technique that delivers the combination of an anticancer agent along with iodized oil to HCC, both having a synergistic effect.[17–19] Conventional TACE or cTACE, is the standard practice of chemoinfusion, via the hepatic artery. Although there is controversy, often-used cancer agents are doxorubicin, with either mitomycin C or cisplatin, or both. Within the United States, there is variance in clinical practice with most IR practitioners using only 1 agent, whereas others combine 2 to 3.[20] Iodized oil serves as the carrier for the chemotherapeutic and embolic substance for the procedure, creating a suspension or emulsion that is locally delivered. Lipiodol is a poppy seed oil that contains ethiodized iodine (ie, combined with ethyl esters of the oil fatty acids). Animal model studies have shown that in suspensions, the therapeutic is uniformly distributed within the iodized oil, which may be preferable to emulsions that undergo more rapid excretion from the body.[21–27] After injection of the drug, 100-μm to 500-μm bland occlusive particles are injected to reduce washout.[28] Patient selection (see **Table 2**) is driven by adequate liver function and performance status without elevated creatinine ($\leq 2.0$ mg/dL), biliary obstruction, hepatofugal flow, or severe systemic infection.[29,30] The procedure itself requires the patient to receive hydration, antiemetics, and narcotics on the morning prior. Computed tomography (CT) is performed after the procedure to confirm the location of the emulsion. Patients can stay overnight for monitoring, and up to 3 days before discharge. Treatments are to be repeated at 60-day to 120-day intervals, tailored to the each patient's response to therapy and disease profile.

TACE is a first-line therapy for intermediate-stage HCC, yielding benefit in patients who have adequate liver function, and is particularly useful in patients who have contraindications to ablation.[31] Intention-to-treat analysis has shown that cTACE can improve survival in unresectable HCC.[32,33] An improvement in survival has been shown in individuals with smaller tumor size, localized disease, lower MELD score, number of TACE procedures, and AFP response after treatment.[34–40] Results of studies by Lewandowski and colleagues[41] and Takayasu and colleagues[42] showed

the importance of appropriate patient selection. In a long-term analysis, in the study by Lewandoski and colleagues,[41] median survival differed significantly among patients with BCLC A (40.0 months), B (17.4 months), and C (6.3 months, $P<.0001$). The study by Takayasu and colleagues[42] evaluated more than 4000 treatment-naïve patients, excluding those who had extrahepatic disease and portal vein invasion, and found a median survival of 39.6 months, showing the value of careful evaluation of a patient's candidacy for cTACE.

Adverse events and complications have been shown to occur in cTACE, led by postembolization syndrome, which presents as nausea, vomiting, and abdominal pain. Liver abscess, biliary duct injury, ulcers of the duodenum or stomach, tumor rupture, and vascular injury leading to spasm are all possible adverse events during or after a cTACE procedure.[43]

A variant of TACE is the use of drug-eluting beads (DEB-TACE) loaded with doxo-rubicin. This is accepted to be a safe delivery method, with improved pharmokinetics when compared with conventional lipiodol-based cTACE.[44–46] The drug-release mechanism, which is dependent on ionic interactions between the drug and bead, results in sustained chemotherapy exposure to the tumor and relatively lower peak systemic levels of drug, in contrast to cTACE.[47] Patient selection is similar to other cather-based therapies; however, clinical trial inclusion for DEB-TACE focuses on HCC that is amenable to selective treatment, rather than lobar (see **Table 2**). Previous guidelines allow for up to 4 treatments within the first 180 days.[48] When compared with bland embolization, DEB-TACE was found to provide a longer time to progression (TTP), showing the synergy of embolization with chemotherapeutics. It is of note that in a recent phase II randomized controlled trial comparing cTACE with DEB-TACE, DEB-TACE did not show a superior therapeutic response.[49] However, patients with advanced disease were found to tolerate DEB-TACE more so than cTACE.[49] In a recent study, hepatotoxicity associated with DEB-TACE, independent of the patient's disease burden, had a significantly worse adverse event profile relative to cTACE ($P<.001$).[50] These results can be contrasted with those of Dhanasekaran and colleagues,[51] who found that DEB-TACE had not only fewer adverse events, but improved survival when compared with cTACE. A recent evaluation of complications in DEB-TACE compared with cTACE found no difference in adverse events, such as vascular injury, pain, nausea, hepatic failure, tumor rupture, and liver abscess.[52,53] However, the data appear mixed with regard to the tolerability of DEB-TACE, and further QoL studies and closer evaluation of the toxicity profile would be beneficial.

In the setting of portal vein invasion by HCC, cTACE has not been shown to improve prognosis or improve mortality, possibly due to rapid liver decompensation.[54] However, the addition of radiation therapy (RT) to TACE in the setting of portal vein tumor thrombus has shown improvement in mortality, and in a retrospective propensity score-matched analysis, potential superiority of combined TACE/RT over sorafenib has been suggested too.[55–57] Another clinical complication that occurs in HCC is arteriovenous (AV) shunting, which can preclude a patient from receiving TACE due to concern for shunting of cancer-killing compounds to vital organs such as the lungs. By blocking the portal veins from the tumor, TACE with portal vein occlusion (TACE-PVO), allows embolization of the entire tumor to be performed, including the arterioportal shunt portions. In the setting of AV shunts in HCC, TACE-PVO has shown promising improvement in survival, which is superior to previous approaches to this pathologic vascular circumstance.[58,59]

Because of the challenges of a dual blood supply to some larger HCC tumors, balloon occlusion of the hepatic vein has been proposed as a viable manipulation for treating the entire tumor area. Selective balloon-occluded TACE (B-TACE) is a

multistep process, with TACE preceding balloon occlusion of the nutrient artery, followed by B-TACE in an effort to completely embolize the area surrounding the tumor, allowing for maximal retention of toxic therapeutic within the targeted tumor area.[60]

TACE can be combined with RFA in an effort to synergistically combine the strengths of each therapy. RFA therapy relies on generating heat to cause cellular damage within the tumor; however, vascular outflow creates a heat-sink effect that may reduce the efficacy of the treatment. Performing cTACE before RFA allows for improved ablation of the tumor, and the resultant hemodynamic alteration allows for retention of thermal energy within the tumor environment. When comparing RFA, TACE, and TACE-RFA combined therapy, in a randomized study, improved median survivals were seen in the combination group (37 months) when compared with the TACE (24 months) and RFA (22 months) groups alone.[61]

TACE combined with sorafenib has been evaluated with mixed results.[62] In a randomized phase III trial, sorafenib given 30 to 90 days after TACE gave no significant survival benefit in CTP-A patients.[63] However, in a phase II study, a shorter period for sorafenib administration after TACE, such as 7 days, drastically improved rates of progression.[64]

### Radioembolization

RE with $^Y90$ represents an alternative to TACE in the treatment of patients with intermediate-stage HCC. RE is the intra-arterial delivery of resin (SIR-Spheres; Sirtex Medical [North Sydney, Australia]) or glass (TheraSphere; BTG plc [Pennsylvania, USA]) microspheres containing $^Y90$, which is a beta-emitting particle that has a localized radius of radiation delivery (2.5–11.0 mm) and a half-life of 60 hours.[65] The delivery of these 30-μm microspheres into the feeding vessels of the tumor eventually leads to their settling in the tumor itself, without affecting the vasculature, in contrast to the other catheter-based locoregional therapies.[66] Because of the absence of vessel occlusion, patients can be discharged within a few hours of the procedure, allowing it to serve as an outpatient therapy, resulting in potentially improved QoL.[67] Radiation-induced cell death in turn induces fibrosis and loss of liver tissue, while compensatory hypertrophy of remaining liver segments allows for sustaining underlying liver function.[68–72] This segmental delivery of $^Y90$ allows for its use in more advanced HCC, because of its acceptable toxicity profile relative to other segmental embolotherapies.[73] Patients receive only 1 RE session initially, and are followed closely to determine if they require further treatment.

Many phase II studies have evaluated long-term outcomes in RE, focusing on toxicity, imaging, and survival, by stratifying patients by United Network for Organ Sharing, BCLC, CTP, and tumor stage. A landmark study was completed with 291 patients to elucidate TTP results for RE, setting the stage for future studies.[74] Thereafter, in a study by Hilgard and colleagues,[75] it was found that RE improved survival at a rate equivalent to cTACE and DEB-TACE, within their cohort of 108 patients, and this was confirmed by a later study with 325 patients.[76] Further studies have led to the design and enrollment of phase III trials comparing RE to sorafenib.[77] There is a dearth of data available comparing TACE and RE in the setting of a randomized controlled trial, but a robust comparative effectiveness analysis found that clinical toxicities, tumor response, adverse events, and TTP were significantly better in the RE group relative to cTACE, without difference in OS.[73] This study brought to light the possibility that TTP may not be an acceptable surrogate for survival, and that approximately 1000 patients would need to be enrolled in a trial to show statistical equivalence between cTACE and RE.[73] Other small retrospective studies have shown no survival difference in intermediate-stage HCC, but cTACE was shown to have significantly higher rates of postprocedural adverse events.[78]

In the setting of portal vein thrombosis (PVT), Kulik and colleagues[79] found that RE can be safely carried out, without risk of hepatic failure, which is opposite to available data regarding cTACE in the same setting.[80] Adverse events found in RE can be fatigue, ischemic ulceration of the stomach or duodenum due to inaccurate delivery of microspheres, cholecystitis, and fibrosis of the liver parenchyma, whereas RILD is rare if patients are appropriately selected for the treatment.[5,81] **Tables 3** and **4** summarize the results of outcomes of embolotherapy, according to HCC stage and case mix.

## ABLATIVE THERAPIES

Ablative therapy is the use of heat, intense cold, or chemicals to induce cancer cell death. Hyperthermal ablation relies on the increase of thermal energy, and encompasses therapies, such as RFA, laser ablation, and MWA. Percutaneous hyperthermal ablative therapies are considered first-line locoregional therapies for early-stage HCC. In contradistinction, cryotherapy relies on cooling of the tumor to induce necrosis. Forms of chemical ablation are PEI and percutaneous acetic acid injection (PAI).

### Radiofrequency Ablation

RFA uses a needle that conducts a high-energy electrical current into the tumor, to induce a rise in temperature that causes necrosis of the tumor tissue.[82] However, as discussed earlier, larger vessels can serve as a heat-sink, preventing complete necrosis of the tumor.[83,84] This issue can be combated by varying approaches in embolization before the procedure.[85] However, some theorize that in patients with cirrhosis, the thickness of liver tissue will allow for retention of heat, acting almost as insulation and a method of protecting surrounding parenchyma.[86] RFA allows for accurate, localized destruction of tissue, without effects on the surrounding liver parenchyma. Long-term evaluation of RFA by Salmi and colleagues[87] showed local tumor progression rates of 4% at 1 year and 14% at 5 years, with survival of 92% at 1 year and 63% at 5 years. Livraghi and colleagues[88] also conducted a trial to determine the efficacy of RFA in large (5.1–9.5 cm) versus medium-size tumors (3.1–5.0 cm), finding significantly higher rates of complete necrosis in medium compared with large tumors. Comparing surgical resection with RFA in one study of more than 5000 patients, there was no significant difference in OS, but rates of recurrence were lower in the surgical arm of the study.[89] Many studies have shown that efficacy of RFA is dependent on the location of the tumor within the liver, and proximity to important nearby structures.[83,84,90] This contrasts to the findings of Ng and colleagues,[91] who found no difference in the success of RFA with regard to tumor progression and survival between perivascular and nonperivascular HCC. The major complication rates of RFA can range from 2.4% to 13.1%, compared with 9.0% to 22.0% for surgical resection.[82,92–95]

### Microwave Ablation

MWA is another hyperthermal ablative technique that alters the polarity of water molecules, thereby generating heat-induced necrosis of HCC. The approach is not limited by charring, thereby reducing the risk of skin burns.[96,97] Relative to RFA, the speed at which a critical level of thermal energy is generated is faster in MWA, requiring fewer insertions, also reducing the heat-sink effects of vascular outflow from the liver.[98] The reduction in heat-sink effects allows for treatment of perivascular HCC as well. Complications due to MWA range from 2.6% to 7.5%, with liver abscess, perforation, and ascites being the more common.[98–101] A key concern of MWA that has been discussed at length by Lee and colleagues[98] is that local tumor progression can occur with MWA, with rates of 42% from possible iatrogenic tumor dissemination when using a large applicator device.

### Irreversible Electroporation

IRE is a locoregional technique that pulses an electrical current through HCC, resulting in trauma that compromises cell membranes, leading to cell death.[102] Similar to other alternatives to RFA, IRE is unaffected by a heat-sink effect, and it has a minimal effect on surrounding vascular and parenchymal structures.[103,104] The absence of fibrosis and scarring reduces the amount of time that must elapse before review of tumor response.[102] However, in contradistinction to other locoregional therapies, IRE requires general anesthesia, even in the percutaneous approach.[105] IRE is a relatively novel HCC treatment that will require further assessment in long-term studies.

### Cryoablation

Cryoablation uses cooled argon gas to reduce temperature below $-20°$Celsius, inducing cell death within the tumor.[106] There is a decreased heat-sink effect relative to RFA, and the procedure allows for dynamic identification of the zone being ablated, via ultrasound, reducing damage to the surrounding viscera.[107–109] Cryotherapy with ultrasound guidance was found to be safe in patients with HCC, with 81.4% survival at 1 year, and 60.3% survival at 3 years, along with disease-free survival at 67.6% and 20.8%, respectively.[110] In another study, by Chang and colleagues,[111] significantly different median survival and TTP were seen with cryotherapy versus controls, with 7.5 months versus 3.2 months, and 3.5 versus 1.5 months, respectively. A meta-analysis evaluating outcomes in cryoablation and RFA found that RFA had an improved rate of local recurrence.[112] Adverse effects may be coagulopathy, disseminated intravascular coagulation, and cryoshock syndrome, which is multiorgan failure in the setting of cryoablation within the liver.[113] There was no HCC stage mentioned, but rather it was evaluating use of cryoablation in liver tumors, via a survey to physicians.

### Percutaneous Ethanol Injection

PEI is a chemical ablation technique via a percutaneous approach that allows for treatment of HCC smaller than 3 cm. Ethanol is injected via a needle, resulting in necrosis of tumor cells through thrombosis, protein damage, and dehydration at the cellular level. Again, cirrhosis has been thought to "wall-in" the ethanol, thereby protecting surrounding tissues.[114] PEI is considered a low-cost and relatively safe approach; however, it requires at least 4 sessions to treat a tumor, even those smaller than 3 cm. In a study comparing PEI, PAI, and RFA, the latter was found to have superior local recurrence and survival at 1 and 3 years, with higher tumor grade and tumor size larger than 2 cm being positively correlated with recurrence.[93] Possible complications for PEI are PVT, liver abscess and necrosis, and gall bladder and bowel injury.[115]

### Locoregional therapy as bridge to transplantation

Downstaging of patients who are listed for transplantation has been proven to be another area of application for previously discussed locoregional therapies, such as RFA, RE, and TACE. Most data in the literature is with regard to TACE, showing potential for downstaging to Milan criteria, whereas others have published data relating to the promise of a synergistic approach of RE or RFA combined with TACE.[116,117] Although there is controversy regarding the topic, EASL has recommended that particular HCCs may warrant downstaging only in the setting of a clinical trial.[12]

## SUMMARY

The purpose of this article was to discuss the variety of different locoregional therapies available for use in treating HCC. Most outcomes addressed were in the setting of

intermediate-stage to advanced-stage HCCs, which account for nearly 70% to 80% of all patients with HCC. As the number of individuals diagnosed with HCC continues to grow, locoregional therapies will play a key role in the future management of HCC. Head-to-head prospective studies should be designed to determine which locoregional therapy is appropriate for a particular patient in light of the stage of their disease and their desired QoL.

## REFERENCES

1. Llovet JM, Burroughs A, Bruix J. Hepatocellular carcinoma. Lancet 2003;362: 1907–17.
2. Cheng AL, Kang YK, Chen Z, et al. Efficacy and safety of sorafenib in patients in the Asia-Pacific region with advanced hepatocellular carcinoma: a phase III randomised, double-blind, placebo-controlled trial. Lancet Oncol 2009;10: 25–34.
3. Llovet JM, Ricci S, Mazzaferro V, et al. Sorafenib in advanced hepatocellular carcinoma. N Engl J Med 2008;359:378–90.
4. Ingold JA, Reed GB, Kaplan HS, et al. Radiation hepatitis. Am J Roentgenol Radium Ther Nucl Med 1965;93:200–8.
5. Gil-Alzugaray B, Chopitea A, Inarrairaegui M, et al. Prognostic factors and prevention of radioembolization-induced liver disease. Hepatology 2013;57: 1078–87.
6. Llovet JM, Bru C, Bruix J. Prognosis of hepatocellular carcinoma: the BCLC staging classification. Semin Liver Dis 1999;19:329–38.
7. Llovet JM, Di Bisceglie AM, Bruix J, et al. Design and endpoints of clinical trials in hepatocellular carcinoma. J Natl Cancer Inst 2008;100:698–711.
8. Mazzaferro V, Regalia E, Doci R, et al. Liver transplantation for the treatment of small hepatocellular carcinomas in patients with cirrhosis. N Engl J Med 1996; 334:693–9.
9. Okuda K, Ohtsuki T, Obata H, et al. Natural history of hepatocellular carcinoma and prognosis in relation to treatment. Study of 850 patients. Cancer 1985;56: 918–28.
10. Salem R, Lewandowski RJ. Chemoembolization and radioembolization for hepatocellular carcinoma. Clin Gastroenterol Hepatol 2013;11:604–11 [quiz: e43–4].
11. Bruix J, Sherman M, American Association for the Study of Liver Diseases. Management of hepatocellular carcinoma: an update. Hepatology 2011;53:1020–2.
12. European Association for the Study of the Liver, European Organisation for Research and Treatment of Cancer. EASL-EORTC clinical practice guidelines: management of hepatocellular carcinoma. J Hepatol 2012;56:908–43.
13. Riaz A, Miller FH, Kulik LM, et al. Imaging response in the primary index lesion and clinical outcomes following transarterial locoregional therapy for hepatocellular carcinoma. JAMA 2010;303:1062–9.
14. Therasse P, Arbuck SG, Eisenhauer EA, et al. New guidelines to evaluate the response to treatment in solid tumors. European Organization for Research and Treatment of Cancer, National Cancer Institute of the United States, National Cancer Institute of Canada. J Natl Cancer Inst 2000;92:205–16.
15. Forner A, Ayuso C, Varela M, et al. Evaluation of tumor response after locoregional therapies in hepatocellular carcinoma: are response evaluation criteria in solid tumors reliable? Cancer 2009;115:616–23.
16. Lencioni R, Llovet JM. Modified RECIST (mRECIST) assessment for hepatocellular carcinoma. Semin Liver Dis 2010;30:52–60.

17. Yoshikawa M, Saisho H, Ebara M, et al. A randomized trial of intrahepatic arterial infusion of 4'-epidoxorubicin with Lipiodol versus 4'-epidoxorubicin alone in the treatment of hepatocellular carcinoma. Cancer Chemother Pharmacol 1994; 33(Suppl):S149–52.

18. Yoon CJ, Chung JW, Park JH, et al. Transcatheter arterial chemoembolization with paclitaxel-lipiodol solution in rabbit VX2 liver tumor. Radiology 2003;229: 126–31.

19. Takayasu K, Shima Y, Muramatsu Y, et al. Hepatocellular carcinoma: treatment with intraarterial iodized oil with and without chemotherapeutic agents. Radiology 1987;163:345–51.

20. Solomon B, Soulen MC, Baum RA, et al. Chemoembolization of hepatocellular carcinoma with cisplatin, doxorubicin, mitomycin-C, ethiodol, and polyvinyl alcohol: prospective evaluation of response and survival in a U.S. population. J Vasc Interv Radiol 1999;10:793–8.

21. Miller DL, O'Leary TJ, Girton M. Distribution of iodized oil within the liver after hepatic arterial injection. Radiology 1987;162:849–52.

22. de Baere T, Dufaux J, Roche A, et al. Circulatory alterations induced by intra-arterial injection of iodized oil and emulsions of iodized oil and doxorubicin: experimental study. Radiology 1995;194:165–70.

23. Ueda T, Murata S, Mine T, et al. Comparison of epirubicin-iodized oil suspension and emulsion for transcatheter arterial chemoembolization in VX2 tumor. ScientificWorldJournal 2012;2012:961986.

24. Mine T, Murata S, Ueda T, et al. Comparative study of cisplatin-iodized oil suspension and emulsion for transcatheter arterial chemoembolization of rabbit VX2 liver tumors. Hepatol Res 2012;42:473–81.

25. Kan Z, Sato M, Ivancev K, et al. Distribution and effect of iodized poppyseed oil in the liver after hepatic artery embolization: experimental study in several animal species. Radiology 1993;186:861–6.

26. Demachi H, Matsui O, Abo H, et al. Simulation model based on non-newtonian fluid mechanics applied to the evaluation of the embolic effect of emulsions of iodized oil and anticancer drug. Cardiovasc Intervent Radiol 2000;23:285–90.

27. Yamamoto K, Shimizu T, Narabayashi I. Intraarterial infusion chemotherapy with lipiodol-CDDP suspension for hepatocellular carcinoma. Cardiovasc Intervent Radiol 2000;23:26–39.

28. Coldwell DM, Stokes KR, Yakes WF. Embolotherapy: agents, clinical applications, and techniques. Radiographics 1994;14:623–43 [quiz: 645–6].

29. Brown DB, Nikolic B, Covey AM, et al. Quality improvement guidelines for transhepatic arterial chemoembolization, embolization, and chemotherapeutic infusion for hepatic malignancy. J Vasc Interv Radiol 2012;23:287–94.

30. Liapi E, Geschwind JF. Transcatheter arterial chemoembolization for liver cancer: is it time to distinguish conventional from drug-eluting chemoembolization? Cardiovasc Intervent Radiol 2011;34:37–49.

31. Bruix J, Sherman M, Practice Guidelines Committee, American Association for the Study of Liver Diseases. Management of hepatocellular carcinoma. Hepatology 2005;42:1208–36.

32. Llovet JM, Real MI, Montana X, et al. Arterial embolisation or chemoembolisation versus symptomatic treatment in patients with unresectable hepatocellular carcinoma: a randomised controlled trial. Lancet 2002;359:1734–9.

33. Lo CM, Ngan H, Tso WK, et al. Randomized controlled trial of transarterial lipiodol chemoembolization for unresectable hepatocellular carcinoma. Hepatology 2002;35:1164–71.

34. Savastano S, Miotto D, Casarrubea G, et al. Transcatheter arterial chemoembolization for hepatocellular carcinoma in patients with Child's grade A or B cirrhosis: a multivariate analysis of prognostic factors. J Clin Gastroenterol 1999;28:334–40.

35. Ji SK, Cho YK, Ahn YS, et al. Multivariate analysis of the predictors of survival for patients with hepatocellular carcinoma undergoing transarterial chemoembolization: focusing on superselective chemoembolization. Korean J Radiol 2008; 9:534–40.

36. Lopez RR Jr, Pan SH, Hoffman AL, et al. Comparison of transarterial chemoembolization in patients with unresectable, diffuse vs focal hepatocellular carcinoma. Arch Surg 2002;137:653–7 [discussion: 657–8].

37. Okuda K, Obata H, Nakajima Y, et al. Prognosis of primary hepatocellular carcinoma. Hepatology 1984;4:3S–6S.

38. Dhanasekaran R, Kooby DA, Staley CA, et al. Prognostic factors for survival in patients with unresectable hepatocellular carcinoma undergoing chemoembolization with doxorubicin drug-eluting beads: a preliminary study. HPB (Oxford) 2010;12:174–80.

39. Farinati F, De Maria N, Marafin C, et al. Unresectable hepatocellular carcinoma in cirrhosis: survival, prognostic factors, and unexpected side effects after transcatheter arterial chemoembolization. Dig Dis Sci 1996;41:2332–9.

40. Berger DH, Carrasco CH, Hohn DC, et al. Hepatic artery chemoembolization or embolization for primary and metastatic liver tumors: post-treatment management and complications. J Surg Oncol 1995;60:116–21.

41. Lewandowski RJ, Mulcahy MF, Kulik LM, et al. Chemoembolization for hepatocellular carcinoma: comprehensive imaging and survival analysis in a 172-patient cohort. Radiology 2010;255:955–65.

42. Takayasu K, Arii S, Kudo M, et al. Superselective transarterial chemoembolization for hepatocellular carcinoma. Validation of treatment algorithm proposed by Japanese guidelines. J Hepatol 2012;56:886–92.

43. Xia J, Ren Z, Ye S, et al. Study of severe and rare complications of transarterial chemoembolization (TACE) for liver cancer. Eur J Radiol 2006;59:407–12.

44. Varela M, Real MI, Burrel M, et al. Chemoembolization of hepatocellular carcinoma with drug eluting beads: efficacy and doxorubicin pharmacokinetics. J Hepatol 2007;46:474–81.

45. Hong K, Khwaja A, Liapi E, et al. New intra-arterial drug delivery system for the treatment of liver cancer: preclinical assessment in a rabbit model of liver cancer. Clin Cancer Res 2006;12:2563–7.

46. Malagari K, Chatzimichael K, Alexopoulou E, et al. Transarterial chemoembolization of unresectable hepatocellular carcinoma with drug eluting beads: results of an open-label study of 62 patients. Cardiovasc Intervent Radiol 2008;31: 269–80.

47. Gonzalez MV, Tang Y, Phillips GJ, et al. Doxorubicin eluting beads-2: methods for evaluating drug elution and in-vitro: in-vivo correlation. J Mater Sci Mater Med 2008;19:767–75.

48. Lencioni R, de Baere T, Burrel M, et al. Transcatheter treatment of hepatocellular carcinoma with Doxorubicin-loaded DC Bead (DEBDOX): technical recommendations. Cardiovasc Intervent Radiol 2012;35:980–5.

49. Lammer J, Malagari K, Vogl T, et al. Prospective randomized study of doxorubicin-eluting-bead embolization in the treatment of hepatocellular carcinoma: results of the PRECISION V study. Cardiovasc Intervent Radiol 2010; 33:41–52.

50. Guiu B, Deschamps F, Aho S, et al. Liver/biliary injuries following chemoembo-lisation of endocrine tumours and hepatocellular carcinoma: lipiodol vs. drug-eluting beads. J Hepatol 2012;56:609–17.
51. Dhanasekaran R, Kooby DA, Staley CA, et al. Comparison of conventional trans-arterial chemoembolization (TACE) and chemoembolization with doxorubicin drug eluting beads (DEB) for unresectable hepatocellular carcinoma (HCC). J Surg Oncol 2010;101:476–80.
52. Vogl TJ, Lammer J, Lencioni R, et al. Liver, gastrointestinal, and cardiac toxicity in intermediate hepatocellular carcinoma treated with PRECISION TACE with drug-eluting beads: results from the PRECISION V randomized trial. AJR Am J Roentgenol 2011;197:W562–70.
53. Malagari K, Pomoni M, Spyridopoulos TN, et al. Safety profile of sequential transcatheter chemoembolization with DC Bead: results of 237 hepatocellular carcinoma (HCC) patients. Cardiovasc Intervent Radiol 2011;34:774–85.
54. Bruix J, Llovet JM, Castells A, et al. Transarterial embolization versus symptom-atic treatment in patients with advanced hepatocellular carcinoma: results of a randomized, controlled trial in a single institution. Hepatology 1998;27:1578–83.
55. Shirai S, Sato M, Suwa K, et al. Feasibility and efficacy of single photon emission computed tomography-based three-dimensional conformal radiotherapy for he-patocellular carcinoma 8 cm or more with portal vein tumor thrombus in combi-nation with transcatheter arterial chemoembolization. Int J Radiat Oncol Biol Phys 2010;76:1037–44.
56. Yoon SM, Lim YS, Won HJ, et al. Radiotherapy plus transarterial chemoemboli-zation for hepatocellular carcinoma invading the portal vein: long-term patient outcomes. Int J Radiat Oncol Biol Phys 2012;82:2004–11.
57. Shim SJ, Seong J, Han KH, et al. Local radiotherapy as a complement to incom-plete transcatheter arterial chemoembolization in locally advanced hepatocellu-lar carcinoma. Liver Int 2005;25:1189–96.
58. Murata S, Tajima H, Nakazawa K, et al. Initial experience of transcatheter arterial chemoembolization during portal vein occlusion for unresectable hepatocellular carcinoma with marked arterioportal shunts. Eur Radiol 2009;19:2016–23.
59. Furuse J, Iwasaki M, Yoshino M, et al. Hepatocellular carcinoma with portal vein tu-mor thrombus: embolization of arterioportal shunts. Radiology 1997;204:787–90.
60. Murata S, Mine T, Sugihara F, et al. Interventional treatment for unresectable he-patocellular carcinoma. World J Gastroenterol 2014;20:13453–65.
61. DeAngelis CD, Fontanarosa PB. Retraction: Cheng B-Q, et al. Chemoembolization combined with radiofrequency ablation for patients with hepatocellular carcinoma larger than 3 cm: a randomized controlled trial. JAMA. 2008;299(14):1669–1677. JAMA 2009;301:1931.
62. Jiang H, Meng Q, Tan H, et al. Antiangiogenic therapy enhances the efficacy of transcatheter arterial embolization for hepatocellular carcinomas. Int J Cancer 2007;121:416–24.
63. Kudo M, Imanaka K, Chida N, et al. Phase III study of sorafenib after transarte-rial chemoembolisation in Japanese and Korean patients with unresectable he-patocellular carcinoma. Eur J Cancer 2011;47:2117–27.
64. Pawlik TM, Reyes DK, Cosgrove D, et al. Phase II trial of sorafenib combined with concurrent transarterial chemoembolization with drug-eluting beads for he-patocellular carcinoma. J Clin Oncol 2011;29:3960–7.
65. Ibrahim SM, Lewandowski RJ, Sato KT, et al. Radioembolization for the treat-ment of unresectable hepatocellular carcinoma: a clinical review. World J Gas-troenterol 2008;14:1664–9.

66. Sato K, Lewandowski RJ, Bui JT, et al. Treatment of unresectable primary and metastatic liver cancer with yttrium-90 microspheres (TheraSphere): assessment of hepatic arterial embolization. Cardiovasc Intervent Radiol 2006;29:522–9.

67. Gates VL, Marshall KG, Salzig K, et al. Outpatient single-session yttrium-90 glass microsphere radioembolization. J Vasc Interv Radiol 2014;25:266–70.

68. Theysohn JM, Ertle J, Muller S, et al. Hepatic volume changes after lobar selective internal radiation therapy (SIRT) of hepatocellular carcinoma. Clin Radiol 2014;69:172–8.

69. Nalesnik MA, Federle M, Buck D, et al. Hepatobiliary effects of 90yttrium microsphere therapy for unresectable hepatocellular carcinoma. Hum Pathol 2009;40:125–34.

70. Jakobs TF, Saleem S, Atassi B, et al. Fibrosis, portal hypertension, and hepatic volume changes induced by intra-arterial radiotherapy with 90yttrium microspheres. Dig Dis Sci 2008;53:2556–63.

71. Kim RD, Kim JS, Watanabe G, et al. Liver regeneration and the atrophy-hypertrophy complex. Semin Intervent Radiol 2008;25:92–103.

72. Gaba RC, Lewandowski RJ, Kulik LM, et al. Radiation lobectomy: preliminary findings of hepatic volumetric response to lobar yttrium-90 radioembolization. Ann Surg Oncol 2009;16:1587–96.

73. Salem R, Lewandowski RJ, Kulik L, et al. Radioembolization results in longer time-to-progression and reduced toxicity compared with chemoembolization in patients with hepatocellular carcinoma. Gastroenterology 2011;140:497–507.e2.

74. Salem R, Lewandowski RJ, Mulcahy MF, et al. Radioembolization for hepatocellular carcinoma using Yttrium-90 microspheres: a comprehensive report of long-term outcomes. Gastroenterology 2010;138:52–64.

75. Hilgard P, Hamami M, Fouly AE, et al. Radioembolization with yttrium-90 glass microspheres in hepatocellular carcinoma: European experience on safety and long-term survival. Hepatology 2010;52:1741–9.

76. Sangro B, Carpanese L, Cianni R, et al. Survival after yttrium-90 resin microsphere radioembolization of hepatocellular carcinoma across Barcelona clinic liver cancer stages: a European evaluation. Hepatology 2011;54:868–78.

77. Available at: http://www.cancer.gov/clinicaltrials/search/view?cdrid=719158&version=HealthProfessional&protocolsearchid=4586421. Accessed November 01, 2014.

78. Lance C, McLennan G, Obuchowski N, et al. Comparative analysis of the safety and efficacy of transcatheter arterial chemoembolization and yttrium-90 radioembolization in patients with unresectable hepatocellular carcinoma. J Vasc Interv Radiol 2011;22:1697–705.

79. Kulik LM, Carr BI, Mulcahy MF, et al. Safety and efficacy of 90Y radiotherapy for hepatocellular carcinoma with and without portal vein thrombosis. Hepatology 2008;47:71–81.

80. Memon K, Kulik L, Lewandowski RJ, et al. Radioembolization for hepatocellular carcinoma with portal vein thrombosis: impact of liver function on systemic treatment options at disease progression. J Hepatol 2013;58:73–80.

81. Riaz A, Lewandowski RJ, Kulik LM, et al. Complications following radioembolization with yttrium-90 microspheres: a comprehensive literature review. J Vasc Interv Radiol 2009;20:1121–30 [quiz: 1131].

82. Gervais DA, Goldberg SN, Brown DB, et al. Society of Interventional Radiology position statement on percutaneous radiofrequency ablation for the treatment of liver tumors. J Vasc Interv Radiol 2009;20:S342–7.

83. McGahan JP, Browning PD, Brock JM, et al. Hepatic ablation using radiofrequency electrocautery. Invest Radiol 1990;25:267–70.

84. Lounsberry W, Goldschmidt V, Linke CA, et al. The early histologic changes following electrocoagulation. J Urol 1961;86:321–9.

85. Pompili M, Mirante VG, Rondinara G, et al. Percutaneous ablation procedures in cirrhotic patients with hepatocellular carcinoma submitted to liver transplantation: assessment of efficacy at explant analysis and of safety for tumor recurrence. Liver Transpl 2005;11:1117–26.

86. Livraghi T, Goldberg SN, Lazzaroni S, et al. Small hepatocellular carcinoma: treatment with radio-frequency ablation versus ethanol injection. Radiology 1999;210:655–61.

87. Salmi A, Turrini R, Lanzani G, et al. Efficacy of radiofrequency ablation of hepatocellular carcinoma associated with chronic liver disease without cirrhosis. Int J Med Sci 2008;5:327–32.

88. Livraghi T, Goldberg SN, Lazzaroni S, et al. Hepatocellular carcinoma: radiofrequency ablation of medium and large lesions. Radiology 2000;214:761–8.

89. Hasegawa K, Makuuchi M, Takayama T, et al. Surgical resection vs. percutaneous ablation for hepatocellular carcinoma: a preliminary report of the Japanese nationwide survey. J Hepatol 2008;49:589–94.

90. Lu DS, Raman SS, Limanond P, et al. Influence of large peritumoral vessels on outcome of radiofrequency ablation of liver tumors. J Vasc Interv Radiol 2003; 14:1267–74.

91. Ng KK, Poon RT, Lam CM, et al. Efficacy and safety of radiofrequency ablation for perivascular hepatocellular carcinoma without hepatic inflow occlusion. Br J Surg 2006;93:440–7.

92. Koffron AJ, Auffenberg G, Kung R, et al. Evaluation of 300 minimally invasive liver resections at a single institution: less is more. Ann Surg 2007;246:385–92 [discussion: 392–4].

93. Lin SM, Lin CJ, Lin CC, et al. Randomised controlled trial comparing percutaneous radiofrequency thermal ablation, percutaneous ethanol injection, and percutaneous acetic acid injection to treat hepatocellular carcinoma of 3 cm or less. Gut 2005;54:1151–6.

94. Curley SA, Izzo F, Ellis LM, et al. Radiofrequency ablation of hepatocellular cancer in 110 patients with cirrhosis. Ann Surg 2000;232:381–91.

95. Livraghi T, Solbiati L, Meloni MF, et al. Treatment of focal liver tumors with percutaneous radio-frequency ablation: complications encountered in a multicenter study. Radiology 2003;226:441–51.

96. Liang P, Wang Y. Microwave ablation of hepatocellular carcinoma. Oncology 2007;72(Suppl 1):124–31.

97. Liu FY, Yu XL, Liang P, et al. Comparison of percutaneous 915 MHz microwave ablation and 2450 MHz microwave ablation in large hepatocellular carcinoma. Int J Hyperthermia 2010;26:448–55.

98. Lee KF, Hui JW, Cheung YS, et al. Surgical ablation of hepatocellular carcinoma with 2.45-GHz microwave: a critical appraisal of treatment outcomes. Hong Kong Med J 2012;18:85–91.

99. Liang P, Wang Y, Yu X, et al. Malignant liver tumors: treatment with percutaneous microwave ablation–complications among cohort of 1136 patients. Radiology 2009;251:933–40.

100. Takami Y, Ryu T, Wada Y, et al. Evaluation of intraoperative microwave coagulonecrotic therapy (MCN) for hepatocellular carcinoma: a single center experience of 719 consecutive cases. J Hepatobiliary Pancreat Sci 2013;20:332–41.

101. Liu Y, Zheng Y, Li S, et al. Percutaneous microwave ablation of larger hepatocellular carcinoma. Clin Radiol 2013;68:21–6.
102. Narayanan G. Irreversible electroporation for treatment of liver cancer. Gastroenterol Hepatol (N Y) 2011;7:313–6.
103. Maor E, Ivorra A, Leor J, et al. The effect of irreversible electroporation on blood vessels. Technol Cancer Res Treat 2007;6:307–12.
104. Charpentier KP, Wolf F, Noble L, et al. Irreversible electroporation of the liver and liver hilum in swine. HPB (Oxford) 2011;13:168–73.
105. Cannon R, Ellis S, Hayes D, et al. Safety and early efficacy of irreversible electroporation for hepatic tumors in proximity to vital structures. J Surg Oncol 2013; 107:544–9.
106. Permpongkosol S, Nicol TL, Link RE, et al. Differences in ablation size in porcine kidney, liver, and lung after cryoablation using the same ablation protocol. AJR Am J Roentgenol 2007;188:1028–32.
107. Permpongkosol S, Nicol TL, Khurana H, et al. Thermal maps around two adjacent cryoprobes creating overlapping ablations in porcine liver, lung, and kidney. J Vasc Interv Radiol 2007;18:283–7.
108. Bilchik AJ, Wood TF, Allegra D, et al. Cryosurgical ablation and radiofrequency ablation for unresectable hepatic malignant neoplasms: a proposed algorithm. Arch Surg 2000;135:657–62 [discussion: 662–4].
109. Sung GT, Gill IS, Hsu TH, et al. Effect of intentional cryo-injury to the renal collecting system. J Urol 2003;170:619–22.
110. Chen HW, Lai EC, Zhen ZJ, et al. Ultrasound-guided percutaneous cryotherapy of hepatocellular carcinoma. Int J Surg 2011;9:188–91.
111. Chang XJ, Lu YY, Bai WL, et al. Clinical efficacy and prognostic factors for cryoablation patients with advanced hepatocellular carcinoma. Zhonghua Gan Zang Bing Za Zhi 2011;19:759–63.
112. Huang YZ, Zhou SC, Zhou H, et al. Radiofrequency ablation versus cryosurgery ablation for hepatocellular carcinoma: a meta-analysis. Hepatogastroenterology 2013;60:1131–5.
113. Seifert JK, Morris DL. World survey on the complications of hepatic and prostate cryotherapy. World J Surg 1999;23:109–13 [discussion: 113–4].
114. Davis CR. Interventional radiological treatment of hepatocellular carcinoma. Cancer Control 2010;17:87–99.
115. Orlando A, Leandro G, Olivo M, et al. Radiofrequency thermal ablation vs. percutaneous ethanol injection for small hepatocellular carcinoma in cirrhosis: meta-analysis of randomized controlled trials. Am J Gastroenterol 2009;104: 514–24.
116. Chapman WC, Majella Doyle MB, Stuart JE, et al. Outcomes of neoadjuvant transarterial chemoembolization to downstage hepatocellular carcinoma before liver transplantation. Ann Surg 2008;248:617–25.
117. Barakat O, Wood RP, Ozaki CF, et al. Morphological features of advanced hepatocellular carcinoma as a predictor of downstaging and liver transplantation: an intention-to-treat analysis. Liver Transpl 2010;16:289–99.

options for patients with HCC are more complex and depend on several factors, including underlying liver disease and tumor characteristics. The impact of the patients' liver reserve and presence of cirrhosis dictates the extent of surgery or whether surgical resection is an option at all. Classifications based on one prognostic parameter, such as tumor size and number (TNM classification) or disease severity (ie the Child-Turcotte-Pugh [CTP] or Model of End-Stage Liver Disease [MELD] scores), are generally not sufficient and have to be used in conjunction with one another to assess patients for the appropriate treatment options.

Assessing hepatic function is the most important aspect in selecting patients for hepatic resection. Clinical staging systems like the CTP score are frequently used to stratify patients who would tolerate a hepatic resection. Resection is generally favored in patients with CTP A cirrhosis (CTP score 5–6) in the absence of portal hypertension. A history of variceal bleeding, finding esophageal varices on endoscopy, or thrombocytopenia (platelet count $<100,000/mm^3$) indicates significant portal hypertension even in CTP A patients. In the absence of these features, CTP A patients typically tolerate a hepatic resection.[5,6] Direct measurement of hepatic venous wedge pressure and gradient provides an accurate estimate of the portal pressure. It is recommended that only patients with hepatic venous wedge pressure of less than 10 mm Hg be considered for hepatic resection.[5,6] Measurement of hepatic venous wedge pressure is an invasive procedure and is generally not required when the clinical picture suggests the presence of portal hypertension. Moreover, splenomegaly and portal venous varices (stigmata of portal hypertension) are easily seen on imaging studies like ultrasound, computed tomography (CT) scan, and MRI. Direct measurement of portal pressure should be reserved for situations when portal hypertension is suspected but cannot be confirmed despite thorough assessment.

Patients with CTP B (CTP score 7–9) and C (CTP score 10–15) cirrhosis are at a high risk of postoperative hepatic decompensation and are generally not considered for hepatic lobar resection. For these patients, liver transplantation offers the best long-term outcome and the only potential cure for both the HCC and underlying liver disease. Patients considered to be unsuitable candidates for liver transplantation because of medical or social reasons should be considered for locoregional therapy (LRT) or chemotherapy.

The MELD score is also a useful tool in assessing patients for hepatic resection. It was originally developed to predict survival of patients with cirrhosis and is currently used worldwide in liver transplant organ allocation. In several studies, the MELD score has been shown to be a strong predictor of postoperative outcomes after hepatic resection. In one report, hepatic resection in patients with a MELD score of 8 or less was associated with no perioperative mortality and minimal morbidity, whereas patients with a MELD score of 9 or greater had a 30% mortality rate.[7]

An important determinant of resectability is careful evaluation of the imaging studies. Multiphasic CT scans as well as MRIs are routinely used to assess tumor size, location, and proximity of the tumor to major hepatic vasculature. Invasion of major portal vein or hepatic vein branches seen on imaging studies is associated with poor outcomes and is considered a contraindication to resection (**Fig. 3**). The size and number of tumors correlates with the risk of recurrence but do not necessarily preclude patients from consideration for resection. Larger tumors are more likely to have vascular invasion but some large encapsulated tumors without vascular invasion can be safely resected without an increased risk of recurrence (**Fig. 4**). In select patients with tumors larger than 10 cm, normal liver parenchyma, and no evidence of vascular invasion, long-term survival has been successfully achieved after hepatic resection.[4,8–10]

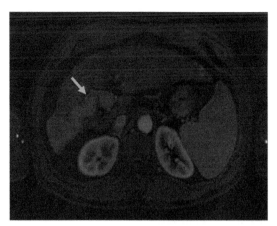

**Fig. 3.** Invasion of the right branch of the portal vein by HCC (*arrow*).

There is no absolute number of lesions that precludes consideration for resection. Multinodular HCC can be either intrahepatic metastasis seen as satellite lesions surrounding a large tumor or separate individual lesions within the liver. Metastatic or multifocal HCC can be safely resected if confined to one hepatic lobe; however, bilobar disease is usually considered a contraindication to resection (**Fig. 5**). Patients with

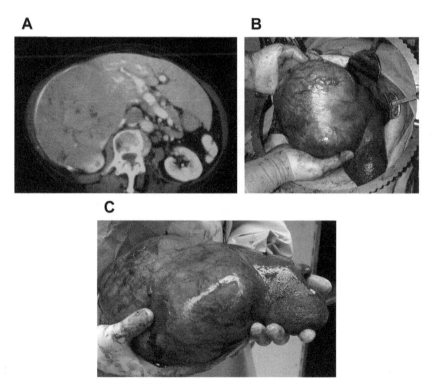

**Fig. 4.** A giant encapsulated HCC in a patient without cirrhosis occupying the right lobe and segment IV requiring extended right hepatectomy. (*A*) CT scan image, (*B*) at operation, (*C*) the resected specimen.

options for patients with HCC are more complex and depend on several factors, including underlying liver disease and tumor characteristics. The impact of the patients' liver reserve and presence of cirrhosis dictates the extent of surgery or whether surgical resection is an option at all. Classifications based on one prognostic parameter, such as tumor size and number (TNM classification) or disease severity (ie the Child-Turcotte-Pugh [CTP] or Model of End-Stage Liver Disease [MELD] scores), are generally not sufficient and have to be used in conjunction with one another to assess patients for the appropriate treatment options.

Assessing hepatic function is the most important aspect in selecting patients for hepatic resection. Clinical staging systems like the CTP score are frequently used to stratify patients who would tolerate a hepatic resection. Resection is generally favored in patients with CTP A cirrhosis (CTP score 5–6) in the absence of portal hypertension. A history of variceal bleeding, finding esophageal varices on endoscopy, or thrombocytopenia (platelet count <100,000/mm$^3$) indicates significant portal hypertension even in CTP A patients. In the absence of these features, CTP A patients typically tolerate a hepatic resection.[5,6] Direct measurement of hepatic venous wedge pressure and gradient provides an accurate estimate of the portal pressure. It is recommended that only patients with hepatic venous wedge pressure of less than 10 mm Hg be considered for hepatic resection.[5,6] Measurement of hepatic venous wedge pressure is an invasive procedure and is generally not required when the clinical picture suggests the presence of portal hypertension. Moreover, splenomegaly and portal venous varices (stigmata of portal hypertension) are easily seen on imaging studies like ultrasound, computed tomography (CT) scan, and MRI. Direct measurement of portal pressure should be reserved for situations when portal hypertension is suspected but cannot be confirmed despite thorough assessment.

Patients with CTP B (CTP score 7–9) and C (CTP score 10–15) cirrhosis are at a high risk of postoperative hepatic decompensation and are generally not considered for hepatic lobar resection. For these patients, liver transplantation offers the best long-term outcome and the only potential cure for both the HCC and underlying liver disease. Patients considered to be unsuitable candidates for liver transplantation because of medical or social reasons should be considered for locoregional therapy (LRT) or chemotherapy.

The MELD score is also a useful tool in assessing patients for hepatic resection. It was originally developed to predict survival of patients with cirrhosis and is currently used worldwide in liver transplant organ allocation. In several studies, the MELD score has been shown to be a strong predictor of postoperative outcomes after hepatic resection. In one report, hepatic resection in patients with a MELD score of 8 or less was associated with no perioperative mortality and minimal morbidity, whereas patients with a MELD score of 9 or greater had a 30% mortality rate.[7]

An important determinant of resectability is careful evaluation of the imaging studies. Multiphasic CT scans as well as MRIs are routinely used to assess tumor size, location, and proximity of the tumor to major hepatic vasculature. Invasion of major portal vein or hepatic vein branches seen on imaging studies is associated with poor outcomes and is considered a contraindication to resection (**Fig. 3**). The size and number of tumors correlates with the risk of recurrence but do not necessarily preclude patients from consideration for resection. Larger tumors are more likely to have vascular invasion but some large encapsulated tumors without vascular invasion can be safely resected without an increased risk of recurrence (**Fig. 4**). In select patients with tumors larger than 10 cm, normal liver parenchyma, and no evidence of vascular invasion, long-term survival has been successfully achieved after hepatic resection.[4,8–10]

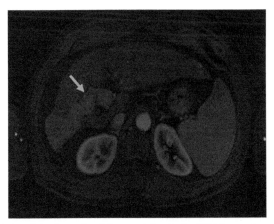

**Fig. 3.** Invasion of the right branch of the portal vein by HCC (*arrow*).

There is no absolute number of lesions that precludes consideration for resection. Multinodular HCC can be either intrahepatic metastasis seen as satellite lesions surrounding a large tumor or separate individual lesions within the liver. Metastatic or multifocal HCC can be safely resected if confined to one hepatic lobe; however, bilobar disease is usually considered a contraindication to resection (**Fig. 5**). Patients with

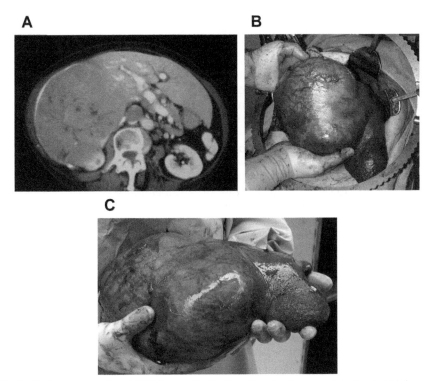

**Fig. 4.** A giant encapsulated HCC in a patient without cirrhosis occupying the right lobe and segment IV requiring extended right hepatectomy. (*A*) CT scan image, (*B*) at operation, (*C*) the resected specimen.

# Systemic Therapy of Hepatocellular Carcinoma

## Current and Promising

Aparna Kalyan, MD[a,b], Halla Nimeiri, MD[a,b], Laura Kulik, MD[b,c],*

### KEYWORDS

- Hepatocellular carcinoma • Systemic therapy • Targeted agents

### KEY POINTS

- Sorafenib is the only approved systemic therapy for hepatocellular carcinoma (HCC).
- Side effects of sorafenib need to be closely monitored.
- Newer agents have failed to show a benefit over sorafenib.
- A personalized approach to HCC to capitalize and inhibit the genes driving hepatocarcinognesis is needed.

## SYSTEMIC THERAPY FOR HEPATOCELLULAR CARCINOMA

The incidence of hepatocellular carcinoma (HCC) continues to increase and although there have been advancements in therapy, HCC has become the second leading cause of cancer-related mortality worldwide.[1] Treatment of HCC is confounded by the competing risk of morbidity and mortality imposed by underlying cirrhosis that is present in nearly 90% of patients with HCC. The treatment of HCC must balance efficacy from an oncologic standpoint with the ability of a diseased liver to tolerate the therapy.

Historically, cytotoxic chemotherapeutic agents have been poorly tolerated in HCC and have not demonstrated a reproducible benefit of improved overall survival (OS).[2] The approval of sorafenib in 2006 ushered in the era of targeted agents.[3] However, the redundant molecular pathways in hepatocarcinogenesis that eventually render the inhibition of the targeted molecular pathway inadequate to control tumor growth have

Disclosure: Dr. Kulik is on the Bayer Advisory Board, Blue Print Advisory Board and is Speaker for Abbvie & Gilead.
[a] Northwestern Medicine Developmental Therapeutics Institute (NMDTI), Chicago, IL, USA; [b] Division of Hematology and Oncology, Robert H. Lurie Medical Research Center, Room 5-121, 303 East Superior, Chicago, IL 60611, USA; [c] Division of Hepatology and Gastroenterology, Northwestern University, 676 North St Clair, 19th Floor, Chicago, IL 60611, USA
* Corresponding author. Division of Gastroenterology and Hepatology, Department of Medicine, Northwestern University, 676 North St Clair, 19th Floor, Chicago, IL 60611.
E-mail address: lkulik@nm.org

limited the sustained efficacy of small molecules. Chronic inflammation leading to fibrosis is a key contributor to hepatocarcinogenesis. As the hepatocytes attempt to regenerate under the ongoing insult of viral hepatitis, alcohol, or oxidative stress related to fatty liver disease, DNA mutations accumulate and lead to the development of cancer. Additionally, fibrogenesis itself contributes to the development of cancer via promotion of angiogenesis and antiapoptotic factors.[4,5] This article reviews systemic therapy for HCC.

## SORAFENIB

Sorafenib remains the only approved systemic therapy available for unresectable HCC. Several questions remain unanswered. The vast majority of patients enrolled in the 2 randomized controlled trials that demonstrated improved OS and prolonged time to progression (TTP) associated with sorafenib compared with placebo were Child–Turcotte–Pugh (CTP) class A with a performance status of 0 or 1.[6,7] The interim analysis of the Global Investigation Of Therapeutic Decision In Hepatocellular Carcinoma And Of Its Treatment With sorafenib (GIDEON), a prospective observational trial of patients treated with sorafenib in real-life clinical practice, highlighted that OS is influenced by CTP status: CTP-A 10.3 versus CTP-B 4.8 months. TTP was similar between CTP-A and CTP-B.[8] Additionally, the development of worsening hepatic function with longer duration of sorafenib has been reported in CTP-B compared with CTP-A.[9] Whether this decline in liver function is attributable to the underlying liver disease itself or related to drug exposure is not known. The final analysis of GIDEON was presented at the American Society for Clinical Oncology (ASCO) meeting in 2013.[10] A total of 3202 patients were evaluated. There was no significant difference in drug-related side effects across CTP classes; however, serious adverse events were more evident in the CTP-B subgroup. Similar to the results of the interim analysis, OS was influence by CTP classification: median OS in CTP-A was 13.6 months (95% CI, 12.8–14.7) and in CTP-B it was 5.2 months (95% CI, 4.6–6.3). The shortest OS was observed in those with CTP-B (score 9) at 3.7 months. TTP was not different according to CTP class: in CTP-A it was 4.7 months (95% CI, 4.3–5.2) and in CTP-B it was 4.4 months (95% CI, 3.5–5.5). The safety and efficacy of sorafenib in CTP-B patients is being examined in an ongoing randomized, controlled trial (RCT), the B Child Patient–Optimization Of Sorafenib Treatment (BOOST) trial (NCT01405573).

The approved dose for sorafenib is 400 mg bid. Dose reductions for side effects, including hand–foot skin reaction (HFSR; **Table 1**), hypertension, diarrhea, and fatigue are often needed in the management of patients on sorafenib. Alternatively, the strategy of initiating sorafenib at 200 bid and titrating up as tolerability allows is often used in clinical practice. Insight into the correlation between drug dosing and duration with OS is limited to a retrospective analysis by Iavarone and colleagues.[9] All patients were started on full-dose sorafenib. However, those patients who required a dose reduction had an overall longer duration of therapy compared with those treated with full dose (6.8 vs 3 months, respectively) and the OS was 21.6 months among those on reduced dose compared with 9.6 months in those continued on full dose. Owing to the retrospective nature of these data, conclusions and therefore recommendations regarding the best dose regimen of sorafenib cannot be drawn. Some experts have hypothesized that the observed improved outcomes with lesser doses of sorafenib may be owing to differences in pharmacodynamics. The suggestion is that in those developing side effects requiring dose reductions, this is an indication of higher kinase inhibition in vivo, compared with those able to tolerate full dose.[11] In line with this idea, side effects such as HFSR have been reported to be associated with a TTP compared with

**Table 1**
**Management of dermatologic toxicity from sorafenib**

| Grade | Occurrence | Dose Modification |
|---|---|---|
| Grade 1 | Any | Continue dose and consider topical therapy. |
| Grade 2 – painful erythema and swelling of hands or feet affecting patient's daily activities | First occurrence | Continue and consider topical therapy for symptomatic relief. If no improvement in 7 d hold therapy until improvement. |
| | No improvement after 7 d or subsequent occurrences | Interrupt therapy until resolution of symptoms. When dose is restarted, decrease dose to 400 mg daily or 400 mg every other day. |
| | Fourth occurrence | Discontinue any further therapy. |
| Grade 3 – Moist desquamation, ulceration, blistering or severe pain of hands and feet affecting patient's daily activities | First or second occurrence | Interrupt therapy until symptoms resolve to grade 0 or 1. When dose is restarted, decrease dose to 400 mg or 400 every other day. |
| | Third occurrence | Discontinue any further therapy. |

Symptoms include dry skin, rash, pruritus, blistering, or desquamation.
*Data from* Bayer AG. Sorafenib [package insert]. Leverkusen, Germany.

those without dermatologic side effects (8.1 vs 4.0 months).[12] However, in another study, there was a failure to find a correlation between the development of HFSR and clinical outcomes, although the development of sorafenib-induced diarrhea was associated with a near doubling of OS compared with those without diarrhea.[13] Additional research to substantiate a potential link between side effects and drug response is needed.

Another unanswered question is what to do once a patient develops progression on sorafenib. In the Sorafenib HCC Assessment Randomized Protocol (SHARP) trial, patients were continued on therapy until there was symptomatic progression. Sorafenib is a cytostatic agent; therefore, the reported radiographic response (RECIST) that has been used traditionally in assessing liver directed therapy is significantly lower at approximately 2% to 3%. In patients who are intolerant of sorafenib or demonstrate tumor progression, the only option is participation in a clinical trial, which is limited generally to those with preserved hepatic function, normal performance status, and adequate hematologic parameters. Limited clinical data are available to answer the question of what to do after tumor progression on sorafenib. However, there is speculation that continuation of sorafenib despite radiographic progression does impart a clinical benefit via tumor suppression. There was improved OS from the time of detection of tumor progression in 23 patients who remained on sorafenib compared with 13 patients in whom drug was discontinued.[14]

Early changes in serum tumor markers associated with sorafenib may be useful. Increased alpha-fetoprotein, defined as a greater than 20% increase from baseline, within 4 weeks of starting sorafenib was an independent predictor of OS (hazard ratio [HR], 4.14). Changes in des-gamma-carboxyl prothrombin (DCP) had no predictive value.[15] In contrast, in another study a 2-fold or greater increase in DCP from baseline that was seen 2 weeks after initiation of sorafenib, was associated with a significant prolongation in TTP compared with those without a change in DCP.[16]

Safety considerations in the clinic when treating with sorafenib are important for providers. Cardiac ischemia in the SHARP trial was reported to be 2.7%. Caution must be exercised in patients who have recently (within 6 months) had a myocardial ischemic event. Furthermore, if a patient experiences myocardial ischemia while on therapy, then temporary discontinuation of sorafenib is recommended. Additional cardiac considerations include monitoring of the electrocardiogram QTc interval. Before starting sorafenib, patients should have an electrocardiogram to assess baseline QT/QTc. It is recommended that patients who have congenital long QT syndrome or prolonged QT at baseline for other reasons should not be treated with sorafenib. When patients are on sorafenib, electrolytes (particularly magnesium, calcium, and potassium) should be checked and maintained at appropriate levels. It is recommended that sorafenib be discontinued if there is greater than a 60-ms increase in QT from baseline or if QT increases to greater than 500 ms.

As with all other tyrosine kinase inhibitors, hypertension is an ensuing side effect. Based on the SHARP trial, approximately 10% of patients develop hypertension. It is recommended that patients undergo weekly monitoring of blood pressure for the first 6 weeks and then as required after the initiation of antihypertensive therapy. In preclinical data, it has been noted that there is a stimulatory effect of vascular endothelial growth factor (VEGF) on endothelial nitric oxide production via upregulation of endothelial nitric oxide synthase expression.[17] As a result, it is hypothesized that VEGF-targeting agents (like ramicirumab and bevacizumab) induce inhibition of VEGF, thereby decreasing nitric oxide synthesis and subsequently increasing vasoconstriction, vascular tone, and sodium retention by renal tubules. As such, it is postulated that in the treatment of anti-VEGF–induced hypertension, calcium channel blockers are the preferred first-line agents.

Perhaps the most common side effect with sorafenib is the HFSR syndrome (see **Table 1**). Management includes topical therapies and discontinuation for severe grade III/IV toxicities (desquamation, ulceration, blistering, and pain) that disrupt activities of daily living. The use of prophylactic urea-based cream has been shown to decrease significantly the incidence of all-grade HFSR compared with best supportive care (56% vs 74%; P<.0001).[18] Rash or desquamation are other dermatologic side effects associated with sorafenib. The use of zinc oxide-based emollients or lanolin-based creams can decrease the incidence of this side effect.[19]

### Combination of Sorafenib with Locoregional Therapy or Resection

The biological plausibility of using sorafenib to blunt the flare of angiogenesis associated with transarterial chemoembolization (TACE) has made combination therapy an attractive option. It is well-known that higher levels of VEGF after TACE portend a poorer prognosis.[20] There have been 3 RCTs that have examined sorafenib plus TACE compared with TACE alone in patients with intermediate HCC.[21–23] The results have been mixed. This may in part be owing to the differences in the strategic approach in terms of the timing of sorafenib administration with TACE performance. Sorafenib can be given after completion of TACE (sequential), before TACE, and held at time of TACE (interrupted) or in a continuous fashion.[24] Because the surge in VEGF occurs within 24 hours of embolization, the approach that would intuitively have the greatest impact would be continuous sorafenib administration before and after TACE.[25] However, in a small retrospective trial from a single center, a cautionary note was reported in the use of sorafenib in a continuous fashion with TACE. Angiographic findings were suggestive of a diminished appearance of HCC lesions owing to intratumoral vascular pruning, leading to suboptimal therapy with TACE.[26] The authors recommended that sorafenib be held for 7 days before TACE to optimize tumor visualization on the angiogram, and then to commence sorafenib immediately after TACE to blunt the angiogenic flare associated with embolization. A metaanalysis of 6 studies (but not including unpublished results of the Sorafenib or Placebo in Combination with TACE for Intermediate HCC [SPACE] trial) deduced that the combination of sorafenib plus TACE improved OS and TTP.[27] Two ongoing RCTs are further exploring the role of TACE with or without sorafenib: Eastern Cooperative Oncology Group (ECOG) 1208 (NCT01004978, US) with TACE given 2 weeks after initiation of sorafenib, or TACE with Drug Eluting Beads (TACE-DEB) with or without sorafenib given 2 to 5 weeks later (NCI01324076; United Kingdom).

The use of a systemic agent to diminish risk of HCC recurrence after an intended curative therapy such as hepatic resection represents a significant clinical interest. The risk of recurrent HCC is estimated to be approximately 70% at 5 years, accounting for the leading cause of mortality after resection. Approximately three-quarters of recurrences are owing to intrahepatic spread. Recurrence generally occurs within 2 years of surgery.[28] An intervention that could impact micrometastatic disease that may be present at the time of resection and inhibit subsequent tumor angiogenesis, could potentially improve outcomes after resection. In vitro, sorafenib leads to apoptosis via inhibition of angiogenesis and tumor cell proliferation.[29] In a nonrandomized, phase II trial of 31 patients, optimistic results were reported; there was a significant decrease in recurrence among those treated with sorafenib 400 mg bid for 4 months compared with control posthepatic resection (29.4% vs 70.7%; $P = .0032$). Furthermore, after a median follow-up of 19 months, the time to recurrence was significantly longer in the adjuvant group (21.5 vs 13.4 months; $P = .006$).[30] The Sorafenib as Adjuvant Treatment in the Prevention of Recurrence of Hepatocellular Carcinoma (STORM) trial was designed to determine the safety and efficacy of sorafenib administered after intended curative therapy with radiofrequency ablation or hepatic resection. Eighty percent of subjects underwent resection, the maximal tumor size was 3.4 cm, and 90% had a solitary lesion. Compared with placebo, sorafenib 400 bid (for up to 4 years after resection until recurrence or discontinuation) did not demonstrate an improvement in recurrence-free survival.[31] Currently, there are no proven adjuvant therapies to decrease postresection HCC recurrence.

### Sorafenib in the Pretransplant Setting

Liver transplantation (LT) offers the best chance for cure in patients with HCC. Priority for LT in the setting of HCC is restricted to those who fulfill the Milan criteria, namely 1 lesion 5 cm or smaller, or 3 lesions with none greater than 3 cm, and no vascular invasion or metastases.[32] Progression of HCC while awaiting LT can lead to dropout from the waiting list; the risk at 1 year ranges from 15% to 30%.[33] Living donor LT is often used in patients who are anticipated to wait longer than 6 months for a transplant in the hope of diminishing tumor progression and hence dropout from the waiting list.[34] Sorafenib has also been used in patients on the waiting list. A Markov analysis concluded that sorafenib is cost effective, compared with no therapy, in patients with an HCC Model of End-stage Liver Disease (MELD) upgrade and who are anticipated to wait less than 6 months.[35] As waiting times increased beyond 6 months, the use of sorafenib became less effective, particularly when living donor LT was incorporated into the model.

The safety and efficacy of sorafenib in the pretransplant setting was examined in a pilot RCT of 20 patients ($^{90}$Y with or without sorafenib). In this study, there was no apparent benefit of sorafenib when added to $^{90}$Y radioembolization, either on explant pathology or clinical outcomes.[36,37] In terms of safety, there was an increased risk of biliary complications ($P = .029$) and acute cellular rejection ($P = .082$) within 30 days, in the sorafenib group. Similarly, in a retrospective trial an increase in biliary complications (67% vs 17%, respectively; $P = .01$) and acute cellular rejection (67% vs 22%, respectively; $P = .04$) was also noted among those treated with sorafenib pretransplantation compared with controls.[38] On the other hand, another single center reported no increased risk of perioperative complications associated with pretransplant sorafenib.[39]

### Sorafenib Combined with Other Agents

Although sorafenib has been shown to improve significantly OS and TTP compared with placebo, these results were marginal. There is interest in combining sorafenib with other agents that may act synergistically and translate into improved outcomes without adverse events that would limit combination therapy.

In a phase II, multinational trial, sorafenib plus doxorubicin was compared with doxorubicin alone. The OS increased to 13.7 months from 6.5 months in the combination arm compared with doxorubicin monotherapy arm.[40] In the phase II study, the major toxicity noted was cardiac. In the combination group left ventricular dysfunction was seen in 19% of patients compared with 2% in the sorafenib arm alone. Although the majority of patients with left ventricular systolic dysfunction were asymptomatic, it is unclear whether increased doxorubicin-associated cardiac toxicity in this study is attributable to a sorafenib-induced increase in doxorubicin area under the curve.[40] There is now an ongoing, phase III, intergroup trial comparing sorafenib plus doxorubicin versus sorafenib alone (NCI01840592).

### Sorafenib and Mammalian Targets of Rapamycin

There are increasing preclinical data suggesting that aberration in the mammalian target of rapamycin pathway is a crucial component of HCC tumors. Recently, a small phase I study of 25 patients in patients with CTP-A and CTP-B HCC were treated with temsirolimus and sorafenib. The maximum tolerated dose was found to be 10 mg/wk and sorafenib was given at 200 mg twice a day. Of the 18 patients treated at the maximum tolerated dose, 8% had a partial response, and a further 60% had stable disease with alpha-fetoprotein having declined by at least 50% in 60% of the assessable patients.[41] These promising preliminary data have led to a phase II study that is recruiting patients currently (NCT01687673).

### Beyond Sorafenib

There is an unmet need in patients who progress on, or become intolerant to, sorafenib. Encouraging results were seen in phase II trials; however, subsequent phase III trials with several other multikinase inhibitors, including brivanib, sunitinib, and linifanib, did not meet their primary endpoints when compared with sorafenib (**Table 2**). This is a very active area of research with more than 50 ongoing agents in clinical investigation.[42]

## SUNITINIB

Sunitinib is an oral multikinase inhibitor that targets receptor tyrosine kinases including VEGF receptor (R)1, VEGFR2, platelet-derived growth factor receptor-alpha/beta, c-KIT, Feline McDonnough Sarcoma Like (FLT)3, and rearranged during transfection (RET) kinases. Despite promising results in several small phase II studies, these were not sustained in a large phase III trial that compared sunitinib at 37.5 mg continuous daily dosing versus sorafenib at 400 mg twice daily in advanced HCC. This large study of 1073 patients was ended prematurely owing to a higher number of adverse events in the sunitinib arm to which 17 patients' death was attributed. Although TTP between the 2 arms was equivalent, sunitinib was associated with a significantly lower

**Table 2**
**Phase III trials with multikinase inhibitors in advanced HCC**

| Trial | Population | Treatment | Results |
|---|---|---|---|
| SHARP | Treatment-naïve advanced HCC | Sorafenib (n = 299) vs placebo (n = 303) | ORR: 2% vs 1% ($P$ = .05)<br>mOS: 10.7 vs 7.9 mo (HR, 0.69; $P$<.01)<br>mTTP: 4.9 vs 4.1 mo (HR, 1.08; $P$ = 0.77) |
| Asia-Pacific | Treatment-naïve advanced HCC | Sorafenib (n = 150) vs placebo (n = 76) | ORR: 3.3% vs 1.3%<br>mOS: 6.5 vs 4.2 mo (HR, 0.68; $P$ = .014)<br>mTTP: 2.8 vs 1.4 mo (HR, 0.57; $P$<.005) |
| BRISK-FL | Treatment-naïve advanced HCC | Brivanib (n = 577) vs sorafenib (n = 578) | ORR: 12% vs 9%<br>mOS: 9.5 vs 9.9 mo (HR, 1.06; $P$ = .373)<br>mTTP: 4.2 vs 4.1 mo (HR, 1.01; $P$ = .853) |
| BRISK-PS | Treatment failure after sorafenib in advanced HCC | Brivanib (n = 263) vs placebo (n = 132) | ORR 10% vs 2%<br>mOS: 9.4 vs 8.2 mo (HR, 0.89; $P$.33)<br>mTTP: 4.2 vs 2.7 mo (HR, 0.56; $P$<.001) |
| SUN 1170 | Treatment-naïve advanced HCC | Sunitinib (n = 530) vs sorafenib (n = 544) | ORR: 6.6% vs 6.1%<br>mOS: 7.9 vs 10.2 mo (HR, 1.30; $P$.999)<br>mTTP: 4.1 vs 3.8 mo (HR, 1.13; $P$ = .8312) |
| NCT01009593 | Treatment-naïve advanced HCC | Linifanib (n = 530) vs sorafenib (n = 544) | ORR: 13% vs 6.9%<br>mOS: 9.1 vs 9.8 mo (HR, 1.046)<br>mTTP: 5.4 vs 4.0 mo |
|  | No prior systemic therapy in advanced HCC | TACE then sorafenib (n = 229) vs sorafenib then placebo (n = 229) | mOS: 29.7 mo vs NE (HR, 1.06; $P$.79)<br>mTTP: 5.4 vs 3.7 mo (HR, 0.87; $P$ = .25) |

*Abbreviations:* HCC, hepatocellular carcinoma; HR, hazard ratio; mOS, median overall survival; mTTP, median time to progression; NE, not estimable; ORR, objective response rate; TACE, transarterial chemoembolization.

OS (7.9 vs 10.2 months; HR, 1.30; 95% 95% CI, 1.13–1.50; $P$ = .0014).[43] Similar to sorafenib, ethnicity and etiology of underlying liver disease seemed to impact OS, which was more prolonged in those with hepatitis C virus–induced HCC compared with hepatitis B virus–induced HCC.

**BRIVANIB**

Brivanib is a multikinase inhibitor with activity against fibroblast growth factor receptor-2 and VEGFR-2. It was hypothesized that, when both pathways are blocked, a better overall response rate could be achieved. Brivanib has since been compared with sorafenib in treatment-naïve patients with advanced HCC in a phase III RCT—Brivanib versus Sorafenib as First-Line Treatment in Patients With Advanced Hepatocellular Carcinoma (BRISK-FL)— as well as a second-line agent among patients who had progressed or were intolerant to sorafenib in the Brivanib Study in HCC Patients at Risk Post-Sorafenib (BRISK-PS).

In a treatment-naïve advanced HCC patient population, brivanib was investigated in a large, international, randomized study (BRISK-FL study).[44] The patients were randomized to receive either sorafenib versus brivanib in a 1:1 fashion, noninferiority trial. The primary endpoint was noninferiority. Unfortunately, not only did the trial not meet its primary endpoint of noninferiority (median OS, 9.9 months with sorafenib and 9.5 months with brivanib), it also demonstrated that brivanib was less well-tolerated compared with sorafenib with a discontinuation rate of 33% for sorafenib and 43% for brivanib.

Brivanib was also investigated in the second-line setting, in advanced HCC patients who had failed or were intolerant of sorafenib in a large, international, phase III study (BRISK-PS study).[45] In BRISK-PS, patients were randomized to receive either sorafenib or placebo in a 2:1 fashion of brivanib 800 mg orally daily versus placebo plus best supportive care for all. Unfortunately, the trial did not meet its primary endpoint either of improvement in OS; the median OS was 9.4 months for brivanib and 8.2 months for placebo (HR, 0.89; $P = .3307$).

### Mammalian Target of Rapamycin Pathway

There have been preclinical data to suggest that the mammalian target of rapamycin pathway is upregulated in HCC patients and inhibition of this aberrant pathway leads to reduced proliferation, impaired angiogenesis, delayed metastases, and improvement in OS.[41,46,47] Recently, the Everolimus for Liver Cancer Evaluation (EVOLVE)-1 study results were presented at ASCO GI 2014. In this large international study, 546 patients were randomized (2:1) to receive everolimus 7.5 mg daily or placebo.[48] All patients received best supportive care with stratification being done geographically (Asia vs rest of the world) and according to the presence or absence of macrovascular invasion. The primary endpoint was OS, but median OS was 7.5 months in the everolimus arm and 7.3 months in the placebo arm (HR, 1.05; $P = .675$), unfortunately demonstrating no improvement in among patients with advanced HCC that have progressed on sorafenib.

### c-Met

There is now increasing evidence that has established that mesothelial epithelial tumor (MET) overexpression is associated with poor prognosis in HCC patients. In a phase I study, tivantinib, a small molecule oral c-met inhibitor, at a dose of 360 mg orally twice daily, was tolerable and did not worsen liver test results in cirrhotic patients.[49] This prompted a randomized, placebo-controlled, phase II study in patients identified as having high tumor MET expression by immunohistochemistry as a possible target population for tivantinib, in the second-line setting. In this study, patients who had progressed on first-line therapy were stratified based on MET expression by immunohistochemistry (high expression was regarded as $\geq$2+ in $\geq$50% of tumor cells), and then were randomized (2:1) to receive tivantinib 360 mg daily or placebo. For patients with high MET expression, median OS was 7.2 months on tivantinib versus 3.8 months on placebo (HR, 0.38; $P = .01$). In addition, this trial also established that 240 mg twice daily was the appropriate dose for HCC patients.[50] Given these promising efficacy data in select MET-high patients, a phase III international study, Metiv-HCC study (NCI01755767), investigating the role of tivantinib versus placebo, is currently enrolling and is anticipated to be completed by mid-2015, with an interim analysis planned when approximately 60% of OS events is reached.

### Antiangiogenesis

Several antiangiogenic agents have been studied in HCC. In general, HCC tumors are characterized by their vascularity. Tumor angiogenesis leads to a pathologic vascularization pattern in HCC.[51] Preclinical and early phase trials have demonstrated that targeting VEGF is a feasible and optimal area in HCC tumors. Recently, ramicirumab, a selective anti–VEGF-2 monoclonal antibody was investigated as monotherapy in advanced HCC patients as first-line therapy.[52] In this study, 42 patients were evaluated with the primary endpoint being progression-free survival and the secondary endpoint being the objective response rate. The median progression-free survival was 4.0 months, with an objective response rate of 9.5%, and median OS of 12.0 months. After treatment with ramicirumab there was an increase in serum VEGF and placental growth factor and a transient decrease in soluble VEGFR, delineating the role of biomarker stratification for anti-VEGF therapy. Ramicirumab is being investigated currently in a large, international, randomized, placebo-controlled, double-blind study in patients who have progressed on first-line sorafenib (NCT01140347). There has been a recent press release from this trial stating that it failed to meet the OS endpoint.

### Personalized Approach in Hepatocellular Carcinoma

Biomarkers are needed to define which subsets of patients will best be served by different systemic agents. To date, serum biomarkers have not met with much success. In the SHARP trial, plasma biomarkers were collected at baseline and 12 weeks after initiation of sorafenib.[53] Although baseline markers (low hepatic growth factor and high c-Kit), demonstrated a trend toward predicting improved OS, none of the 10 biomarkers that were measured were actually able to predict the response to sorafenib. Tumor biopsies may be helpful to determine driver genes in an individual's tumor; however, this is performed inconsistently in clinical practice and generally only routinely done to qualify for participation in a clinical trial. The importance of tumor tissue is highlighted in a metaanalysis that reported that tumor tissue VEGF expression correlated with OS.[54]

## SUMMARY

Treating patients with advanced hepatocellular cancer requires a multidisciplinary approach. Although sorafenib remains the only approved agent in this setting, there are some promising results from newer targeted agents. Of the new agents available to date, MET expression and associated specific c-MET inhibitor, tivantinib, is perhaps one of the most exciting agents in the clinical trial realm. The question of potentially combining therapies like tivantinib with sorafenib is a potential option and requires further exploration. Biomarkers are needed to define which subsets of patients will be served best by different systemic agents and unfortunately this remains difficult to delineate to date.

## REFERENCES

1. Altekruse SF, McGlynn KA, Reichman ME. Hepatocellular carcinoma incidence, mortality, and survival trends in the United States from 1975 to 2005. J Clin Oncol 2009;27:1485–91.
2. Yeo W, Mok TS, Zee B, et al. A randomized phase III study of doxorubicin versus cisplatin/interferon alpha -2b/doxorubicin/fluorouracil (PIAF) combination chemotherapy for unresectable hepatocellular carcinoma. J Natl Cancer Inst 2005;97: 1532–8.
3. Available at: www.nexavar-us.com. Accessed October 1, 2014.
4. Farazi PA, Depinho RA. Hepatocellular carcinoma pathogenesis: from genes to environment. Nat Rev Cancer 2006;6:674–87.

5. Zhang DY, Friedman SL. Fibrosis-dependent mechanisms of hepatocarcinogenesis. Hepatology 2012;56:769–75.
6. Llovet JM, Ricci S, Mazzaferro V, et al. Sorafenib in advanced hepatocellular carcinoma. N Engl J Med 2008;359(4):378–90.
7. Cheng AL, Kang YK, Chen Z, et al. Efficacy and safety of sorafenib in patients in the Asia-Pacific region with advanced hepatocellular carcinoma: a phase III randomised, double-blind, placebo-controlled trial. Lancet Oncol 2009;10(1):25–34.
8. Marrero J, Lencioni R, Kudo M, et al. Global investigation of therapeutic decisions in hepatocellular carcinoma and of its treatment with sorafenib (GIDEON) second interim analysis in more than 1,500 patients: clinical findings in patients with liver dysfunction. J Clin Oncol 2011;29(20 Suppl):4001.
9. Iavarone M, Cabibbo G, Piscaglia F, et al. Field-practice study of sorafenib therapy for hepatocellular carcinoma: a prospective multicenter study in Italy. Hepatology 2011;54:2055–63.
10. Marrero JA, Lencioni R, Ye SL, et al. Final analysis of GIDEON (Global investigation of therapeutic decisions in hepatocellular carcinoma [HCC] and of its treatment with sorafenib [Sor]) in >3000 Sor-treated patients (pts): clinical findings in pts with liver dysfunction. ASCO 2013 Annual Meeting. J Clin Oncol 2013;31(Suppl) [abstract: 4126].
11. Abou-Alfa GK. Sorafenib use in hepatocellular carcinoma: more questions than answers. Hepatology 2014;60:15–7.
12. Vincenzi B, Santini D, Russo A, et al. Early skin toxicity as a predictive factor for tumor control in hepatocellular carcinoma patients treated with sorafenib. Oncologist 2010;15(1):85–92.
13. Bettinger D, Schultheiss M, Knuppel E, et al. Diarrhea predicts a positive response to sorafenib in patients with advanced hepatocellular carcinoma. Hepatology 2012;56(2):789–90.
14. Miyahara K, Nouso K, Morimoto Y, et al. Efficacy of sorafenib beyond first progression in patients with metastatic hepatocellular carcinoma. Hepatol Res 2014;44:296–301.
15. Nakazawa T, Hidaka H, Takada J, et al. Early increase in $\alpha$-fetoprotein for predicting unfavorable clinical outcomes in patients with advanced hepatocellular carcinoma treated with sorafenib. Eur J Gastroenterol Hepatol 2013;25(6):683–9.
16. Ueshima K, Kudo M, Takita M, et al. Tatsumi C, Des-$\gamma$-carboxyprothrombin may be a promising biomarker to determine the therapeutic efficacy of sorafenib for hepatocellular carcinoma. Dig Dis 2011;29(3):321–5.
17. Syrigos K, Boura P, Manegold C, et al. Bevacizumab-induced hypertension: pathogenesis and management. BioDrugs 2011;25(3):159–69.
18. Ren Z, Zhu K, Kang H, et al. A randomized controlled phase II study of the prophylactic effect of urea-based cream on the hand-foot skin reaction associated with sorafenib in advanced hepatocellular carcinoma. J Clin Oncol 2012;30(15):4008.
19. Zhang L, Zhou Q, Ma L, et al. Meta-analysis of dermatological toxicities associated with sorafenib. Clin Exp Dermatol 2011;36(4):344–50.
20. Sergio A, Cristofori C, Cardin R, et al. Transcatheter arterial chemoembolization (TACE) in hepatocellular carcinoma (HCC): the role of angiogenesis and invasiveness. Am J Gastroenterol 2008;103:914–21.
21. Kudo M, Imanaka K, Chida N, et al. Phase III study of sorafenib after transarterial chemoembolisation in Japanese and Korean patients with unresectable hepatocellular carcinoma. Eur J Cancer 2011;47(14):2117–27.

22.  Sansonno D, Lauletta G, Russi S, et al. Transarterial chemoembolization plus sorafenib: a sequential therapeutic scheme for HCV-related intermediate-stage hepatocellular carcinoma: a randomized clinical trial. Oncologist 2012;17(3):359–66.

23.  Lencioni R, Llovet JM, Han G. Sorafenib or placebo in combination with transarterial chemoembolization (TACE) with doxorubicin-eluting beads (DEBDOX) for intermediate-stage hepatocellular carcinoma (HCC): phase II, randomized, double-blind SPACE trial. J Clin Oncol 2012;30(4 Suppl) [abstract: LBA154].

24.  Strebel BM, Dulfour JF. Combined approach to hepatocellular carcinoma: a new treatment concept for nonresectable disease. Expert Rev Anticancer Ther 2008; 8:1743–9.

25.  Li X, Feng GS, Zheng CS, et al. Expression of plasma vascular endothelial growth factor in patients with hepatocellular carcinoma and effect of transcatheter arterial chemoembolization therapy on plasma vascular endothelial growth factor level. World J Gastroenterol 2004;10:2878–82.

26.  Haydar AA, Mukherji D, Faraj W, et al. Challenges in combining antiangiogenic therapy with transarterial chemoembolization for hepatocellular carcinoma. Gastrointest Cancer Res 2014;7:98–102.

27.  Zhang L, Hu P, Chen X, et al. Transarterial chemoembolization (TACE) plus sorafenib versus TACE for intermediate or advanced stage hepatocellular carcinoma: a meta-analysis. PLoS One 2014;9(6):e100305.

28.  Imamura H, Matsuyama Y, Tanaka E, et al. Risk factors contributing to early and late phase intra hepatic recurrence of hepatocellular carcinoma after hepatectomy. J Hepatol 2003;38:200–7.

29.  Wilhelm SM, Carter C, Tang L, et al. BAY 43-9006 exhibits broad spectrum oral antitumor activity and targets the RAF/MEK/ERK pathway and receptor tyrosine kinases involved in tumor progression and angiogenesis. Cancer Res 2004;64:7099–109.

30.  Wang SN, Chuang SC, Lee KT. Efficacy of sorafenib as adjuvant therapy to prevent early recurrence of hepatocellular carcinoma after curative surgery: a pilot study. Hepatol Res 2014;44:523–31.

31.  ASCO presented by Briux J at ASCO 06/14.

32.  Mazzaferro V, Regalia E, Doci R, et al. Liver transplantation for the treatment of small hepatocellular carcinomas in patients with cirrhosis. N Engl J Med 1996; 334:693–9.

33.  Yao FY, Bass NM, Nikolai B, et al. Liver Transplantation for hepatocellular carcinoma: analysis of survival according to intention-to-treat principle and dropout from the waiting list. Liver Transpl 2002;8:873–83.

34.  Clavien P, Lesurtel M, Bossuyt PM, et al. Recommendations for liver transplantation for hepatocellular carcinoma: an international consensus conference report. Lancet Oncol 2012;13:e11–22.

35.  Vitale A, Volk ML, Pastorelli D, et al. Use of sorafenib in patients with hepatocellular carcinoma before liver transplantation: a cost-benefit analysis while awaiting data on sorafenib safety. Hepatology 2010;51:165–73.

36.  Vouche M, Kulik L, Atassi R, et al. Radiological-pathological analysis of WHO, RECIST, EASL, mRECIST and DWI: Imaging analysis from a prospective randomized trial of Y90 +/− sorafenib. Hepatology 2013;58(5):1655–66.

37.  Kulik L, Vouche M, Koppe S, et al. Prospective randomized pilot study of Y90 +/− sorafenib as bridge to transplantation in hepatocellular carcinoma. J Hepatol 2014;61(2):309–17.

38.  Truesdale AE, Caldwell SH, Shah NL, et al. Sorafenib therapy for hepatocellular carcinoma prior to liver transplant is associated with increased complications after transplant. Transpl Int 2011;24(10):991–8.

39. Frenette C, Boktourn M, Burroughs SG, et al. Sorafenib prior to liver transplant does not result in increased surgical complications. Transpl Int 2013;26(7):734–9.

40. Abou-Alfa GK, Johnson P, Knox JJ, et al. Doxorubicin plus sorafenib vs doxorubicin alone in patients with advanced hepatocellular carcinoma: a randomized trial. JAMA 2010;304:2154–60.

41. Kelley R, Nimeiri HS, Munster PN, et al. Temsirolimus combined with sorafenib in hepatocellular carcinoma: a phase I dose-finding trial with pharmacokinetic and biomarker correlates. Ann Oncol 2013;24(7):1900–7.

42. Miyahara K, Nouso K, Yamamoto K, et al. Chemotherapy for advanced hepatocellular carcinoma in the sorafenib age. World J Gastroenterol 2014;20(15): 4151–9.

43. Cheng AL, Kang YK, Lin DY, et al. Sunitinib versus sorafenib in advanced hepatocellular cancer: results of a randomized phase III trial. J Clin Oncol 2013;31: 4067–75.

44. Johnson PJ, Qin S, Park JW, et al. Brivanib versus sorafenib as first-line therapy in patients with unresectable, advanced hepatocellular carcinoma: results from the randomized phase III BRISK-FL study. J Clin Oncol 2013;31(28):3517–24.

45. Llovet JM, Decaens T, Raoul JL, et al. Brivanib in patients with advanced hepatocellular carcinoma who were intolerant to sorafenib or for whom sorafenib failed: results from the randomized phase III BRISK-PS study. J Clin Oncol 2013;31(28):3509–16.

46. Semela D, Piguet AC, Kolev M, et al. Vascular remodeling and antitumoral effects of mTOR inhibition in a rat model of hepatocellular carcinoma. J Hepatol 2007; 46(5):840–8.

47. Villanueva A, Chiang DY, Newell P, et al. Pivotal role of mTOR signaling in hepatocellular carcinoma. Gastroenterology 2008;135(6):1972–83, 1983.e1–11.

48. Zhu AX, Kudo M, Assenat E, et al. EVOLVE-1: phase 3 study of everolimus for advanced HCC that progressed during or after sorafenib. ASCO Meeting Abstracts 2014;32(3 Suppl):172.

49. Santoro A, Simonelli M, Rodriguez-Lope C, et al. A Phase-1b study of tivantinib (ARQ 197) in adult patients with hepatocellular carcinoma and cirrhosis. Br J Cancer 2013;108(1):21–4.

50. Rimassa L, Porta C, Borbath I, et al. Tivantinib (ARQ 197) versus placebo in patients (Pts) with hepatocellular carcinoma (HCC) who failed one systemic therapy: results of a randomized controlled phase II trial (RCT). J Clin Oncol 2012; 30(Suppl) [abstract: 4006].

51. Patel A, Sun W. Molecular targeted therapy in hepatocellular carcinoma: from biology to clinical practice and future. Curr Treat Options Oncol 2014;15(3): 380–94.

52. Zhu AX, Finn RS, Mulcahy M, et al. A phase II and biomarker study of ramucirumab, a human monoclonal antibody targeting the VEGF receptor-2, as first-line monotherapy in patients with advanced hepatocellular cancer. Clin Cancer Res 2013;19(23):6614–23.

53. Llovet JM, Pena CE, Lathia CD, et al. Plasma biomarkers as predictors of outcome in patients with advanced hepatocellular carcinoma. Clin Cancer Res 2012;18:2290–300.

54. Zhan P, Qian Q, Yu LK. Prognostic significance of vascular endothelial growth factor expression in hepatocellular carcinoma tissue: a meta-analysis. Hepatobiliary Surg Nutr 2013;2:148–55.

# Hepatocellular Carcinoma in Children

Deirdre Kelly, FRCPCH, FRCP, FRCPI, MD[a],*, Khalid Sharif, FRCS Paed, FCPS Paed Surg (Pak)[a],
Rachel M. Brown, MBChB, FRCPath[b], Bruce Morland, MBChB, MRCP, DM, FRCPCH[c]

## KEYWORDS

- Hepatocellular • Carcinoma • Pediatrics • Epidemiology • Histopathology
- Transplant • Outcome

## KEY POINTS

- The spectrum of background liver disease predisposing to hepatocellular carcinoma (HCC) in children is different from that in adults.
- In children younger than 5 years the differential diagnosis of hepatoblastoma (HB) should be considered.
- The fibrolamellar variant preferentially affects teenagers and young adults.

## HEPATOCELLULAR CARCINOMA IN CHILDREN

Liver tumors are relatively rare in childhood, but may be associated with a range of diagnostic, genetic, therapeutic, and surgical challenges sufficient to tax even the most experienced clinician. This article outlines the epidemiology, etiology, pathology, initial workup, and management of HCC in children and adolescents.

### Epidemiology

Primary pediatric liver malignancies comprise 1% to 2% of all pediatric tumors. HB is the commonest primary hepatic malignancy (48%); HCC is the second most common primary liver malignancy of childhood (27%) with vascular tumors and sarcomas making up the rest.[1] HCC has an incidence of 0.3 to 0.45 cases per million per year (23%) and represents an increasingly common indication for liver transplant (LT) in children. Although HCC is more common in adolescents (10–14 years), histologically

The authors have nothing to disclose.
[a] The Liver Unit, Birmingham Children's Hospital, Steelhouse Lane, Birmingham B4 6NH, UK;
[b] Department of Cellular Pathology, Queen Elizabeth Hospital Birmingham, University Hospitals Birmingham NHS Foundation Trust, Mindelsohn Way, Edgbaston, Birmingham B15 2WB, UK; [c] Oncology Department, Birmingham Children's Hospital, Steelhouse Lane, Birmingham B4 6NH, UK
* Corresponding author.
E-mail address: deirdre.kelly@bch.nhs.uk

confirmed HCC has been reported in children younger than 5 years. HCC is more common in males than in females with 3:1 preponderance and tends to present with more advanced disease in children than in adults. Childhood HCC incidence increases significantly with age; however, it has remained stable over the past few decades. Data collected from the West Midlands Regional Children's Tumour Registry[2] have indicated the incidence of liver tumors to be 1.2 per million person-years: the incidence of HCC was 0.09, somewhat lower than that reported in published series.

### Cause

HCC is primarily an adult-onset disease, with only 0.5% to 1% of cases occurring before the age of 20 years. Many etiologic factors worldwide have been linked with the development of HCC including cirrhosis (due to various causes including alcohol intake), hepatitis B and C, and ingestion of aflatoxins in contaminated food. These factors produce significant geographic variation, with HCC being most common in sub-Saharan Africa and southeast Asia, where its incidence may reach 90 to 100 per 100,000 population largely as a result of hepatitis B virus (HBV) infection. There is a strong link between HCC and infection with the HBV. The incidence of HCC in chronic HBV carriers is approximately100-fold greater than that in the HBV-negative population[3] and is commoner in areas with high endemic HBV infection rates. Chen and colleagues[4] reported 100% positivity for HBV infection in Taiwan, and Chan and colleagues[5] reported 64% positivity in children with HCC in Hong Kong. Although integration of the HBV genome into the HCC genome can be demonstrated at the molecular level,[6] this event in itself is not necessarily oncogenic and a secondary, as yet unidentified, promoter is probably necessary for the development of tumor.[7] This secondary promoter could be environmental influences or genetic variations. The decrease of HBV because of neonatal vaccination has led to a reduction of cases in childhood, which will, in time, be reflected in the adult population.[8] Although hepatitis C is a known risk factor for HCC in adults, it is rare in children and there is only a single case report of this occurrence requiring transplant.[9]

Tyrosinemia I (fumarylacetoacetate hydrolase deficiency) is an autosomal recessive inborn error of tyrosine metabolism that produces liver failure in infancy or chronic liver disease with cirrhosis. Before therapy, there was a high risk of HCC in childhood or early adolescence. The development of therapy with nitisinone (2-[2-nitro-4-(trifluoro-methyl)benzoyl] cyclohexane-1,3-dione), which prevents the production of cytotoxic tyrosine metabolites in combination with a tyrosine- and phenylalanine-restricted diet, has transformed the natural history of tyrosinemia and has reduced, but not eliminated the risk of HCC.[10,11] HCC is also associated with glycogen storage disease types 1 and IV.[12]

The link between cirrhosis and HCC is unclear; however, the association of cirrhosis of any origin and dysplastic regenerating nodules have long been considered as precursors of HCC. Only about 30% of pediatric cases of HCC are associated with cirrhosis or preexisting liver abnormality, in contrast to adult HCC in which cirrhosis is present in 70% to 90%. Similarly, alpha-1-antitrypsin deficiency exhibits a different mechanism for carcinogenesis, where liver injury results from abnormal and chronic regenerative signaling from the sick cells to younger less-sick hepatocytes: chronic regeneration in the presence of tissue injury leading to adenomas and ultimately to carcinomas. It is suggested that the latter mechanism may explain hepatocarcinogenesis in other chronic liver diseases, that is, genetic disorders, viral hepatitis or nonalcoholic steatohepatitis, and glycogen storage disease type III. It has been recently suggested that progressive familial intrahepatic cholestasis type 2 (PFIC 2), associated with a mutation of the ABCB11 gene resulting in deficiency of bile salt export pump (BSEP; a membrane canalicular bile acid transporter), represents a specific and previously unrecognized risk for HCC in young children.[13]

In cases associated with tyrosinemia type I, cirrhosis is an invariable finding. In cases associated with biliary atresia, the development of HCC is not universally associated with cirrhosis, and in cases of Wilson disease or cholestatic syndromes that may not be associated with cirrhosis (eg, Alagille syndrome and PFIC 1 and PFIC 3), there seems to be no predisposition to malignant transformation.[14] Thus, while the development of cirrhosis clearly has a part to play in oncogenesis, the exact relationship remains unclear.

## Clinical Features

The classic symptoms of HCC in noncirrhotic individuals are similar to symptoms of those with other liver tumors, the common presentation being an abdominal mass and pain; in advanced cases children may have cachexia or jaundice. Symptoms and signs of liver insufficiency may be present if the tumor arises in the context of liver disease, and thus signs of underlying liver disease (splenomegaly from portal hypertension, spider nevi, etc.) should be sought as a possible clue to underlying etiologic factors.

The rare fibrolamellar type of HCC is usually seen in the older age group (median age 26.4 years) and generally occurs in noncirrhotic livers. The commonest presentation is with an abdominal mass without any other systemic symptoms. These tumors are thought to have a more favorable prognosis because these tend not to spread early.

## Diagnostic Investigations

### Laboratory tests

There are no specific diagnostic findings on full blood count associated with HCC; however, liver function tests frequently give abnormal results especially in children in whom HCC has occurred in cirrhotic livers. In children with PFIC 2, gamma glutamyltransferase levels are low.

Exclusion of known risk factors, such as serology for hepatitis B and C, plasma and urine amino acid and urinary succinyl acetone for tyrosinemia, as well as level and phenotype for alpha-1 antitrypsin, should be performed. If suspected, genetic confirmation of PFIC 2, tyrosinemia, and Alagille syndrome should be done.

### Alphafetoprotein

Alphafetoprotein (AFP) is a useful diagnostic and prognostic marker of HCC and its level is elevated in nearly 50% to 70% patients with HCC.[15,16] However, it should be noted that cirrhosis may also lead to persistent AFP elevation because of hepatic regeneration. Most investigators agree that AFP levels greater than 400 to 500 ng/mL in a patient with cirrhosis strongly suggest the diagnosis of HCC, whereas some propose an even lower cutoff between 200 and 300 ng/mL. Levels tend to be higher in patients with more bulky disease and with metastases. AFP levels are used as a useful prognostic marker, with return of AFP levels to normal after treatment indicating remission, whereas persistently abnormal results should alert the clinician to the possibility of residual tumor or relapse.

### Other markers

The fibrolamellar variant of HCC is usually associated with normal values of AFP, but elevation of levels of vitamin-$B_{12}$-binding proteins, especially transcobalamin I, makes this a useful marker that may also be used to monitor disease response and progression.

### Radiologic Investigations

The radiologic assessment of HCC aims to determine the site and characteristics of the tumor, establish the presence of any metastases, and help to assess the suitability for surgical resection. In children without cirrhosis, it is difficult to distinguish HCC from HB on imaging grounds alone. Both tumors are typically large (unless detected by screening) and are often multifocal. In both tumors there may be evidence of calcification, venous invasion, and lung metastases.

### Ultrasonography

The typical sonographic appearance of HCC is of a large, heterogeneous (usually predominantly hyperechoic), and vascular mass. The use of ultrasonographic contrast agents in children is currently experimental, but the results in adults suggest that they may be helpful for identifying and characterizing liver lesions.[17]

### Computed tomography scan

Computed tomographic (CT) scanning gives detailed information on the anatomic limits of liver tumors. Triphasic CT scan, after administration of intravenous contrast typically shows HCCs to be hypervascular in the arterial phase and isodense or hypodense in the portal venous phase. This technique is widely used for the detection of HCC in adults with cirrhosis, but it is relatively insensitive to small tumors, especially when cirrhosis is present, with an overall sensitivity and specificity of about 80% to 85% and 90% to 95%, respectively.[18,19]

### MRI scanning

MRI scanning is now considered as the investigation of choice because it gives good definition of the tumor and surrounding infiltration, enabling accurate assessment of segmental involvement. MRI findings of HCC tend to be of a heterogeneous (but predominantly hypointense) mass on T1-weighted images, and mildly hyperintense in comparison with normal liver on T2-weighted images. Contrast-enhanced T1-weighted images show a pattern similar to CT, with early arterial enhancement and reduced signal intensity in the portal venous phase.[20] This observation has important implications for clinical staging and any proposed surgical interventions. The vascular anatomy can also be demonstrated and may avoid the need for hepatic angiography.

In the adult with a chronically deranged liver, radiologic staging of HCC is based on conventional criteria endorsed by the European Association for Study of the Liver and the American Association for the Study of Liver Disease.[21] While these staging criteria can be adopted for staging of HCC in children, prospective series using these systems have not been validated.

### PET scan imaging

Areas of high metabolism may help to find extrahepatic sites that may not be detected by other imaging modalities. PET has been proved to be useful for localizing relatively early some metastases or recurrence of disease before any mass effect per se was detectable on routine checks.

### Biopsy

Although clinical and laboratory clues can lead to a presumptive diagnosis in most children with liver tumors, caution must be exercised at all times. Unless primary surgery is feasible, biopsy is necessary in all patients without cirrhosis. In the setting of cirrhosis, HCC can often be diagnosed by imaging and elevated AFP level; however, biopsy may still be required in equivocal cases, especially with small lesions (<2 cm). Image-guided needle biopsy is generally preferred to open biopsy because of the multifocal nature of tumor.[22] The purpose of the biopsy is to obtain enough representative tumor tissue for an accurate diagnosis, without causing immediate complications (hemorrhage) or tumor seeding.

Three important precautions may reduce the risk of tumor seeding in pediatric patients.

1. The tumor should not be approached directly, but instead along a short path through unaffected liver, taking care to cross only those segments that will be removed at subsequent surgery.
2. A coaxial biopsy system should be used, and this allows several cores of tissue to be obtained with a single puncture. A recent retrospective review of 128 adult HCC biopsies performed with a 17- or 18-gauge coaxial technique showed no tumor seeding at a mean follow-up of 410 days.[23]
3. The needle tract should be plugged, either with gelatin foam or with slurry of collagen.

### Pathology of Hepatocellular Carcinoma in Children

Pathologic aspects of HCC have been reviewed by Brunt EM and Pittman ME elsewhere in this issue. Three topics relevant to the pediatric situation are discussed here:

### Pathology of the background liver

As already discussed HCC can arise in children without background liver disease but cirrhosis remains a predisposing factor to HCC in childhood as it is in adulthood. Viral hepatitis is a risk factor in both age groups, but otherwise the spectrum of predisposing disease is different in children. Tyrosinemia is an important example. Early histologic changes include a distinctive rosetting cholestasis and steatosis. Regenerative nodules are an early feature containing more fat and less hemosiderin than the adjacent parenchyma.[24]

Fibrosis and cirrhosis develop later if the child is not treated with nitisinone and diet. Although nitisinone has reduced the risk of developing HCC, it is still an important risk factor. The HCCs tend to be well differentiated. Trabecular and solid architecture is more prevalent than an acinar architecture. Steatosis and in particular clear cell change have been observed.[13,25] The expression of heat shock proteins and antiapoptotic proteins have been described as a mechanism whereby transformed cells maintain a survival advantage in a murine model of tyrosinemia.[26] If the child undergoes LT, the explant liver is examined for the presence of dominant nodules, which are extensively sampled (**Fig. 1**). It may be difficult to differentiate between regenerative/dysplastic nodules and HCC in a child with cirrhosis.

As indicated above, risk factors in children also include glycogen storage disease type 1 and PFIC II (ABCB11 disease). The absence of the canalicular BSEP by immunohistochemistry correlates well with ABCB11 mutations.[27] A recent report of a case with preserved BSEP staining but ABCB11 mutations implicated activating mutations in β-catenin (CTNNB1) and nuclear factor erythroid 2-related factor 2 (NFE2L2) in the carcinogenic pathway.[28] The toxic effects of intracellular bile salts have also been postulated as a mechanism of causing genomic modifications. Excessive gene amplification has been described with targeting of the mitogen-activated protein kinase pathway.[29]

Cytogenetic and molecular characteristics of HCC have been much more extensively investigated in adults. López-Terrada and colleagues,[30] the investigators of a recent pediatric liver tumor consensus classification,[30] think that future collaborative studies will be better able to define pediatric HCC in terms of molecular pathology. It will be of interest to see if pediatric HCCs are different from those occurring in adults

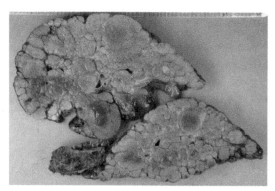

**Fig. 1.** Sections through a liver removed at the time of transplant from a patient with tyrosinemia. The larger nodules seen here could represent HCC and should be extensively sampled.

and whether those occurring in a background of chronic disease are different from those arising in normal liver. It will also be important to define the targets of potentially therapeutic biological agents discussed later in this article. From a morphologic point of view, with the exception of HCC arising in tyrosinemia, childhood HCCs have a similar appearance to those in adults. Epithelial cell adhesion molecule expression seems to be far stronger in pediatric than adult HCC.[13]

### The differential diagnosis between hepatoblastoma and HCC

When HB has embryonal-type epithelial, or mesenchymal, elements, it is easily recognized. When it assumes a macrotrabecular architecture and/or is composed of purely well-differentiated fetal epithelial cells, the differential diagnosis is acknowledged to be occasionally "virtually impossible."[31]

The age of the child is helpful; HB is unusual after 5 years of age. HB can occur in very-low-birth-weight children or as part of a multisystemic syndrome such as the Beckwith-Wiedemann overgrowth disorder that predisposes the child to an increased risk of several childhood malignancies. The presence of underlying liver disease, especially with a known risk factor, favors HCC. The inclusion of liver in a tumor biopsy showing chronic liver disease (changes over and above those expected in liver close to a space-occupying lesion of any kind) should prompt serious consideration of HCC. As therapy is so dramatically different, every attempt should be made to differentiate these tumors. Immunohistochemical profiles are frustratingly similar. Known cytogenetic and molecular abnormalities are heterogeneous and overlap. Gene expression studies do show a different pattern for HB when compared with HCC. Insulinlike growth factor 2 and mitogen-inducible gene 6 have been shown to have an increased expression; 3 of 7 cases showed delta-like 1 homolog overexpression. Transforming growth factor β level is increased; the same is true in HCC, but in this case the increase is not over and above that seen in adjacent background liver.[32]

The recent pediatric liver tumor consensus classification[30] has introduced a category of "hepatocellular neoplasm not otherwise specified" to acknowledge this difficulty. This category encompasses a set of tumors described in older children previously hypothesized to be arising from cells that are transitional between hepatoblasts and hepatocytes.[33]

### Fibrolamellar carcinoma

This rare variant of HCC affects adolescents and young adults preferentially. This variant is a distinctive neoplasm arising in noncirrhotic liver (**Fig. 2**). The level of AFP

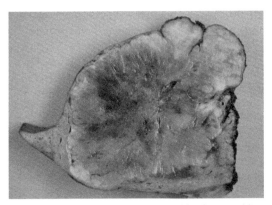

**Fig. 2.** This large fibrolamellar HCC is arising in normal background liver.

is typically not elevated. This neoplasm is composed of large cells with copious eosinophilic oncocytic cytoplasm (**Fig. 3**) in a lamellated sometimes hyalinized stroma. The oncocytic appearance is secondary to mitochondrial accumulation. The cytoplasm sometimes contains inclusionlike structures. Fibrolamellar areas can be seen within otherwise conventional HCCs, but this mixed pattern is usually seen in adults. The immunohistochemical profile is interesting with expression of both hepatocellular and biliary markers. In comparison with conventional HCC the fibrolamellar variant shows fewer genetic alterations. Methylation of the promoters of tumor suppressor genes is also less frequent in fibrolamellar variants.[34]

### Clinical Staging

There is no uniformly accepted staging system for HCC in children. The Barcelona Clinic Liver Cancer score is becoming the most widely accepted system in adults, because it takes into consideration not only the state of the tumor but also the condition of the patient and the liver. The tumor node metastasis (TNM) staging system does not seem to be particularly suited for predicting prognosis in HCC, despite recent amendments.

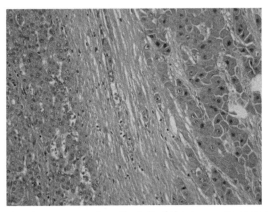

**Fig. 3.** Normal hepatocytes are present on the left of this image. In comparison, the cells on the right, from a fibrolamellar HCC, are large with copious eosinophilic cytoplasm and large nucleoli (H&E, original magnification ×200).

Other systems that have claimed a predictive value in HCC are the Cancer of the Liver Italian Program scale and the Okuda system (already referenced in relevant sections). In the late 1980s the Children's Oncology Group adopted a system based mostly on surgical findings. The pretreatment extent of disease (PRETEXT) system, developed in 1988/1989 by the International Society of Paediatric Oncology Liver Tumour Study (SIOPEL) Group, and revised in 2005, may be the best way of comparing the results of studies conducted in children by different organizations. This surgically oriented system divides patients with liver tumors into 4 categories according to the number of liver sections not involved by tumor.[35] Extrahepatic extension (including involvement of the portal and hepatic veins and inferior vena cava) and metastatic disease are separately classified. The interobserver reliability of the system has been shown to be high, and a recent version of the system, especially suited to HCC in children and young adults, has been established. The PRETEXT staging has the advantage that it stratifies patients for the most effective treatment, surgical resection.

## Treatment

The classic management of all malignant liver tumors consists of a combination of chemotherapy and surgical resection, with the highest cure rates being associated with complete surgical resection. The various modalities currently used in the management of HCC can be summarized as follows:

### Local treatment

**Liver resection** When an older child or a young adult with a predisposing condition presents with a resectable tumor, likely to be HCC, primary resection is recommended without any attempt at biopsy. Although all studies have confirmed the importance of complete tumor resection for obtaining cure, less than 20% of patients are amenable to initial surgery. PRETEXT I and II tumors (defined by there being 3 or 2 adjacent sectors, respectively, free of tumor) are quite easily removed by surgery, but PRETEXT III tumors (in which only 1 sector or 2 nonadjacent sectors are tumor free) require specialized experience of liver surgery including transplant and intensive care facilities. PRETEXT IV tumors (in which there are no tumor-free sectors) are considered unresectable because of extensive liver involvement. The ultimate goal of surgical resection of HCC is to achieve complete tumor clearance with margins of at least 1 cm, although several reports in the adult population showed that any clear margin (even <1 cm) may be acceptable, which implies that all options should be explored before declaring a tumor unresectable. In this regard, patients should be referred to units with all facilities for major hepatic resections and also access to LT. Intraoperative ultrasound examination is mandatory for determining segmental hepatic removal and safe resection planes.[36] The volume of the liver that can be removed with major hepatic resections can be predicted by CT- or MRI-based calculations. In children the usual limit for resection (a ratio obtained by dividing the remnant liver volume in milliliters by the patient body weight in kilograms) can safely exceed the usual 0.8 mL/kg value to 0.6 mL/kg. Sampling of lymph nodes from the hepatoduodenal ligament should be performed in every case because involvement has a significant effect on prognosis. After liver resection, the 5-year survival is reported to be in the range 35% to 50%. The recurrence rate is about 20% to 30% at the same interval, with little change in the past decade.

**Liver transplantation** The role of orthotopic liver transplant (OLT) in the treatment strategy for HCC remains undecided. The criteria for LT in adult cirrhotic candidates with HCC has changed over time, from a period with unrestricted tumor limits to precise tumor burden, that is, the conventional Milan criteria (CMC). Using CMC (single tumor smaller than 5 cm, or in case of many tumors, no more than 3, and each not exceeding 3 cm in diameter) as the safe limit for LT, a predicted 5-year survival rate of about 70% has been reported.

There have been no prospective randomized studies comparing liver resection and OLT for HCC in children. The published experience with OLT in pediatric HCC is quite limited.[37] Two earlier reports, by Tagge and colleagues[38] and Iwatsuki and colleagues[39] showed low survival, in the range of 29% to 35% in young patients with unresectable tumors. A more recent report from Pittsburgh (19 cases) and some unpublished experience from other centers[40] show improved survival, in the range of 60% at 5 years, and confirm the negative influence of tumor size and vascular invasion on prognosis, very much as in adults. Because of the possible differences in biology between pediatric (noncirrhotic) and adult (cirrhotic) HCC, it is not known whether the adult experience can be extrapolated to children. In general, contraindications for LT include extrahepatic disease and fibrolamellar tumors. In view of the varied outcome, decisions need to be made on a case-by-case basis.

**Ablative therapies** *Radiofrequency ablation (RFA) and percutaneous ethanol injection* are the most common methods for tumor ablation.[41] These techniques have been well investigated in the adult setting and have been proved to be comparable to surgery for tumors less than or equal to 3 cm, whereas their effect on HCC up to 5 cm or more is not proven to be better than tumor removal. However, little is known about the efficacy of RFA in children with HCC, in whom the tumors tend to be larger than 5 cm.

*Chemoembolization: Transfemoral hepatic artery chemoembolization (TACE)* is an established method of treatment of HCC in adults, with evidence of improved survival in randomized controlled trials.[42] Indications for TACE in children and adolescents with HCC have been similar to those in adults, a bridge to LT (while waiting for a liver donor to become available) or to resection (attempted conversion of nonresectable tumors to resectability). The potential advantages of TACE include the delivery of a higher concentration of cytotoxic drugs to the tumor, which is mostly vascularized by hepatic artery branches, prolonged dwell time of drug in the tumor, and reduced systemic toxicity. TACE may be safe in children and adolescents with HCC who do not have cirrhosis, although it may require a high degree of technical expertise.

Although promising, experience with TACE in children with HCC is limited, with only anecdotal experiences reported in the literature. A marked reduction in tumor size has been reported in 2 cases of fibrolamellar HCC in adolescents treated with TACE using lipiodol as embolizing agent and doxorubicin, carboplatin, or cisplatin as chemotherapeutic agents. TACE rendered HCC resectable in 2 of 3 children in one series. TACE served successfully as a bridge to LT in 3 other children, 1 of whom was alive 14 months after transplant. Severe complications may occur. Pulmonary embolism has been reported after a significant response to TACE in one child with HCC. Although the available data are scanty, it seems that the use of TACE should be explored further, especially in children with highly vascularized HCC after systemic chemotherapy, as a bridge to resection or transplant.

As TACE may be associated with thrombosis of some of the hepatic artery branches, or even of the main (right, left, or both) arterial branches, it may interfere with further surgical resection: TACE should thus be considered after multidisciplinary discussion and taking into account the surgical options to consider at the end of the treatment.

**Chemotherapy** There is extensive experience with the medical management of HCC in adults. Despite the extensive use of neoadjuvant and adjuvant chemotherapy, there is no convincing published evidence to suggest that this translates to a benefit in survival. Even if some evidence of activity (in terms of response rates) has been shown in phase 2 studies with anthracyclines, only 10% to 20% of adults with HCC are suitable for primary resection.

The North American Intergroup Hepatoma study (INT-0098) and the International Childhood Liver Tumor Study Group (SIOPEL 1) study investigated the effect of chemotherapy in increasing surgical resectability, the ultimate foundation for curative therapy for liver tumors, in children and adolescents with HCC. In the North American Intergroup Hepatoma study patients, were randomized after initial surgery or biopsy to receive cisplatin with either doxorubicin or 5-fluorouracil (5-FU) and vincristine. There was no difference in response or survival rates between the 2 treatment regimens. Of the 8 patients with complete tumor excision at time of diagnosis (stage I) followed by adjuvant cisplatin-based chemotherapy, 7 survived (88%) compared with 12 of 33 patients (36%) with initially unresectable tumors. This result suggests that adjuvant chemotherapy may be of benefit for patients with completely resected HCC. In contrast, outcome was uniformly poor for patients with advanced-stage disease, with a 5-year event-free survival (EFS) for patients with stage III and IV HCC of 23% and 10%, respectively. Tumor resection after neoadjuvant chemotherapy was only feasible in 2 patients, and although they did have a prolonged survival, they eventually died of recurrent disease.

The SIOPEL 1 study showed similar disappointing results (5-year EFS of 17%). Of these, 2 had complete resection of the tumor at diagnosis followed by chemotherapy and 37 had preoperative chemotherapy with cisplatin and doxorubicin (PLADO). Although partial tumor shrinkage was observed in 49% of the patients, tumor resection was achieved in only 36% of them (14/39). Long-term survival occurred only after complete surgical excision confirmed at pathologic examination, reinforcing the importance of surgical clearance for achieving cure. The SIOPEL 2 trial investigated the concept of a dose-intensified chemotherapy strategy of PLADO plus carboplatin.[43] Of the 17 patients 15 received preoperative chemotherapy. Partial response to preoperative chemotherapy was observed in 5 of 15 cases (33%); 10 patients underwent tumor resection including 1 undergoing LT and 2 being operated, primarily giving a total resection rate of 59%. Seven tumors (41%) never became operable. Four of the patients whose tumors were resected were alive at a median follow-up of 8 years (88–99 months). Twelve patients died because of progressive disease and 1 from surgical complications. The overall survival for this study was only 24%, and thus despite the increased intensity of preoperative and postoperative chemotherapy in SIOPEL 2 compared with SIOPEL 1, there was no improvement in treatment results for HCC.

In the 3 cooperative studies of the German Society for Pediatric Oncology and Hematology (GPOH), HCC has been treated with the same regimens as HB, with surgery recommended as the primary treatment in all patients. The chemotherapy in HB89 consisted of ifosfamide, cisplatin, and doxorubicin (IPA), whereas HB94 added carboplatin and etoposide to IPA.[44] The results were not satisfactory, with a disease-free survival of only 32% in HB94. In the current study, high-dose carboplatin and etoposide is given for nonresectable HCC. Some initial effect in terms of tumor regression and achievement of a surgical resection with microscopic residual tumor (termed an R1 resection) has been observed: all 7 patients with complete resection are tumor free, as well as 1 of 2 with primary microscopic residual tumor and all 6 with presumed tumor spillage at primary operation. Although encouraging responses to carboplatin and etoposide have been seen, this again does not seem to translate into significant improvement in survival.

In common with experience in adult HCC, there is interest in exploring newer targeted therapies in pediatric groups. In a placebo-controlled randomized trial, sorafenib (a multikinase inhibitor that targets vascular endothelial growth factor [VEGF] and the Raf kinase pathway) in combination with doxorubicin has been shown to be beneficial in adult patients with advanced HCC, yielding improved progression-free survival and tumor shrinkage. In a recent publication, GPOH has presented a series of patients receiving PLADO in combination with sorafenib used as first-line therapy in pediatric patients with HCC. Of 12 patients with histologically confirmed HCC, 6 (50%) achieved complete remission at a median follow-up of 20 months. Of these 6 patients, 4 received PLADO/sorafenib and had a liver resection and 2 underwent transplant after a localized relapse. Of the 7 patients with unresectable disease, chemotherapy induced a partial response in 4 patients and stable disease in 2; 1 patient had progressive disease. Of these patients, 3 were alive after complete resection following alternate salvage therapy. Of the 5 patients with primary resection, 1 was alive and free of disease at 27 months postdiagnosis and 4 had local or metastatic relapse (2 of whom were rescued with LT).

Alternate approaches with first- and second-line chemotherapy regimens have been described in the adult literature, although pediatric data are scarce. These regimens include treatment with gemcitabine/oxaliplatin (GemOx), 5-FU/cisplatin, capecitabine/cisplatin, 5-FU/mitomycin, 5-FU/oxaliplatin, gemcitabine/cisplatin, 5-FU/interferon, and monotherapy with sorafenib.

Small single-institution studies in children have described objective responses with the combination of irinotecan, vincristine, temozolomide, and bevacizumab; oxaliplatin, irinotecan, and gemcitabine; and gemcitabine and oxaliplatin. While data on GemOx in pediatric HCC are scarce, the adult experience suggests it has efficacy and tolerable toxicity in the setting of relapsed/refractory disease, suggesting some potential for use in front-line therapy.

Finally, as the biological pathways that lead to oncogenesis and proliferation in HCC are better elucidated, the potential for deploying targeted therapies, either as single agents or in combination with other chemotherapy/targeted agents, will increase. One example is the VEGF/VEGF receptor pathway and its role in mediating initiation, proliferation, and dissemination of HCC via angiogenesis. Agents such as sorafenib, bevacizumab, brivanib, and sunitinib take advantage of this mechanism to inhibit tumor growth both in vitro and in vivo. Similarly, erlotinib, which targets the epidermal growth factor pathway, is currently in phase 2 trials both as a single agent and in combination with sorafenib. The mammalian target of rapamycin pathway inhibitor everolimus has also shown antitumor activity in early clinical trials in adult HCC. An ongoing randomized placebo-controlled trial is investigating everolimus as a single agent in adult patients pretreated with sorafenib. Perhaps of greatest potential benefit are agents that target cMET, a tyrosine kinase receptor for the hepatocyte growth factor, which is implicated in neoplasia and proliferation in both HB and HCC. Recently, a randomized phase 2 study of the cMET inhibitor tivantinib has demonstrated activity in a subset of patients with advanced HCC who had progressed on sorafenib. Similarly, agents such as cabozantinib, which have dual activity against cMET and VEGF pathways, offer the promise of disabling multiple mechanisms by which HCC cells proliferate.

The fibrolamellar variant of HCC is usually a slow-growing tumor, which metastasizes late and can often be treated surgically without the need for adjuvant chemotherapy. It was at one time thought that this variant of HCC had a more favorable outcome, but studies from the US and SIOPEL groups suggest that in patients with advanced disease, response to chemotherapy and outcome does not differ from that in conventional HCC.

**Response to therapy** The response to therapy may be monitored by the following serial measurements:

- Radiology. Repeat CT scans or ultrasonography document shrinkage of the hepatic tumor, whereas chest radiograph or chest CT scans monitor progress of pulmonary metastases.
- AFP levels in tumors secreting AFP. Patients with a good response to chemotherapy have a rapid decrease in serum AFP levels, whereas a failure to return to normal limits in the absence of radiological disease is highly suspicious of minimal residual disease. An increase in AFP levels after initiation of chemotherapy is usually a sensitive marker of relapse or treatment failure.
- A fall in transcobalamin I levels in fibrolamellar HCC may be a guide to response.

**Long-term outcome** McAteer and colleagues[45] reported unadjusted 5- and 10-year survival varies across demographic variables and treatment characteristics. Survival for the younger children (0–4 year) was better than that for older children, with an unadjusted 5-year survival of 53% compared with 32% for those aged 5 to 19 years. Overall 5-year survival was better in males (40%) compared with females (26%). Asian children were reported to have worse survival (13%), compared with 33% for white and 46% for black children.

Recently, Allan and colleagues[46] reported the results of Surveillance, Epidemiology and End Results database with a large series of 218 pediatric HCC cases. There was no significant difference in the overall survival by gender, age at diagnosis, race, ethnicity, or use of radiation. Overall survival was greater for fibrolamellar compared to nonfibrolamellar subtypes of HCC. An overall 5-year survival for the entire cohort of 24% and 20-year survival of 8% was reported.

In contrast, in a recent study from SIOPEL, the investigators did not find that children with fibrolamellar HCC had a more favorable prognosis because 31% responded to chemotherapy compared with 53% of patients with HCC, although there was no difference in the 3-year survival.[47]

Children with initially resectable HCC have a good prognosis irrespective of histologic subtype with survival rates in excess of 50%, although children with HCC do less well than those with HB.[48]

**Survival post-liver transplant** Most series of LT for primary liver tumors focus on survival posttransplant for HBs, but a review from the United Network for Organ Sharing demonstrated that of 152 transplants in 135 pediatric patients for liver tumors, there were 43 transplants in 41 pediatric patients for HCC. The respective 1-, 5-, and 10-year patient survivals after LT were 86%, 63%, and 58%, respectively, for HCC. The primary cause of death was metastatic or recurrent disease, accounting for 86% of the children with HCC.[49]

## SUMMARY

HCC is a rare but important tumor in childhood. The incidence may decrease because of effective vaccination of HBV and therapy for tyrosinemia. Although the diagnosis remains challenging and the prognosis variable, early diagnosis and complete resection of the tumor is associated with a good prognosis. LT remains a viable option for selected children without extrahepatic spread.

## REFERENCES

1. Moore SW, Davidson A, Hadley GP, et al. Malignant liver tumors in South African children: a national audit. World J Surg 2008;32(7):1389–95.
2. Mann JR, Kasthuri N, Raafat F, et al. Malignant hepatic tumours in children: incidence, clinical features and aetiology. Paediatr Perinat Epidemiol 1990;4: 276–89.
3. Hall AJ, Winter PD, Wright R. Mortality of hepatitis B positive blood donors in England and Wales. Lancet 1985;1:91–3.
4. Chen WJ, Lee JC, Hung WT. Primary malignant tumour of liver in infants and children in Taiwan. J Pediatr Surg 1988;23:457–61.
5. Chan KL, Fan ST, Tam PK, et al. Paediatric hepatoblastoma and hepatocellular carcinoma: retrospective study. Hong Kong Med J 2002;8:13–7.
6. Brechot C, Pourcel C, Louise A, et al. Presence of integrated hepatitis-B virus DNA in cellular DNA of human hepatocellular carcinoma. Nature 1980;286: 533–5.
7. Perilongo G, Pontisso P, Basso G. Can primary cancer of the liver in Western countries be prevented? Pediatric point of view. Med Pediatr Oncol 1990;18: 57–60.
8. Chang MH. Hepatitis B virus and cancer prevention. Recent Results Cancer Res 2011;188:75–84.
9. Malik S, Dekio F, Wen JW. Liver transplantation in a child with multifocal hepatocellular carcinoma hepatitis C & management of post-transplant viral recurrence using boceprevir. Pediatr Transplant 2014;18(2):E64–8.
10. Holme E, Lindstedt S. Nontransplant treatment of tyrosinemia. Clin Liver Dis 2000; 4:805–14.
11. McKiernan PJ. Nitisinone in the treatment of hereditary tyrosinaemia type 1. Drugs 2006;66:743–50.
12. Manzia TM, Angelico R, Toti L, et al. Glycogen storage disease type Ia and VI associated with hepatocellular carcinoma: two case reports. Transplant Proc 2011;43(4):1181–3.
13. Zen Y, Vara R, Portmann B, et al. Childhood hepatocellular carcinoma: a clinicopathological study of 12 cases with special reference to EpCAM. Histopathology 2014;64(5):671–82.
14. Bhadri VA, Stormon MO, Arbuckle S, et al. Hepatocellular carcinoma in children with Alagille syndrome. J Pediatr Gastroenterol Nutr 2005;41(5):676–8.
15. Weinberg AG, Finegold MJ. Primary hepatic tumors of childhood. Hum Pathol 1983;14:512–37.
16. Katzenstein HM, Krailo MD, Malogolowkin MH, et al. Hepatocellular carcinoma in children and adolescents: results from the Pediatric Oncology Group and the Children's Cancer Group intergroup study. J Clin Oncol 2002;20:2789–97.
17. Dietrich CF, Ignee A, Trojan J, et al. Improved characterisation of histologically proven liver tumours by tumours by contrast enhanced ultrasonography during the portal venous and specific late phase of SHU 508A. Gut 2004;53(3):401–5.
18. Kojiro M, Roskams T. Early hepatocellular carcinoma and dysplastic nodules. Semin Liver Dis 2005;25:133–42.
19. Burrel M, Llovet JM, Ayuso C, et al. MRI angiography is superior to helical CT for detection of HCC prior to liver transplantation: an explant correlation. Hepatology 2003;3:1034–42.
20. Taouli B, Losada M, Holland A, et al. Magnetic resonance imaging of hepatocellular carcinoma. Gastroenterology 2004;127(5 Suppl 1):S144–52.

21. Bruix J, Sherman M, Llovet JM, et al. Clinical management of hepatocellular carcinoma. Conclusions of the Barcelona-2000 EASL conference. European Association for the Study of the Liver. J Hepatol 2001;35:421–30.

22. Postovsky S, Elhasid R, Ben Arush MW, et al. Local dissemination of hepatocellular carcinoma in a child after fine-needle aspiration. Med Pediatr Oncol 2001; 26(6):667–8.

23. Mauren KE, Nghiem HV, Marrero JA, et al. Lack of tumor seeding after percutaneous biopsy of hepatocellular carcinoma using coaxial cutting needle technique [abstract]. AJR Am J Roentgenol 2005;184(Suppl 4):37.

24. Portmann BC. Liver biopsy in the diagnosis of inherited metabolic disorders. In: Anthony PP, MacSween RN, editors. Recent advances in histopathology, vol. 13. Churchill Livingstone; 1987. p. 139–59.

25. Seda Neto J, Leite KM, Porta A, et al. HCC prevalence and histopathological findings in liver explants of patients with hereditary tyrosinemia type 1. Pediatr Blood Cancer 2014;61(9):1584–9.

26. Angileri F, Morrow G, Roy V, et al. Heat shock response associated with hepatocarcinogenesis in a murine model of hereditary tyrosinemia type I. Cancers (Basel) 2014;6(2):998–1019.

27. Knisely AS, Strautnieks SS, Meier Y, et al. Hepatocellular carcinoma in ten children under five years of age with bile salt export pump deficiency. Hepatology 2006;44(2):478–86.

28. Vilarinho S, Erson-Omay EZ, Harmanci AS, et al. Paediatric hepatocellular carcinoma due to somatic CTNNB1 and NFE2L2 mutations in the setting of inherited bi-allelic ABCB11 mutations. J Hepatol 2014;61(5):1178–83.

29. Iannelli F, Collino A, Sinha S, et al. Massive gene amplification drives paediatric hepatocellular carcinoma caused by bile salt export pump deficiency. Nat Commun 2014;5:3850.

30. López-Terrada D, Alaggio R, de Dávila MT, et al. Towards an international pediatric liver tumor consensus classification: proceedings of the Los Angeles COG liver tumors symposium. Mod Pathol 2014;27(3):472–91.

31. Tanaka Y, Inoue T, Horie H. International pediatric liver cancer pathological classification: current trend. Int J Clin Oncol 2013;18(6):946–54.

32. Luo JH, Ren B, Keryanov S, et al. Transcriptomic and genomic analysis of human hepatocellular carcinomas and hepatoblastomas. Hepatology 2006;44(4): 1012–24.

33. Prokurat A, Kluge P, Kościesza A, et al. Transitional liver cell tumors (TLCT) in older children and adolescents: a novel group of aggressive hepatic tumors expressing beta-catenin. Med Pediatr Oncol 2002;39(5):510–8.

34. Ward SC, Waxman S. Fibrolamellar carcinoma: a review with focus on genetics and comparison to other malignant primary liver tumors. Semin Liver Dis 2011; 31(1):61–70.

35. Aronson DC, Schnater JM, Staalman CR, et al. Predictive value of the pretreatment extent of disease system in hepatoblastoma: results from the International Society of Pediatric Oncology Liver Tumor Study Group SIOPEL-1 study. J Clin Oncol 2005;23(6):1245–52.

36. Silberhumer GR, Steininger R, Laengle F, et al. Intraoperative ultrasonography in patients who undergo liver resection or transplantation for hepatocellular carcinoma. Surg Technol Int 2004;12:145–51.

37. Achilleos O, Buist LJ, Kelly DA, et al. Unresectable hepatic tumors in children and the role of liver transplantation. J Pediatr Surg 1996;31:1563–7.

38. Tagge EP, Tagge DU, Reyes J, et al. Resection, including transplantation, for hepatoblastoma and hepatocellular carcinoma: impact on survival. J Pediatr Surg 1992;27:292–7.
39. Iwatsuki S, Starzl TE, Sheahan DG, et al. Hepatic resection vs. transplantation for hepatocellular carcinoma. Ann Surg 1991;214:221–9.
40. Reyes JD, Carr B, Dvorchik I, et al. Liver transplantation and chemotherapy for hepatoblastoma and hepatocellular cancer in childhood and adolescence. J Pediatr 2000;136:795–804.
41. Ikeda M, Okada S, Ueno H, et al. Radiofrequency ablation and percutaneous ethanol injection in patients with small hepatocellular carcinoma: comparative study. Jpn J Clin Oncol 2001;31:297–8.
42. Lo CM, Ngan H, Tso WK, et al. Randomized controlled trial of transarterial lipiodol chemoembolization for unresectable hepatocellular carcinoma. Hepatology 2002;35:1164–71.
43. Perilongo G, Shafford E, Maibach R, et al. Risk-adapted treatment for childhood hepatoblastoma. Final report of the second study of the International Society of Pediatric Oncology - SIOPEL 2. Eur J Cancer 2004;40:411–21.
44. von Schweinitz D, Burger D, Bode U, et al. Results of the HB-89 Study in treatment of malignant epithelial liver tumors in childhood and concept of a new HB-94 protocol. Klin Padiatr 1994;206:282–8.
45. McAteer JP, Goldin AB, Healey PJ, et al. Hepatocellular carcinoma in children: epidemiology and the impact of regional lymphadenectomy on surgical outcomes. J Pediatr Surg 2013;48:2194–201.
46. Allan BJ, Wang B, Davis JS, et al. A review of 218 pediatric cases of hepatocellular carcinoma. J Pediatr Surg 2014;49:166–71.
47. Weeda VB, Murawski M, McCabe AJ, et al. Fibrolamellar variant of hepatocellular carcinoma does not have a better survival than conventional hepatocellular carcinoma–results and treatment recommendations from the Childhood Liver Tumour Strategy Group (SIOPEL) experience. Eur J Cancer 2013;49(12):2698–704.
48. Pham TH, Iqbal CW, Grams JM, et al. Outcomes of primary liver cancer in children: an appraisal of experience. J Pediatr Surg 2007;42(5):834–9.
49. Austin MT, Leys CM, Feurer ID, et al. Liver transplantation for childhood hepatic malignancy: a review of the United Network for Organ Sharing (UNOS) database. J Pediatr Surg 2006;41(1):182–6.

# Moving?

## Make sure your subscription moves with you!

To notify us of your new address, find your **Clinics Account Number** (located on your mailing label above your name), and contact customer service at:

**Email: journalscustomerservice-usa@elsevier.com**

**800-654-2452** (subscribers in the U.S. & Canada)
**314-447-8871** (subscribers outside of the U.S. & Canada)

**Fax number: 314-447-8029**

**Elsevier Health Sciences Division
Subscription Customer Service
3251 Riverport Lane
Maryland Heights, MO 63043**

*To ensure uninterrupted delivery of your subscription, please notify us at least 4 weeks in advance of move.